OVARIAN HYPERSTIMULATION SYNDROME

REPRODUCTIVE MEDICINE
& ASSISTED REPRODUCTIVE TECHNIQUES SERIES

Series Editors

David K Gardner DPhil
Colorado Center for Reproductive Medicine, Englewood, CO, USA

Jan Gerris MD PhD
Professor of Gynecology, University Hospital Ghent, Ghent, Belgium

Zeev Shoham MD
Director, Infertility Unit, Kaplan Hospital, Rehovot, Israel

Forthcoming Titles

1. *Gerris, Delvigne and Olivennes:* Ovarian Hyperstimulation Syndrome
2. *Sutcliffe:* Health and Welfare of ART Children
3. *Keck, Tempfer and Hugues:* Conservative Infertility Management
4. *Pellicer and Simón:* Stem Cells in Reproductive Medicine
5. *Tan, Chian and Buckett:* In-vitro Maturation of Human Oocytes
6. *Elder and Cohen:* Human Embryo Evaluation and Selection
7. *Tucker and Liebermann:* Vitrification in Assisted Reproduction

OVARIAN HYPERSTIMULATION SYNDROME

Edited by

Jan Gerris MD PhD
Division of Gynecology
University Hospital Ghent
Ghent, Belgium

Annick Delvigne MD PhD
Center for Reproductive Medicine
St Pierre Hospital
Brussels, Belgium

François Olivennes MD PhD
Unit of Reproductive Medicine
Obstetrics and Gynecology Service II, Cochin Hospital
Paris, France

CRC Press
Taylor & Francis Group
Boca Raton London New York

CRC Press is an imprint of the
Taylor & Francis Group, an **informa** business

First published 2006 by Informa Healthcare

Published 2018 by CRC Press
Taylor & Francis Group
6000 Broken Sound Parkway NW, Suite 300
Boca Raton, FL 33487-2742

ISBN 13: 978-1-84214-328-5 (hbk)

A CIP record for this book is available from the British Library.

Library of Congress Cataloging-in-Publication Data

Data available on application

Composition by Parthenon Publishing

Contents

Contributors

Rina Agrawal MD DGO MRCOG
Clinical Director
Centre of Reproductive Medicine
Park Road, London
UK

Gautam N Allahbadia MD DNB FNAMS
Rotunda – The Center for Human Reproduction
Bandra, Mumbai
India

Rob E Bernardus MD PhD
Department of Ob-Gyn-Fert
Hospital Gooi-Noord
Blaricum
The Netherlands

Didi D M Braat MD PhD
Professor and Chair, Department of Obstetrics and Gynecology
Department of Ob-Gyn-Fert
Radboud University Nijmegen Medical Center
Nijmegen
The Netherlands

Mats Brännström MD PhD
Department of Obstetrics and Gynecology
Sahlgrenska Academy at Göteborg University
Göteborg
Sweden

Sabine Costagliola PhD
Institut de Recherche Interdisciplinaire en Biologie Humaine et Moléculaire (IRIBHM)
Faculté de Médecine, Campus Erasme
Université Libre de Bruxelles
Brussels
Belgium

Anne Delbaere MD PhD
Laboratory of Research on Human Reproduction
Faculté de Médecine, Campus Erasme
Université Libre de Bruxelles
and Fertility Clinic
Hôpital Erasme
Brussels
Belgium

Annick Delvigne MD PhD
Clinical Director IVF Unit
Department of Ob-Gyn-Fert
CHU St Pierre
Brussels
Belgium

Diane De Neubourg MD
Center for Reproductive Medicine
Department of Ob-Gyn-Fert
Middelheim Hospital
Antwerp
Belgium

Petra De Sutter MD PhD
Centre for Reproductive Medicine
Department of Ob-Gyn-Fert
University Hospital Ghent
Ghent
Belgium

Marc Dhont MD PhD
Head of Department of Obstetrics and Gynecology
University Hospital Ghent
Ghent
Belgium

Anders Enskog MD PhD
Department of Anesthesia and Intensive Care
Sahlgrenska Academy at Göteborg University
Göteborg
Sweden

Margo R Fluker MD FRCSC
Co-Director, Genesis Fertility Centre
Clinical Professor, Department of Obstetrics and Gynaecology
University of British Colombia
Vancouver
Canada

Shevach Friedler MD
IVF and Infertility Unit
Assaf Harofeh Medical Center
Tel-Aviv University
Zerifin
Israel

Isabel Hernández García
Profesora Titular de Fisiología
Departmento de Fisiología
Facultad de Medicina
Universidad de Murcia
Murcia
Spain

Juan A García-Velasco MD
Instituto Valenciano de Infertilidad
University of Valencia
Valencia
Spain

Jan Gerris MD PhD
Division of Gynecology
University Hospital Ghent
Ghent
Belgium

Oya Gökmen
Associate Professor, Medical Director and Scientific Coordinator
Centrum Clinic
Ankara Women's Health and Reproductive Technologies Center
Gaziosmanpaşa
Ankara
Turkey

Raul Gómez PhD
Instituto Valenciano de Infertilidad
University of Valencia
Valencia
Spain

Juliette Guibert
Unité de Médecine de la Reproduction
Service de Gynécologie Obstétrique II
Hôpital Cochin
Paris
France

A Zeki Isik
Associate Professor and Scientific Coordinator
Ankara IVF Center
Ovacler
Ankara
Turkey

Shahar Kol MD
IVF Unit
Department of Obstetrics and Gynecology
Rambam Medical Center
Haifa
Israel

Zalman Levine MD
Assistant Professor of Obstetrics and Gynecology
Division of Reproductive Endocrinology and Infertility
New York Medical College
and The Fertility Institute of NJ and NY
New York, NY
USA

Lucia Montanelli PhD
Institut de Recherche Interdisciplinaire en Biologie Humaine et Moléculaire (IRIBHM)
Faculté de Médecine, Campus Erasme
Université Libre de Bruxelles
Brussels
Belgium

Randy S Morris MD
Medical Director, IVF 1
Naperville, IL
USA

Daniel Navot MD
Professor of Obstetrics and Gynecology
Chief, Division of Reproductive Endocrinology and Infertility
New York Medical College
and The Fertility Institute of NJ and NY
New York, NY
USA

Joseph Neulen
University Clinic for Gynecological Endocrinology and Reproductive Medicine
University Clinic
RWTH Aachen
Aachen
Germany

François Olivennes MD PhD
Clinical Director
Unité de Médecine de la Reproduction
Service de Gynécologie Obstétrique II
Hôpital Cochin
Paris
France

Antonio Pellicer MD
Clinical Director
Instituto Valenciano de Infertilidad
Valencia
Spain

Arieh Raziel MD
IVF and Infertility Unit
Assaf Harofeh Medical Center
Tel-Aviv University
Zerifin
Israel

José Remohi MD
Instituto Valenciano de Infertilidad
University of Valencia
Valencia
Spain

Botros Rizk MD MA FACOG FACS HCLD FRCOG FRCS(C)
Professor and Director
Division of Reproductive Endocrinology and Infertility
University of South Alabama
Mobile, AL
USA

Raphael Ron-El MD
Head of IVF and Infertility Unit
Assaf Harofeh Medical Center
Tel-Aviv University
Zerifin
Israel

Morey Schachter MD
IVF and Infertility Unit
Assaf Harofeh Medical Center
Tel-Aviv University
Zerifin
Israel

Gamal I Serour FRCOG FRCS
Professor of Obstetrics and Gynecology
Al-Azhar University
Clinical Director of the Egyptian IVF Center
Maadi, Cairo
Egypt

Carlos Simon MD
Instituto Valenciano de Infertilidad
University of Valencia
Valencia
Spain

Guillaume Smits MD PhD
Institut de Recherche Interdisciplinaire en Biologie Humaine et Moléculaire (IRIBHM)
Faculté de Médecine, Campus Erasme
Université Libre de Bruxelles
and Medical Genetics Department
Hôpital Erasme
Brussels
Belgium

Jane A Stewart MD BSc MBChB MRCOG
Consultant in Reproductive Medicine
Newcastle Fertility Centre at LIFE
Bioscience Centre, International Centre for Life
Newcastle upon Tyne
UK

Maria José Teruel
Departmento de Fisiología
Facultad de Medicina
Universidad de Murcia
Murcia
Spain

Peter van Dop MD PhD
Head of Department Ob-Gyn-Fert
Catharina-Ziekenhuis
Eindhoven
The Netherlands

Gilbert Vassart MD PhD
Institut de Recherche Interdisciplinaire en Biologie Humaine et Moléculaire (IRIBHM)
Faculté de Médecine, Campus Erasme
Université Libre de Bruxelles
and Medical Genetics Department
Hôpital Erasme
Brussels
Belgium

Ralf Zimmermann MD
Department of Obstetrics and Gynecology
Colombia University
New York, NY
USA

Preface

Multiple pregnancies and the ovarian hyperstimulation syndrome (OHSS) are the two most important complications of assisted reproductive technologies (ART). In contrast to multiple pregnancies, OHSS has been openly recognized as a major problem from the very first years that gonadotropins were utilized to induce ovulation. There is a bulk of knowledge about its physiopathology, its genetics and its endocrine, immunological and epidemiological aspects, and many expert clinicians have devised approaches to minimize its occurrence or reduce its major risk, i.e. thromboembolism. Nevertheless, OHSS seems to occur unabated in our daily practice. The treacherous thing about OHSS is that it appears less of a problem than it is. There are two major reasons for this. First, lethal cases, although very rare, do occur from time to time and are certainly underreported. Second, severe OHSS occurs relatively rarely (around 1% of all *in vitro* fertilization (IVF) stimulations) and does not always come to the attention of the practitioner treating the patient, giving to the individual physician the impression of a rare event indeed. Furthermore, OHSS in non-IVF cycles has become very rare because stimulations have become less aggressive since the 1980s; serious OHSS occurs almost exclusively in IVF treatment cycles.

To date, there is no easy, acceptable and feasible solution to avoid all OHSS, although complete avoidance of human chorionic gonadotropin (hCG) as ovulation trigger should and has been given serious thought. Replacement of hCG by other triggers of ovulation, however, is in the hands of the industry, not treating physicians. Health-economic considerations, although favoring less aggressive ovulation-triggering methods, seem to weigh less heavily on the balance than in the case of, for example, prevention of multiples by single embryo transfer. It is likely that for some time to come, and as long as we use the existing urinary hCG preparations as ovulation trigger, we will have to live with a risk for OHSS.

The contributions in this book are written by senior authors from around the world who have made original clinical and/or scientific contributions to our understanding and management of the syndrome. Authors from Europe, America and the East synthesize the balance of their experience, dictated in part by differences in medical culture and cost considerations – although, undoubtedly, no cost is too high to avoid a young woman dying from an artificial and purely iatrogenic disease.

As a rainbow unfolds its many-colored splendor, so the subsequent chapters, radiating from a common starting point, unfold their different scopes and visions, each highlighting one specific aspect of the syndrome. What will emerge is the insight that in OHSS there is definitely more than meets the eye, literally and metaphorically: literally, a seemingly innocuous hyperstimulation may quickly and unexpectedly turn into disaster; metaphorically, OHSS is more than just 'the ovaries reacting a bit more like usual'. It is truly a disease state, triggered by ovarian hyperstimulation, probably occurring in genetically predisposed women, inducing a cascade of disruptions that affect many regulatory systems, mainly blood clotting and kidney function, holding the killing dagger of multiorgan failure under its wings.

This book also serves as an indirect plea for prospective registration of OHSS, at least of serious cases, and certainly of lethal cases. This is easier said than done. In a world where doctors are under great medicolegal pressure, cases tend to be minimized. However, starting with registration on a national basis could be a first step in the right direction. Just as many national registries of deliveries do register the equally sensitive issue of maternal mortality, ART registries should ask for patient mortalities, irrespective of the cause of death. In the end, this may result only in a more robust consolidation of the quality and safety of our profession.

Short, practical OHSS guidelines for daily use on the working floor have been added to Chapter 6, and a longer summary of the most important aspects of OHSS is provided at the end of the book. It will be clear that, as is the case for many clinical situations, personal opinions and management strategies differ somewhat. This is richness, not poverty. But clearly, the guidelines and the summary should be considered as a plausible possibility among others which may differ slightly.

OHSS represents one of the intensive-care aspects of gynecological practice. Giving correct pretreatment information to patients is an unattractive option, comparable to a car salesman showing his customers the bodies of crash victims. Yet, this is where the true challenge lies: all health-care professionals working in reproductive medicine should be acquainted with the theoretical and practical aspects of this syndrome, both from a prophylactic point of view and once it has developed. OHSS needs to be taken seriously, without discrediting the huge advantages that our modern reproductive technologies offer. Therefore, a book focused on the clinically relevant aspects of the syndrome should be useful for all who take their reproductive job seriously. Decreasing the risk for OHSS in the first place, correct recognition of the condition and professional management avoiding the most serious complications and eventually death of the patient will definitely contribute to an increased safety of ART treatments.

Jan Gerris

Foreword

Cars collide, trains derail, airplanes crash, big ships break and sink, and nuclear as well as industrial plants fail and pollute. Humankind has always been compelled to pay a heavy tribute to technological advancement. This inexorable law applies no less to medical practice, in which almost every significant investigative or therapeutic progress has entailed untoward side-effects and sometimes dramatic consequences. Strictly speaking, this paradox is in opposition with the old Hippocratic aphorism: *primum non nocere*. The ovarian hyperstimulation syndrome (OHSS) appears as the utmost stereotype of this contradiction. This explains why this iatrogenic entity has – rather amazingly to the outside observer – become the object of as much thorough investigation and care as the infertile situations from which it originates indirectly.

In the middle of the last century, gonadotropins already being on the market, OHSS was a rare but much feared complication of anovulation treatment. Its physiopathological mechanism remained a mystery and, all too often, serious forms of this syndrome resulted in bilateral ovariectomy and pregnancy loss. By strongly boosting the ovarian response, assisted reproductive technologies (ART) have vastly increased the numbers of OHSS cases. As ART are not vital to the physical health of patients, it was thus imperative that the most dangerous and sometimes life-threatening complication of this treatment should be prevented at all costs. Therefore, it its hardly surprising that the search for prevention and treatment of OHSS should have rapidly evolved in several directions. Clinical, pharmacological, molecular, genetic and even economic areas relevant to this syndrome have all been tackled and are currently explored.

Artificial transformation of the mono-ovulatory human female into the equivalent of a polytocous species entails a cataclysmic rupture of the subtle neuroendocrine and para-autocrine balance which enables the human ovary to release generally no more than one egg per cycle.

As explained in certain chapters of the present book, it is fascinating to learn that the homeostatic conditions prevailing in women with stimulated ovaries depend on a delicate equilibrium existing between antagonistic types of receptors for VEGF (vascular epithelial growth factor) and between divergent actions of ovarian and renal RAS (renin–angiotensin systems).

A vast array of prevention modes and of therapeutic attack angles for the OHSS has likewise emerged from a host of clinical studies, which are thoroughly analyzed in the present volume. However, prospective and well-planned multicentric studies are still needed to ensure proper assessment of the results. Hopefully, future genetic investigations will also help in understanding why some patients develop OHSS while others, although showing similar basic conditions as well as an equally high estrogenic response, do not. These are only a few examples of the many new insights offered by the various experts who have contributed to this book.

From the ethical point of view, the OHSS situation remains a most problematic one. This is especially true in the presence of a so-called 'critical case', when the physician will feel that he is treading the razor's edge, asking himself if he should put an end to an ongoing pregnancy or pursue a very risky gamble indeed. Under such conditions, the extreme solution of pregnancy termination obviously represents a catastrophic failure of treatment threatening to entail indelible psychological sequelae. A series of excellent guidelines are offered here that will enable practicing fertility specialists to avoid becoming entrapped in such hair-raising dilemmas and to prevent high-risk situations for their patients.

Finally, it is to be hoped that the pharmaceutical industry will be able to resume investigations into recombinant gonadotropins in order to produce an efficient ovulatory molecule not burdened with a long half-life such as that of hCG.

Fernand Leroy
Honorary Professor of
Obstetrics and Gynecology
Free University Brussels (ULB)

CHAPTER 1

General definition of the ovarian hyperstimulation syndrome

Annick Delvigne

Ovarian hyperstimulation syndrome (OHSS) is a potentially fatal iatrogenic complication of the luteal phase in ovulation stimulation. This syndrome is characterized by an increased size of the ovaries due to multiple cysts, and by an increase in the vascular permeability causing ascites, pleural effusion and sometimes even pericardial effusion. Severe forms are also accompanied by electrolyte disturbances and cardiopulmonary, hepatic, renal and hemodynamic disturbances associated with increased thromboembolic risk.

There is currently no specific treatment for OHSS.

The prevalence of the severe form of OHSS is fortunately small, varying according to the literature between 0.5 and 5%. Nevertheless, since this is an iatrogenic complication of a non-vital treatment with a potential fatal outcome, the syndrome remains a serious problem for specialists dealing with infertility, leading to important clinical questions:

(1) Is it possible to identify patients at risk?

(2) Which are the most adequate stimulation schemes and follow-up methods for patients with an identified risk (primary prevention)?

(3) Which preventive method should be applied when an exaggerated ovarian response occurs (secondary prevention)?

(4) Which symptoms are pathognomonic and which are rare but essential to be accurately identified?

(5) What is the physiopathology of this syndrome?

(6) Which is the most adequate treatment according to the severity of OHSS?

HISTORICAL PERSPECTIVE

The ovarian hyperstimulation syndrome is a rare iatrogenic complication of ovarian stimulation occurring during the luteal phase or during early pregnancy. This syndrome has been known since gonadotropins (gonadotropic preparations made from the serum of pregnant mares or extracts of sheeps' pituitary glands and the urine of pregnant women) were first used to induce ovulation in 1943[1,2]. The first fatal cases were described in 1951 by Gotzsche[3] and in 1958 by Figueroa-Casas[4]. In 1957, Le Dall[5] described this syndrome in his thesis. This author reported acute cases necessitating a laparotomy and unilateral or bilateral ovariectomy, or puncture and suture of ruptured cysts. Further subacute situations are also mentioned, characterized by pain and healing in 58% of the cases after bedrest and antispasmodic treatment. Oliguria and renal failure were the principal complications leading to death at that time.

Later on, OHSS appeared to be a possible complication of the induction of ovulation by almost every agent used for this purpose. The presentation and severity of this clinical syndrome have evolved with time in relation to stimulation protocols. For instance, the development of *in vitro* fertilization (IVF) and other techniques such as cryopreservation has led to more and more aggressive treatment schemes aimed at obtaining sufficient numbers of oocytes and embryos, but consequently leading to an increased risk of OHSS.

Thus, historical descriptions of OHSS diagnosed using elevated urinary estradiol excretion are now obsolete, since new techniques aim at obtaining hyperstimulation *per se*.

DEFINITION

Nowadays, it is the loss of control over hyperstimulation that constitutes the 'ovarian hyperstimulation syndrome'.

The *most common form* occurs a few days after follicular rupture or puncture, when follicular growth has been medically induced utilizing either clomiphene citrate or gonadotropins, sometimes in conjunction with gonadotropin-releasing hormone (GnRH) agonists or antagonists and following final follicular maturation and luteinization achieved by the administration of human chorionic gonadotropin (hCG).

Some other *particular forms* of OHSS have also been reported: spontaneous OHSS, sometimes occurring repeatedly in the same patient or family[6–17]; or OHSS subsequent to a flare-up effect of a GnRH agonist, whether or not in conjunction with gonadotropins[18–22].

Apart from these rare events, OHSS generally happens only after ovarian stimulation and exposure to hCG.

This iatrogenic complication is very particular, because it is not the consequence of a treatment that is vital or mandatory for the patient's health. However, it can be fatal: the OHSS mortality rate has been estimated at 1/45 000–500 000, with a morbidity even higher but not accurately quantified[23].

CLINICAL DESCRIPTION

In the initial form, the increase in size of the ovaries is accompanied by abdominal discomfort. In a more advanced form, the ovaries become cystic, and this will often result in abdominal distension and pain, nausea, vomiting and sometimes diarrhea.

These digestive symptoms may be present as soon as 48 h after hCG administration, but they become most severe between days 7 and 10 after hCG.

The following clinical signs are likely to result from a circulatory dysfunction corresponding to increased vascular permeability and marked arterial dilatation[24]. The first sign of OHSS is the formation of a small amount of ascites, which is sometimes only visualized through vaginal ultrasound. It is difficult to distinguish this from the frequent bleeding occurring after oocyte pick-up (Figure 1). In more severe forms, ascites is echographically obvious (Figure 2) and clinically identifiable, but is very uncommon before day 7 after hCG administration. The cystic ovaries are enlarged, sometimes reaching a size even greater than 12 cm. Cases of rupture and/or hemorrhage of ovarian cysts have been observed, sometimes masking an ectopic pregnancy.

Compression by enlarged ovaries can induce hydroureter. A series of other complications may occur, some of them ending in complex end-organ failure.

Ascites fluid is characterized by a high concentration in proteins (4.8 g/100 ml), a low leukocyte count and the presence of relatively high numbers of red blood cells.

The extravascular protein-rich exudate accumulated in the peritoneum, in the pleura (hydrothorax) (Figure 3) and even in the pericardiac space is associated with intravascular volume depletion and hemoconcentration, activation of vasoconstrictor and antinatriuretic factors, severe hypoalbuminemia and sometimes vulvar or generalized edema (anasarca). The cardiovascular effects include arterial hypotension, reduced fluid volume, low central venous pressure, tachycardia, increased cardiac output, low peripheral resistance, increased vascular stasis, hemoconcentration and hypercoagulation.

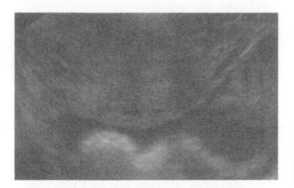

Figure 1 Thin line of ascites hardly discernible from usual discrete intra-abdominal bleeding as the result of ovarian puncture

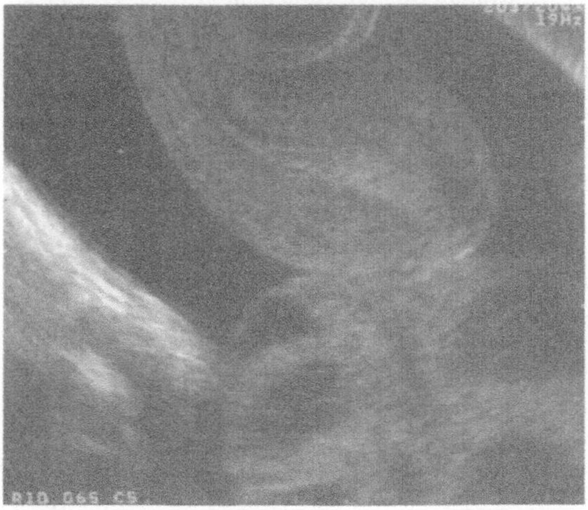

Figure 2 Uterus floating in echographically obvious large quantity of ascites

The associated hypovolemia can induce oliguria and electrolyte imbalance. Oliguria exists in about 30% of cases, and renal failure secondary to hypoperfusion or to compressive obstruction occurs in about 1.4% of the severe forms of OHSS[21,25]. Decreased renal perfusion induces stimulation of renal tubules and resorption of sodium and water, resulting in clinical manifestations of oliguria and sodium retention. Electrolyte imbalance is then observed, typically hyponatremia and hyperkalemia.

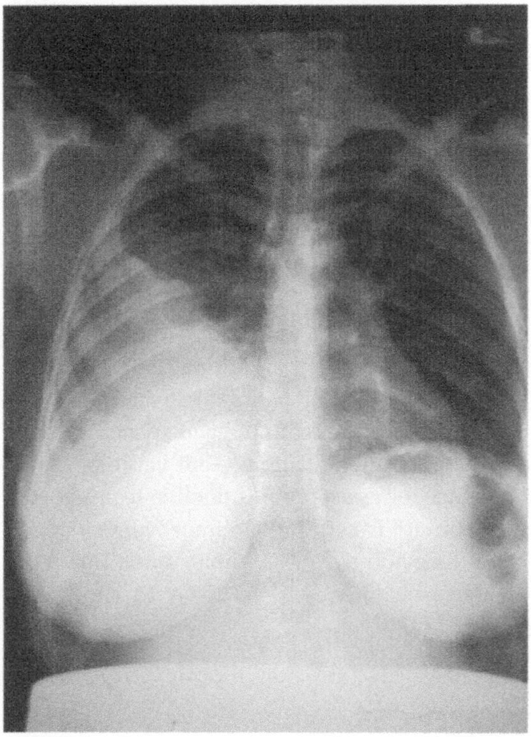

Figure 3 Hydrothorax (usually right-sided)

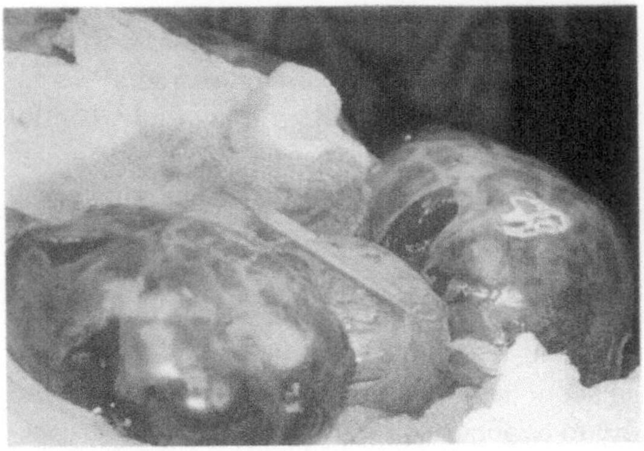

Figure 4 Two severely enlarged ovaries in OHSS patient undergoing laparotomy. Courtesy Dr G I Serour, Egypt

Together with ascites, the associated paralytic ileus can impair diaphragmatic movement to such an extent that respiratory problems ensue. If pleural effusion also develops, lung function may be seriously affected, leading to adult respiratory distress syndrome (ARDS).

Pleural effusion can complicate massive ascites or exist as an isolated manifestation of OHSS without peritoneal fluid accumulation. Liver dysfunction can also occur. Thromboembolic phenomena constitute the ultimate complication of OHSS and are capable, despite appropriate treatment, of killing the patient[26].

Such an array of potential severity of side-effects is rarely encountered, especially for a treatment applied for non-lethal pathology. The challenge for assisted reproductive technologies in the future is certainly an improvement of the baby take-home rate without impairment of women's health and their long- or short-term quality of life.

REFERENCES

1. Rydberg E, Pedersen-Bjergaard K. Effect of serum gonadotrophin and chorionic gonadotrophin on the human ovary. JAMA 1943; 121: 1117–22.
2. Davis E, Hellebaum AA. Observations on the experimental use of gonadotropic extracts in the human female. J Clin Endocrinol 1944; 4: 400–9.
3. Esteban-Altirriba J. Le syndrome d'hyperstimulation massive des ovaires. Rev Franç Gynécol Obstet 1961; 56: 555–64.
4. Rotmensch S, Scommegna A. Spontaneous ovarian hyperstimulation syndrome associated with hypothyroidism. Am J Obstet Gynecol 1989; 160: 1220–2.
5. Le Dall R. Le syndrome d'hyperlutéinisation massive des deux ovaires par injection intempestive d'hormones gonadotropes. Thesis (no. 915), Paris, 1957
6. Zalel Y, Katz Z, Caspi B, et al. Spontaneous ovarian hyperstimulation syndrome concomitant with spontaneous pregnancy in a woman with polycystic ovary disease. Am J Obstet Gynecol 1992; 167: 122–4.
7. Ayhan A, Tuncer ZS, Aksu AT. Ovarian hyperstimulation syndrome associated with spontaneous pregnancy. Hum Reprod 1996; 11: 1600–1.
8. Lipitz S, Grisaru D, Achiron R, et al. Spontaneous ovarian hyperstimulation mimicking an ovarian tumour. Hum Reprod 1996; 11: 720–1.
9. Olatunbosun OA, Gilliland B, Brydon LA, et al. Spontaneous ovarian hyperstimulation syndrome in four consecutive pregnancies. Clin Exp Obstet Gynecol 1996; 23: 127–32.
10. Abu-Louz SK, Ahmed AA, Swan RW. Spontaneous ovarian hyperstimulation syndrome with pregnancy. Am J Obstet Gynecol 1997; 177: 476–7.
11. Di Carlo C, Bruno P, Cirillo D, et al. Increased concentrations of renin, aldosterone and Ca125 in a case of spontaneous, recurrent, familial, severe ovarian hyperstimulation syndrome. Hum Reprod 1997; 12: 2115–17.
12. Nappi RG, Di Naro E, D'Aries AP. Natural pregnancy in hypothyroid woman complicated by spontaneous ovarian hyperstimulation syndrome. Am J Obstet Gynecol 1998; 178: 610–11.

13. Todros T, Carmazzi CM, Bontempo S, et al. Spontaneous ovarian hyperstimulation syndrome and deep vein thrombosis in pregnancy: case report. Hum Reprod 1999; 14: 2245–8.

14. Pentz-Vidovic I, Skoric T, Grubisic G, et al. Evolution of clinical symptoms in a young woman with a recurrent gonadotroph adenoma causing ovarian hyperstimulation. Eur J Endocrinol 2000; 143: 607–14.

15. Jung BG, Kim H. Severe spontaneous ovarian hyperstimulation syndrome with MR findings. J Comput Assist Tomogr 2001; 25: 215–17.

16. Hee-Dong C, Eun-Joo P, Sung-Hoon K, et al. Ovarian hyperstimulation complicating a spontaneous singleton pregnancy: case report. J Assist Reprod Genet 2001; 18: 120–3.

17. Smits G, Olatunbosun O, Delbaere A. Ovarian hyperstimulation syndrome due to a mutation in the follicle-stimulation hormone receptor. N Engl J Med 2003; 349: 753–9.

18. Hampton HL, Whitworth NS, Cowan BD. Gonadotrophin-releasing hormone agonist (leuprolide acetate) induced ovarian hyperstimulation syndrome in a woman undergoing intermittent hemodialysis. Fertil Steril 1991; 55: 429–31.

19. Weissman A, Barash A, Shapiro H, et al. Ovarian hyperstimulation following the sole administration of agonistic analogues of gonadotrophin releasing hormone. Hum Reprod 1998; 13: 3421–4.

20. Letterie GS. Ovarian hyperstimulation caused by a gonadotrophin agonist. Am J Obstet Gynecol 2000; 182: 747.

21. Khalaf Y, Anderson H, Taylor A, et al. Two rare events in one patient undergoing assisted conception: empty follicle syndrome and ovarian hyperstimulation with the sole administration of a gonadotrophin-releasing hormone agonist. Fertil Steril 2000; 73: 171–2.

22. Campo S, Bezzi I, Garcea N. Ovarian hyperstimulation after administration of triptorelin therapy to a patient with polycystic ovary syndrome. Fertil Steril 2000; 73: 1256–8.

23. Brinsden PR, Wada I, Tan SL, et al. Diagnosis, prevention and management of ovarian hyperstimulation syndrome. Br J Obstet Gynaecol 1995; 102: 767–72.

24. Fabregues F, Balasch J, Manau D, et al. Haematocrit, leucocyte and platelet counts and the severity of the ovarian hyperstimulation syndrome. Hum Reprod 1998; 13: 2406–10.

25. Abramov Y, Elchalal U, Schenker JG. Pulmonary manifestations of severe ovarian hyperstimulation syndrome: a multicenter study. Fertil Steril 1999; 71: 645–51.

26. Cluroe AD, Synek BJ. A fatal case of ovarian hyperstimulation syndrome with cerebral infarction. Pathology 1995; 27: 344–6.

CHAPTER 2

Epidemiology and primary risk factors for ovarian hyperstimulation syndrome

Peter van Dop

In this chapter, risk factors for ovarian hyperstimulation syndrome (OHSS) are restricted to so-called controlled ovarian hyperstimulation (COH). The primary risks for OHSS in ovulation induction (OI) are not dealt with, since the aim of OI (preferably obtaining one follicle) is different from that of COH (obtaining multiple follicles), and a low number of follicles excludes OHSS.

Epidemiology is a science that deals with the incidence, distribution and control of disease in a population. Incidence is the rate of occurrence of new cases of a particular disease in a population being studied (*Webster's Unabridged Dictionary*, 1976). To avoid semantic hair-splitting in this area, we keep only to the incidence of OHSS.

DIFFICULTIES IN DEFINITION OF OHSS

OHSS is an iatrogenic condition characterized by cystic enlargement of the ovaries and a fluid shift from the intravascular to the third space following increased capillary permeability[1]. Hence, the main features of OHSS are cystic enlargement of the ovaries and a fluid shift. Both the size of the ovaries and the amount of fluid may (independently) vary in a quantitative way. These variations – and other features – are the basic concepts of grading (the severity of) OHSS. The grading of OHSS is extensively discussed in a subsequent chapter.

Difficulties in analysis of the *quantitative* parts of the definition of OHSS (ovarian enlargement and amount of peritoneal fluid) still exist. Measurement of the size to which ovaries can develop is much more exact than measurement of the amount of peritoneal fluid. Owing to its sharply recognizable borders, ovarian size can be measured by ultrasound in an exact and reproducible way. Owing to the nature of the fluid and its dispersion between other intraperitoneal organs, this is not true for the ultrasound measurement of peritoneal fluid. Precision in ultrasound measurement of the amount of peritoneal fluid has not been assessed. Intra- and interobserver errors of the ultrasound measurement of peritoneal fluid in OHSS are not known. The accumulation of peritoneal fluid in larger (more than 1 litre) quantities may be assessed most accurately by weighing every luteal day on the same weighing scale under the same conditions. Weighing should be performed every morning after voiding of the early-morning urine.

FLUID SHIFT, OVARIAN SIZE AND OHSS

In the natural monofollicular ovulatory cycle, the occurrence of a certain amount of peritoneal fluid is a normal phenomenon[2]. At present, no reliable prospective data on ultrasound measurement of the size of ovaries during COH and its relationship to the risk of ovarian hyperstimulation as a *syndrome* are available. No studies are available addressing the question of whether the degree of ovarian enlargement *without* considerable fluid shift in the intraperitoneal space has any relation to the incidence of OHSS. Even the quantitative relationship between ovarian size and the amount of peritoneal fluid has not been studied in depth. However, in daily practice two facts are clear: a substantial enlargement of the ovaries during COH is possible without signs of OHSS, and OHSS is not likely without a substantial fluid shift to the peritoneal space. In this latter situation enlargement of the ovaries is present, but may be seen as an epiphenomenon.

INCIDENCE OF OHSS

The main classifications of OHHS are by Golan *et al.*[3] and by Navot and co-workers[4]. The incidence of OHSS varies with the degree or the grade of OHSS. The incidence of mild OHSS may vary between 8 and 23% and may be of little clinical relevance; the incidence lies between < 1 and 7% for moderate grades and the severe form is reported to vary between < 1 and 10%. A report from Israel[5] suggests an increase in the severe form over the years. The main characteristic of the incidence of OHSS is its large variation. It may be concluded that OHSS from a quantitative point of view is an ill-defined condition, and this impairs reliable epidemiological studies on the incidence of the disease.

PRIMARY RISK FACTORS

Within the scope of this chapter, a primary risk factor is defined as a factor that entails a greater risk for developing OHSS apart from the risk caused by controlled ovarian hyperstimulation. In the November 2003 issue of *Fertility and Sterility*, the Practice Committee of the American Society for Reproductive Medicine (ASRM) discussed a guideline on OHSS[6]. The following risk factors were enumerated: young age, low body weight, polycystic ovarian syndrome (PCOS), higher doses of exogenous gonadotropins, high absolute or rapidly rising estradiol levels and previous episodes of OHSS. The first three features can be considered as primary risk factors and are discussed in this chapter, whereas other risks of OHSS are reviewed by other authors.

Assessing clinical risks

To assess risks in clinical practice, tools used in evidence-based medicine (EBM) are helpful. Already in 1985, Sackett, Haynes and Tugwell[7] described the principles and tools to assess risks for a target disorder, which in the context of this chapter is OHSS. The sensitivity and specificity of a test are calculated from the well-known 2×2 table of a target disorder (OHSS) being present or absent versus a positive or negative test. Receiver operating characteristic (ROC) curves show the interrelation between sensitivity and specificity. Odds ratios may be used to compare incidences due to risk factors. To determine the power of diagnostic tools for assessing the risk of OHSS, a likelihood ratio (LR) is best used in EBM. The LR = the post-test odds/the pre-test odds for the target disorder. A cut-off point for the test (e.g. a certain age for the risk of OHSS) and a 'gold standard' to assess the disease are indispensable, but not available. Stolwijk and co-workers[8] used other sophisticated tools for prediction of the outcome of *in vitro* fertilization (IVF). This group[9] also dealt with the issue of external validation of factors predicting IVF outcome. External validation of primary risk factors for OHSS has not been performed.

Young age as a primary risk factor

In the above-mentioned OHSS guideline of the ASRM, five references to the literature concerning the subject of primary risks are given. Neither the ASRM paper, nor any of these references, presents quantitative data on age, let alone an EBM analysis to assess the risk of age. In a retrospective Belgian study[10] including 128 cases of OHSS and 256 controls, the mean age of OHSS patients was 30.2 ± 3.5 years versus 32.0 ± 4.5 years in controls. This small difference between the means combined with the wide spread expressed by relatively large standard deviations permits the concern that a usable cut-off point for age as a risk factor is not available. Similar small differences with a wide variation in age have been shown in two prospective studies[10,11]. Finding differences for a possible risk factor between different groups of patients does not necessarily mean that these risk factors can be used to predict the risk for a certain disease.

Proper tools used in EBM are necessary for risk assessment in clinical practice. Internal and external validations of a possible risk factor are a necessary next step to validate its clinical value. So, the conclusion can be that young age as a risk factor for developing OHSS is mentioned in many papers, book chapters and presentations, but has not been evaluated in a robust, scientifically sound way. Moreover, the fact that older patients have a greater risk of being poor responders during COH, and hence have a lower risk for OHSS, does not necessarily imply that patients with a young age are at greater risk.

Low body weight as a risk factor

Low weight is an obsolete notion, since it does not consider height. A better and more useful concept is the body mass index (BMI), since with BMI weight is related to height. IVF stimulation protocols do not usually correct the dose of gonadotropins for BMI or weight. This means that patients with a low BMI or weight receive relatively higher doses of gonadotropins. Merely due to a relatively higher dose, a higher risk of OHSS is likely, but has not been proved.

A recent Medline search performed by the author utilizing OHSS and weight or body mass as the search terms yielded 11 hits, from which only two hits were usable, since they had body weight or mass in the title of the study. Lashen *et al.*[12] studied extreme body mass, which is not relevant to this chapter. Enskog *et al.*[11] and Delvigne *et al.*[10] found no correlation between lean body mass and OHSS, whereas only the study of Navot and co-workers[13] described a positive correlation. Danninger and co-workers[14] found a lower body weight in women developing OHSS during COH in IVF. Unfortunately they presented their data only as the p value ($p = 0.011$) of the difference.

The conclusion can be that, at present, a low body mass index is not a scientifically sound proven risk factor for developing OHSS.

PCOS as a risk factor for OHSS

PCOS is notorious not only in OI but also in COH for its narrow therapeutic range. In the study of Delvigne *et al.*[10], 37% of their OHSS patients suffered from PCOS versus 15% in the controls. PCOS-like ovarian ultrasound features (more than ten follicles) are a predictive factor for OHSS in IVF[15].

Delvigne and co-workers[16], as well as Bodis *et al.*[17], showed an increased risk for OHSS in patients with a luteinizing hormone/follicle stimulating hormone (LH/FSH) ratio of more than 2. The same was shown[17] for patients with elevated levels of androstenedione not related to PCOS.

PCOS seems to be a risk factor to develop OHSS, but quantitative analysis of the risk must be improved by tools used in EBM.

Ovarian volume as a risk factor for OHSS

Danninger and co-workers[14] measured baseline ovarian volume in patients who underwent IVF with COH using three-dimensional ultrasound. This volume was significantly greater (11.3 ml vs. 8.9 ml) in patients who subsequently developed OHSS. They did not elaborate their data. The cut-off was 'roughly estimated' to be 10 ml. In patients with an ovarian volume < 10 ml, 10% had OHSS, whereas, of patients with an ovarian volume > 10 ml, 23.5% developed the syndrome. They did not mention the cut-off value for ovarian volume for which no or very few patients showed OHSS. Hence, their data are not applicable to the individual patient.

Other primary risk factors

Patients who have suffered previous severe OHSS, patients with a high initial antral follicle count and patients with an allergic disposition (see Chapter 12) may also be considered at an increased primary risk to develop severe OHSS.

CONCLUSIONS

OHSS is an iatrogenic condition and may be life-threatening. When applying so-called controlled ovarian hyperstimulation, OHSS is a condition that is difficult to avoid, since the etiology and risk factors for patients are not sufficiently known. Due to lack of insight into the etiology, no therapy, but only management, is available for OHSS. The early recognition of patients at risk is mandatory, but a scientifically sound risk assessment is still lacking, despite the fact that young age and low weight are often mentioned as primary risk factors. PCOS as a primary risk factor is better described from a quantitative point of view, but needs further analysis with EBM tools. For a robust risk analysis, tools employed in EBM must be used.

At present it is incomprehensible why not all patients undergoing COH and showing completely non-physiological numbers of follicles develop OHSS. Even under these non-physiological circumstances the incidence of severe OHSS can be considered as low, but nevertheless it remains dangerous. Thus, it might be helpful to identify patients at risk. Unfortunately this is currently not possible utilizing primary risk factors such as young age and low body weight or BMI, despite that these factors are mentioned in many publications. Low BMI and young age need robust scientific analysis before they can be assigned the status of primary risk factors for OHSS.

Every patient undergoing COH should be considered at (primary) risk for OHSS. All co-workers, medical and non-medical, in an IVF team should be taught to recognize OHSS. This must be evident in protocols relating to both patients and those working in an IVF setting.

REFERENCES

1. Beerendonk CC, van Dop PA, Braat DD, et al. Ovarian hyperstimulation syndrome: facts and fallacies. Obstet Gynecol Surv 1998; 53: 439–49.
2. Maathuis JB, Van Look PF, Michie EA. Changes in volume, total protein and ovarian steroid concentrations of peritoneal fluid throughout the human menstrual cycle. J Endocrinol 1978; 76: 123–33.
3. Golan A, Ron-el R, Herman A, et al. Ovarian hyperstimulation syndrome: an update review. Obstet Gynecol Surv 1989; 44: 430–40.
4. Navot D, Bergh PA, Laufer N. Ovarian hyperstimulation syndrome in novel reproductive technologies: prevention and treatment. Fertil Steril 1992; 58: 249–61.
5. Abramov Y, Elchalal U, Schenker JG. Severe OHSS: an 'epidemic' of severe OHSS: a price we have to pay? Hum Reprod 1999; 14: 2181–3.

6. The Practice Committee of the American Society for Reproductive Medicine. Ovarian hyperstimulation syndrome. Fertil Steril 2003; 80: 1309–14.

7. Sackett DL, Haynes RB, Tugwell P. Clinical Epidemiology – A Basic Science for Clinical Medicine. Boston: Little, Brown and Company, 1985.

8. Stolwijk AM, Zielhuis GA, Hamilton CJ, et al. Prognostic models for the probability of achieving an ongoing pregnancy after in-vitro fertilization and the importance of testing their predictive value. Hum Reprod 1996; 11: 2298–303.

9. Stolwijk AM, Straatman H, Zielhuis GA, et al. External validation of prognostic models for ongoing pregnancy after in-vitro fertilization. Hum Reprod 1998; 13: 3542–9.

10. Delvigne A, Demoulin A, Smitz J, et al. The ovarian hyperstimulation syndrome in in-vitro fertilization: a Belgian multicentric study. I. Clinical and biological features. Hum Reprod 1993; 8: 1353–60.

11. Enskog A, Henriksson M, Unander M, et al. Prospective study of the clinical and laboratory parameters of patients in whom ovarian hyperstimulation syndrome developed during controlled ovarian hyperstimulation for in vitro fertilization. Fertil Steril 1999; 71: 808–14.

12. Lashen H, Ledger W, Bernal AL, et al. Extremes of body mass do not adversely affect the outcome of superovulation and in-vitro fertilization. Hum Reprod 1999; 14: 712–15.

13. Navot D, Relou A, Birkenfeld A, et al. Risk factors and prognostic variables in the ovarian hyperstimulation syndrome. Am J Obstet Gynecol 1988; 159: 210–15.

14. Danninger B, Brunner M, Obruca A, et al. Prediction of ovarian hyperstimulation of baseline volume prior to stimulation. Hum Reprod 1996; 8: 1597–9.

15. Tibi C, Alvarez S, Cornet D, et al. Prédiction des hyperstimulations ovariennes. Contracept Fertil Sex 1989; 17: 751–2.

16. Delvigne A, Dubois M, Battheu B, et al. The ovarian hyperstimulation syndrome in in-vitro fertilization: a Belgian multicentric study. II. Multiple discriminant analysis for risk prediction. Hum Reprod 1993; 8: 1361–6.

17. Bodis J, Török A, Tinneberg HR. LH/FSH ratios as a predictor of ovarian hyperstimulation syndrome. Hum Reprod 1996; 11: 1597–9.

CHAPTER 3

Secondary risk factors for ovarian hyperstimulation syndrome during stimulation

Annick Delvigne, Rina Agrawal and Gautam Allahbadia

INTRODUCTION

The ovarian hyperstimulation syndrome (OHSS) is a serious and potentially life-threatening iatrogenic complication, typically encountered in patients who undergo so-called controlled ovarian hyperstimulation (COH). The syndrome is usually associated with regimens of exogenous gonadotropins, but can also be seen, albeit rarely, during the administration of clomiphene citrate for ovulation induction, and, moreover, exceptional spontaneous OHSS may also occur. Although the full clinical manifestation of the syndrome occurs in the postovulatory (or post-oocyte retrieval) phase of a stimulated cycle, signs and symptoms predictive of OHSS can be observed earlier in the stimulation phase of the treatment cycle. At this stage of our knowledge of the etiology of OHSS, we have to base our decisions about preventive strategies on the identification of risk factors that have been associated with OHSS and are thought to have predictive value, as there is currently no specific treatment for the condition.

The scope of this chapter is to discuss the secondary risk factors for OHSS.

Secondary risk factors are by definition those that come to the surface once controlled ovarian stimulation has started[1].

ESTRADIOL

Many investigators have shown that an elevated *serum estrogen concentration at the day of human chorionic gonadotropin (hCG) administration* constitutes a (secondary) risk factor for OHSS[2,3]. Already in 1970, a correlation was demonstrated between preovulatory urinary estrogen and the incidence of severe OHSS[4], while in a series of 70 ovulation induction cycles with menotropins, the serum estradiol (E_2) level was found to be the only predictive factor for OHSS[5]. Others attempted to identify a high-risk group among 637 *in vitro* fertilization (IVF) patients, with six (0.94%) suffering from severe OHSS[6]. In this group, none of the patients with serum E_2 levels < 3500 pg/ml developed OHSS, while 1.5% of those with E_2 levels of 3500 ± 5999 pg/ml and 38% with serum E_2 levels > 6000 pg/ml developed OHSS. These authors identified a sensitivity of 83% and a specificity of 99%, but the positive predictive value was only 38%. Another group discussed the predictive value of E_2, and found only 8.8% of OHSS cases among patients with E_2 levels of over 6000 pg/ml ($n = 34$)[7]. This rather low incidence was probably due to the mixed population studied, which also included oocyte donors. When a more homogeneous group of

IVF cycles with embryo transfer was considered, the incidence was 17% ($n = 18$). An additional group, using a cohort of 78 early- and late-OHSS patients, determined the oocyte number and peak E_2 level that best discriminated cycles with and without OHSS[8]. These authors calculated the sensitivity and specificity for different cut-off limits: only a moderately significant positive likelihood ratio (LR; 6.37) was obtained for an E_2 level > 2642 pg/ml, while a moderately significant negative LR (0.13) was obtained for an E_2 level < 1847 pg/ml.

Although mean serum E_2 levels are significantly higher in patients who develop OHSS compared with controls, serum E_2 alone is not a sufficiently predictive factor. Indeed, an extensive overlap of serum E_2 values was found between controls and OHSS patients in two series of 54 OHSS patients[2] and 128 patients[9] (Figure 1).

Some authors studied the predictive value of measuring the *early cycle serum E_2 level* to estimate cycle outcome in IVF. E_2 was measured in the mid-follicular phase (day 9) during COH (long gonadotropin-releasing hormone (GnRH) agonist and human menopausal gonadotropin (hMG) started on day 3), and excessive ovarian responsiveness was defined by E_2 > 4000 pg/ml on the day of hCG administration or the necessity for coasting based on E_2 > 3000 pg/ml before the day of hCG injection. With a serum E_2 level > 800 pg/ml on cycle day 9, 55.8% of patients fulfilled the criteria for excessive ovarian responsiveness, but none of the patients with a serum E_2 level < 300 pg/ml met the criteria. According to these previous data, the authors recommended decreasing the hMG dose on day 9 in order to tailor the ovarian response[10].

D'Angelo *et al.* studied the predictive value of different serum E_2 cut-off levels on days 11 and 8 of COH in a retrospective case–control study of 80 patients[11]. A serum E_2 of 3354 pg/ml on day 11 of COH gave a sensitivity and specificity of 85% for the detection of women at risk for OHSS (only mild and moderate OHSS were recorded in the studied patients). Moreover,

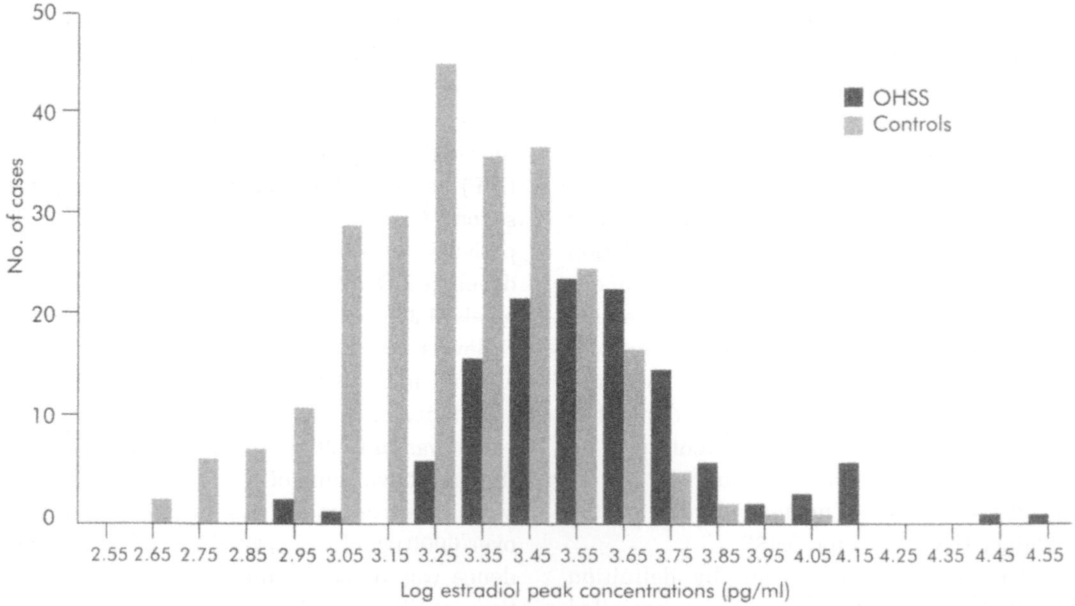

Figure 1 Overlap of estradiol values between OHSS and control patients[9]

they found that all women who developed OHSS had elevated E_2 on day 11 but only 60% had a high E_2 level on day 8. The authors recommended using E_2 level on day 11 as an 'early warning' sign to apply subsequent preventive measures[11].

The rate of E_2 increase during stimulation is also a (secondary) risk factor, as has been shown in a multicentric study evaluating 128 OHSS cases[9]. The discriminant analysis selects the increase in E_2 expressed semi-logarithmically for the mathematical model (β) (Tables 1 and 2). Some authors also take this measure into consideration when deciding on preventive measures[12,13].

Severe OHSS has been observed in patients with very low serum E_2 levels of 475 and 29 pg/ml[14–16]; likewise, five atypical cases of severe OHSS characterized by a mean serum E_2 level of only 2138 pg/ml have been reported[17]. Severe OHSS was also reported for patients with partial 17,20-desmolase deficiency with very low E_2[18]. These observations underscore the inadequacy of serum E_2 as the sole predictive factor.

The role of elevated serum E_2 levels to predict OHSS remains somewhat controversial, but lowering the serum E_2 level by coasting helps to prevent OHSS[19,20]. Moreover, monitoring serum E_2 was found to be effective in reducing the

Table 1 Discriminant analysis by progressive introduction of data for all ovarian hyperstimulation syndrome (OHSS) cases: post-oocyte retrieval conditions

Variables studied	*No. of cases*		*False values (%)*		*Cases correctly classified (%)*
	OHSS	*Controls*	*Positive*	*Negative*	
Log estradiol, β^a, hMG[b], OR[c]	96	200	22.0	19.8	78.7
+ age (years)	96	198	21.7	21.9	78.2
+ log estradiol m[d]	33[h]	95[h]	24.2	30.3	74.2
+ ooc. m[e]	33[h]	97[h]	21.6	30.3	76.1
+ endocrinopathy	96	199	21.1	22.9	78.3
+ LH/FSH > 2[f]	94	199	23.1	18.1	78.5
+ necklace sign[g]	86	172	20.3	22.1	79.1
+ hyperandrogenism	96	200	22.5	20.8	78.0
+ anovulation	94	200	22.5	19.1	78.6

[a]Slope of estradiol increment; [b]no. of human menopausal gonadotropin (hMG) ampoules administered; [c]no. of oocytes retrieved; [d]logarithm of mean estradiol concentrations of previous trials; [e]mean no. of oocytes retrieved during previous trials; [f]LH/FSH, luteinizing hormone/follicle stimulating hormone ratio; [g]polycystic ovaries at ultrasound examination; [h]low numbers of cases

Predictive formula for post-oocyte retrieval conditions

The best prediction for post-oocyte retrieval conditions obtained false-negative value 18.1% and prediction rate 78.5%

(LH/FSH ratio with score of 1 if LH/FSH > 2 and 0 if LH/FSH < 2)

$\Delta = (2.89 \times \log \text{ estradiol}) + (0.32 \times \beta) - (0.77 \times 10^{-2} \times \text{hMG dose}) + (0.07 \times \text{number of oocytes retrieved}) + (0.23 \times \text{LH/FSH}) - 10.86$

$\Delta > 0.26$ in OHSS cases

Table 2 Discriminant analysis by progressive introduction of data for all ovarian hyperstimulation syndrome (OHSS) cases: preovulation-triggering conditions

Variables studied	*No. of cases*		*False values (%)*		*Cases correctly classified (%)*
	OHSS	*Controls*	*Positive*	*Negative*	
Log estradiol, β[a]	96	200	27.0	18.8	75.7
+ age (years)	96	198	28.8	18.8	74.5
+ log estradiol m[b]	33[f]	95	26.3	24.2	74.2
+ ooc. m[c]	33[f]	97	26.8	24.2	73.8
+ endocrinopathy	96	199	25.6	19.8	76.3
+ LH/FSH > 2[d]	94	199	26.6	18.1	76.1
+ necklace sign[e]	86	172	26.2	19.8	76.0
+ hyperandrogenism	96	200	27.0	19.8	75.3
+ anovulation	94	200	27.0	19.1	75.5

[a–e]See Table 1; [f]low numbers of cases

Predictive formula under preovulation-triggering conditions

The best prediction for preovulation-triggering conditions obtained prediction rate 76.1% and false-negative rate 18.1%

$\Delta = (4.44 \times \log \text{estradiol}) + (1.38 \times \beta) + (0.09 \times \text{LH/FSH}) - 15.54$

$\Delta > 0.24$ in OHSS cases

incidence of OHSS[3,21]. The reasons why coasting is effective in preventing OHSS are speculative, and are elaborated in more depth in Chapters 22 and 23. Tortoriello *et al.*[22] hypothesized that coasting may diminish the functional granulosa cell cohort, resulting in the gradual decline in circulating levels of serum E_2, and of the chemical mediators or precursors of fluid extravasation. The size of the granulosa cell population available for luteinization following hCG determines both the incidence and the severity of OHSS[20]. Moreover, the findings of Tozer *et al.* suggest that coasting has an effect on the functional capacity of the granulosa cells and the duration of their function[23]. The E_2 level can be considered as a good marker of the granulosa cell population available to produce this vasoactive mediator.

The threshold of serum E_2 level above which there is a considerable risk of OHSS varies widely among different investigators. Most studies selected a serum E_2 of 3000 pg/ml as a safe value for hCG administration[20] (Figure 2).

A recent prospective cohort study evaluated the predictive value of *E_2 in antagonist cycles*[24]. None of the E_2 thresholds could predict severe, late or early OHSS in this type of COH[24].

In conclusion, it is believed that, irrespective of the debatable role of E_2 itself in the pathogenesis of OHSS, there is a general agreement that serial serum E_2 assays are an important marker for detecting the majority of patients at risk for OHSS and deciding whether to apply a preventive method such as coasting, for example[19].

FOLLICLE NUMBER AND SIZE DURING STIMULATION AND OOCYTES COLLECTED

Most studies have found that a large number of preovulatory follicles during stimulation

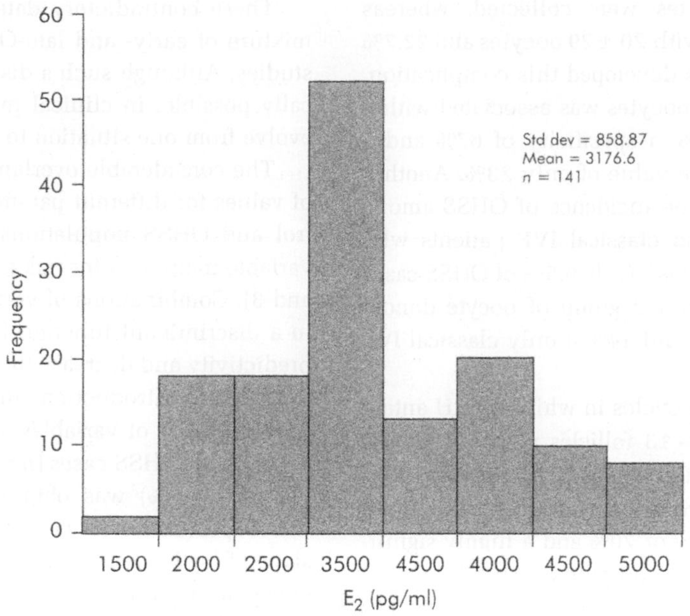

Figure 2 Frequency histogram of estradiol (E_2) value (pg/ml) which was chosen by physicians ($n = 141$) as value for administration of human chorionic gonadotropin (hCG) when applying coasting as preventive measure

constitute a risk factor for OHSS. Moreover, according to different authors, the size of follicles which should be considered a threshold value for risk is variable. Blankstein *et al.*[25] in 1987 evaluated a cohort of 65 patients treated with COH and found that patients with OHSS had significantly more follicles at the time of hCG than did patients without OHSS. In moderate to severe OHSS, 95% of the preovulatory follicles were < 16 mm and 55% < 9 mm; in contrast, in mild OHSS, 69% were follicles of intermediate size (9–15 mm). Although this study is often cited as a reference, its results should be distinguished from those of other reports, because the stimulation conditions were quite different. For example, hCG was administered to all patients when their 24-h urinary excretion of E_2 was between 80 and 180 μg, independent of any maturation criteria assessed by ultrasound.

A significant correlation was found between the presence of multiple (> 4.2) secondary follicles of size 14–16 mm and severe OHSS[26], while others[2,27] found that during ovarian induction and IVF cycles, respectively, follicles of 12–14 mm or < 18 mm were associated with an increased risk of OHSS.

Finally, it was observed that, during IVF, OHSS patients had more follicles > 15 mm in size[15].

The discussion regarding follicular size may be obsolete, because stimulation criteria are totally different according to whether ovarian induction or IVF is applied. Furthermore, the error in follicle measurement and counting is related to their number[6]. Hence, the risk of OHSS is often related to the total number of developing follicles and to the number of collected oocytes (90% of follicles seen)[6]. In the latter study, no patient developed severe OHSS when < 20 oocytes were collected, whereas 1.4% of patients with 20 ± 29 oocytes and 22.7% with > 30 oocytes developed this complication. Retrieval of > 30 oocytes was associated with a sensitivity of 83%, a specificity of 67% and a positive predictive value of only 23%. Another group evaluated the incidence of OHSS among oocyte donors and classical IVF patients who yielded > 30 oocytes[7]. Only 6.5% of OHSS cases were in the combined group of oocyte donors and classical IVF, and 14% if only classical IVF was considered.

If we consider cycles in which GnRH antagonists are used, > 13 follicles with a diameter above 11 mm on the day of hCG administration predict all OHSS cases with a sensitivity of 100%, a specificity of 70% and a highly significant negative likelihood ratio of 0.01[24].

COMBINATION OF DATA TO PREDICT OHSS

Serum E_2 level and number of follicles and/or oocytes collected are often used together to predict OHSS occurrence: according to one group, for patients with a serum E_2 level > 6000 pg/ml and > 30 oocytes collected, the incidence of severe OHSS was 80%[6].

Morris *et al.*[7] in 1995 reported an incidence of 20% of cases of OHSS when they considered only classical IVF and excluded oocyte donors. Once more, markedly elevated serum estradiol concentrations and/or numerous oocytes may predispose to, but are not sufficient for the development of, OHSS. Some oocyte donors did not develop OHSS even in the presence of high serum levels of E_2 (maximum 9590 pg/ml) and when large numbers of oocytes (maximum 58) were collected.

According to one investigation, early OHSS is predicted by E_2 and the number of oocytes retrieved, while late OHSS is related to the number of gestational sacs seen at ultrasound[28].

These contradictory data may be due to a mixture of early- and late-OHSS cases in most studies. Although such a distinction is theoretically possible, in clinical practice, many cases evolve from one situation to the other.

The considerable overlap of the distribution of values for different parameters between control and OHSS populations makes any single variable inefficient for risk prediction (Figures 1 and 3). Combinations of variables were studied in a discriminant function in order to increase predictivity and decrease the false-negative rate. Progressive introduction and automated stepwise selection of variables were applied to IVF patients, all OHSS cases ($n = 128$). The best prediction (78.5%) was obtained in OHSS cases under post-retrieval conditions using log E_2, slope of log E_2 increment, hMG dosage, number of oocytes retrieved and ratio of luteinizing hormone/follicle stimulating hormone (LH/FSH) in the formula, with a corresponding false-negative rate of 18.1% (Table 1). However, effective prevention of OHSS implies the ability to withhold hCG injection. Therefore, a formula for pre-oocyte retrieval conditions was established yielding a prediction rate of 76.1%, with a false-negative rate of 18.1% (Table 2). To be validated, such formulae would have to be applied to another population of IVF cases used as a 'testing-set'[29].

OVARIAN VOLUME

Total ovarian volume on transvaginal sonography before hCG administration was found to be higher in women who develop moderate or severe OHSS compared with controls, and may therefore be used as an additional parameter in the preventive strategy for ovarian hyperstimulation syndrome[30]. Using ovarian volume measurement, one group found a significant correlation between baseline ovarian volume (measured by three-dimensional ultrasonography) and the development of OHSS in 101

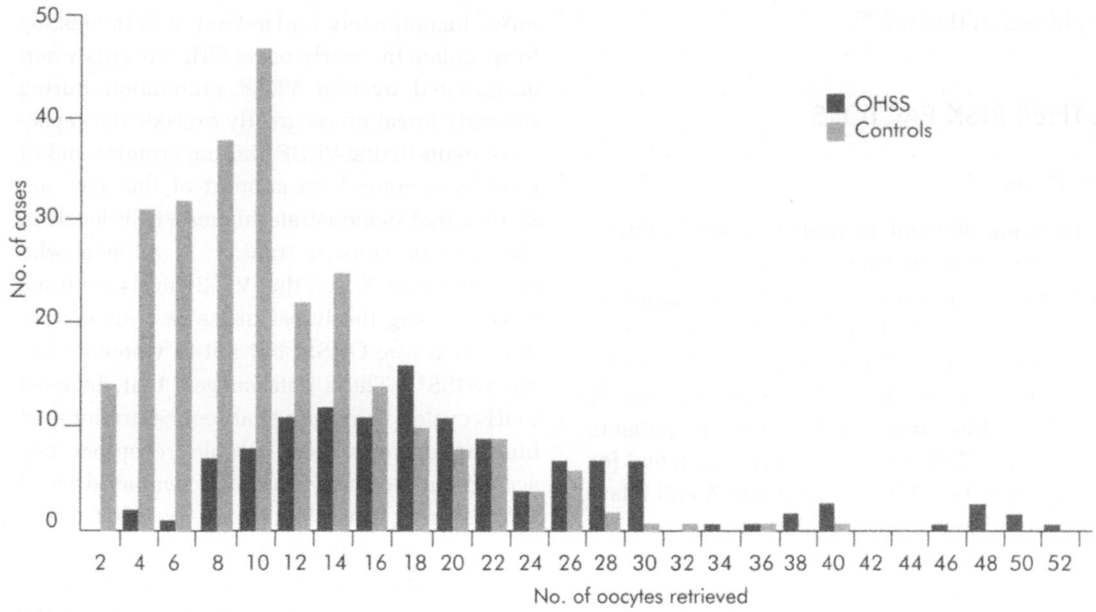

Figure 3 Overlap of number of oocytes retrieved between OHSS and control patients[20]

patients who underwent IVF[31]. In addition, a significant correlation was found between the baseline number of follicles, the number of oocytes retrieved and OHSS.

Some investigators furthermore evaluated the intraovarian blood flow, and identified a close correlation between OHSS severity and lowered resistance to blood flow in the stimulated ovaries[32]. However, the predictive value of these data should be validated in larger series. Agrawal *et al.* suggested that within ovarian and uterine blood vessels, blood flow velocities were higher in the early follicular phase and on the day of hCG administration in women with polycystic ovaries/polycystic ovarian syndrome (PCO/PCOS)[33]. A positive correlation was observed between serum vascular endothelial growth factor (VEGF) and E_2 concentrations on the days of hCG administration and oocyte retrieval, and between serum VEGF concentration and Doppler blood flow velocities throughout the IVF cycle[33]. Quantification of the Doppler signal in PCOS using three-dimensional power Doppler ultrasonography was recently published by Pan *et al.*[34]. These authors found that mean ovarian volume was significantly higher ($p < 0.05$) in women with PCOS compared with women with normal ovaries. The vascularization flow index (VFI), flow index (FI) and vascularization index (VI) were significantly higher ($p < 0.05$) in women with PCOS compared with women with normal ovaries. The authors concluded that this observation may help to explain the excessive response often seen during gonadotropin administration in women with PCOS[34]. However, other investigators have concluded that polycystic ovaries are not associated with an inherent disturbance in blood flow dynamics of the uterine and ovarian arteries, as measured by color Doppler, and that an increased sensitivity of polycystic ovaries to stimulation with gonadotropins cannot be explained in this way[35].

OTHER RISK FACTORS

Inhibins

A common element in most theories of OHSS has been endothelial activation by ovarian products and an increase in capillary permeability leading to fluid shifting to third spaces[36]. Several such products have been studied as putative predictors of OHSS, including inhibins A and B[37]. These were evaluated in 15 patients with severe OHSS and 15 controls matched for age and number of follicles. Inhibin A and B levels were followed from the start of ovarian stimulation until at least 3 days post-embryo transfer. Inhibin A, in the OHSS group, showed a continuous increase during stimulation to embryo transfer, but this elevation was significantly higher than in the controls only at the point where OHSS had developed. Inhibin B levels also rose from the start of the stimulation, with peak values 3 days prior to oocyte retrieval, and then declined. This elevation was significantly higher in OHSS patients as well as on the day of oocyte retrieval. The authors suggest that inhibin levels may serve as indicators of OHSS risk, but threshold levels have still to be defined[37].

Vascular endothelial growth factor

Serum VEGF levels are higher in women at risk for OHSS, and correlate with the clinical course of the syndrome[38]. In addition, anti-VEGF antibodies neutralize the vascular permeability activity of follicular fluids and of ascitic fluid obtained in women with OHSS[39]. In contrast to the natural cycle, COH cycles are associated with an exaggerated ovarian production of VEGF that results in an increase in circulating levels of free VEGF during the early luteal phase in women at risk for OHSS. Why some women develop OHSS during COH cycles and others do not is incompletely understood. It is interesting to speculate that early-onset OHSS occurs when exaggerated ovarian VEGF production during the early luteal phase greatly exceeds the capacity of neutralizing VEGF binding proteins and/or soluble receptors[8]. In support of this idea are studies that demonstrate higher VEGF levels at the time of embryo transfer in women who develop OHSS[40], and that VEGF levels continue to rise during the luteal phase in women who develop severe OHSS, but not in women without OHSS[41]. These data suggest that, in most COH cycles, physiological concentrations of binding proteins and soluble receptors can accommodate rising levels of ovarian-derived VEGF during the luteal phase, but that OHSS may occur when free/total VEGF ratios are dramatically altered. Whether other angiogenic factors contribute or modify VEGF actions in the pathogenesis of OHSS is currently unknown, but represents an important area of future investigation.

Today, VEGF measurement is not recommended to predict OHSS in individual patients even if its role in the etiopathology of OHSS seems more and more accepted.

Rising FSH levels

Agrawal *et al.*[41] found that FSH stimulated VEGF production to a similar degree, compared with hCG. This emphasizes the importance of circulating FSH levels in the pathogenesis of OHSS and correlates nicely with results of a study showing that circulating FSH levels were much higher during the days before hCG in anovulatory women treated with FSH who had marked enlargement of the ovaries after hCG[42]. It was not clear whether those increased circulating levels of FSH were due to increased endogenous release, to decreased clearance of FSH or both. It has been empirically observed that tapering of the FSH dose later in the course of ovarian stimulation for IVF reduces the risk of

OHSS despite a higher starting dose of stimulation. This approach may also be more physiological and has been empirically associated with a better IVF outcome. Reduction of circulating FSH may be the mechanism through which coasting reduces the incidence of OHSS. Al-Shawaf *et al.*[43] showed that circulating FSH fell to the normal range over this period of time. The adverse effects of FSH may also indicate that recombinant LH is a better approach as a surrogate LH surge than use of a GnRH agonist, which releases large amounts of both FSH and LH.

Erythrocyte aggregation

Increased capillary leak brought about by the elevation of erythrocyte aggregation could be a newly discovered mediator in the pathophysiology of OHSS and an independent risk factor[44]. An increase in erythrocyte aggregation is associated with unfavorable hemorrheological effects in terms of microcirculatory slow flow, tissue hypoxemia and microcirculatory occlusions[45]. These changes alter the peripheral resistance, reduce capillary perfusion and oxygen transfer to tissues and bring about a degeneration of the vascular wall, leading to capillary leak[46]. A recent study clearly showed that enhanced erythrocyte aggregation can be detected in the peripheral blood of women following gonadotropin administration. This phenomenon of erythrocyte aggregability can have a deleterious effect on the microcirculatory flow[46,47]. Levin *et al.* believe that increased erythrocyte aggregation in patients with COH and OHSS after the administration of gonadotropins is brought about by hyperfibrinogenemia[44]. It has been shown that fibrinogen has a major role in the induction and/or maintenance of increased erythrocyte aggregation in the peripheral blood[47]. The enhanced synthesis of this macromolecule is probably a result of the presence of enhanced interleukin-6 (IL-6) concentrations in the peripheral blood[48].

C-reactive protein

C-reactive protein (CRP) is a biological marker of systemic inflammation, produced by the liver. It was recently demonstrated to have a strong prognostic value for cardiovascular events[49]. CRP levels have no diurnal variation, are stable over long periods[50] and increase after estrogen administration[51]. Orvieto *et al.* observed a 60% increase in CRP levels from the initial day of stimulation to the day of hCG administration, which is in accordance with the positive effect of the serum E_2 level on the CRP level[52]. The finding in a recent study of an observed increase in serum CRP, which reflects a state of systemic inflammatory response, may further substantiate the role of systemic inflammation in the pathophysiology of OHSS and may designate increasing levels of CRP as a risk factor for OHSS during ovarian stimulation[53].

CONCLUSIONS

The most frequently used and studied predictive factors reflect the amplitude of the ovarian response to COH (E_2 level and number of follicles). This is based on the fact that most women who develop OHSS also have an exaggerated response to stimulation. Different threshold levels and a combination of these predictive factors have been proposed, but no optimal prediction currently exists. Indeed, these parameters do not reflect the physiopathology of OHSS.

Therefore, other parameters linked to the etiology and pathology of the syndrome are evaluated (VEGF, erythrocyte aggregation, CRP) but have not yet been validated in clinical use.

In clinical practice, in the mean time, absolute serum E_2 level and the rate of its increase, and the number of follicles or the number of oocytes collected, remain the factors that should be used to monitor COH and initiate preventive measures (Table 3).

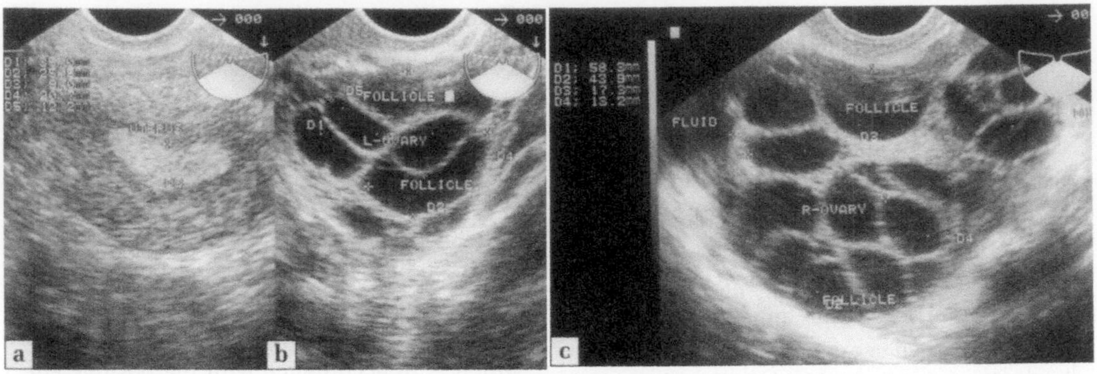

Figure 4 (a) Thickened endometrium during ovarian stimulation. (b, c) Multifollicular ovarian development in left and right ovaries accompanied by small quantities of free abdominal fluid. Courtesy Dr D Navot and Dr Z Levine, USA

Table 3 Secondary risk factors predicting OHSS

Serum estradiol > 3000 pg/ml at hCG injection
Serum estradiol > 800 pg/ml at day 9
Serum estradiol > 3354 pg/ml at day 11
> 20 follicles at the end of the follicular phase of COH with GnRH agonist
> 13 follicles at the end of the follicular phase of COH with GnRH antagonist
> 15 oocytes retrieved

hCG, human chorionic gonadotropin; COH, controlled ovarian hyperstimulation; GnRH, gonadotropin-releasing hormone

REFERENCES

1. Delvigne A, Rozenberg S. Epidemiology and prevention of ovarian hyperstimulation syndrome (OHSS): a review. Hum Reprod 2002; 6: 559–77.

2. Navot D, Relou A, Birkenfeld A, et al. Risk factors and prognostic variables in the ovarian hyperstimulation syndrome. Am J Obstet Gynecol 1988; 159: 210–15.

3. Haning RV Jr, Austin CW, Carlson LH, et al. Plasma estradiol is superior to ultrasound and urinary estriol glucuronide as a predictor of ovarian hyperstimulation during induction of ovulation with menotropins. Fertil Steril 1983; 40: 31–6.

4. Crooke AC. Induction of ovulation with gonadotrophins. Br Med Bull 1970; 26: 17–21.

5. Diamond MP, Wentz AC. Ovulation induction with human menopausal gonadotropins. Obstet Gynecol Surv 1986; 41: 480–90.

6. Asch RH, Li HP, Balmaceda JP, et al. Severe ovarian hyperstimulation syndrome in assisted reproductive technology: definition of high risk groups. Hum Reprod 1991; 6: 1395–9.

7. Morris RS, Wong IL, Kirkman E, et al. Inhibition of ovarian-derived prorenin to angiotensin cascade in the treatment of ovarian hyperstimulation syndrome. Hum Reprod 1995; 10: 1355–8.

8. Mathur RS, Akande AV, Keay SD, et al. Distinction between early and late ovarian hyperstimulation syndrome. Fertil Steril 2000; 73: 901–7.

9. Delvigne A, Demoulin A, Smitz J, et al. The ovarian hyperstimulation syndrome in in-vitro fertilization: a Belgian multicentric study. I. Clinical and biological features. Hum Reprod 1993; 8: 1353–60.

10. Ho H-Y, Lee RK, Lin MH, Hwu YM. Estradiol level on day 9 as a predictor of risk for ovarian hyperresponse during controlled ovarian hyper-

stimulation. J Assist Reprod Genet 2003; 20: 222–6.

11. D'Angelo A, Davies R, Salah E, et al. Value of the serum estradiol level for preventing ovarian hyperstimulation syndrome: a retrospective case control study. Fertil Steril 2004; 81: 332–6.

12. Fluker MR, Hooper WM, Yuzpe AA, et al. Withholding gonadotropins ('coasting') to minimize the risk of ovarian hyperstimulation during superovulation and in vitro fertilization–embryo transfer cycles. Fertil Steril 1999; 71: 294–301.

13. Enskog A, Henriksson M, Unander M, et al. Prospective study of the clinical and laboratory parameters of patients in whom ovarian hyperstimulation syndrome developed during controlled ovarian hyperstimulation for in vitro fertilization. Fertil Steril 1999; 71: 808–14.

14. Orvieto R. Prediction of ovarian hyperstimulation syndrome. Hum Reprod 2003; 18: 665–7.

15. Levy T, Orvieto R, Homburg R, et al. Severe ovarian hyperstimulation syndrome despite low plasma oestrogen concentrations in a hypogonadotrophic, hypogonadal patient. Hum Reprod 1996; 11: 1177–9.

16. Shimon I, Rubinek T, Bar-Hava L, et al. Ovarian hyperstimulation without elevated serum estradiol associated with pure follicle-stimulating hormone-secreting pituitary adenoma. J Clin Endocrinol Metab 2001; 86: 3635–40.

17. Delvigne A, Vandromme J, Demeestere I, et al. Unpredictable cases of complicated ovarian hyperstimulation in IVF. Int J Fertil Womens Med 1997; 42: 268–70.

18. Pellicer A, Miro F, Sampaio M, et al. In vitro fertilization as a diagnostic and therapeutic tool in a patient with partial 17,20-desmolase deficiency. Fertil Steril 1991; 55: 970–5.

19. Aboulghar M. Prediction of ovarian hyperstimulation syndrome (OHSS). Hum Reprod 2003; 18: 1140–1.

20. Delvigne A. Preventive attitude of physicians to avoid ovarian hyperstimulation syndrome in IVF patients. Hum Reprod 2001; 16: 2491–5.

21. Golan A, Ron-El R, Herman A, et al. Ovarian hyperstimulation syndrome: an update review. Obstet Gynecol Surv 1989; 44: 430–40.

22. Tortoriello DV, McGovern PG, Colon JM, et al. Coasting does not adversely affect cycle outcome in a subset of highly responsive in vitro fertilization patients. Fertil Steril 1998; 69: 454–60.

23. Tozer AJ, Iles RK, Iammarrone E, et al. Characteristics of populations of granulosa cells from individual follicles in women undergoing 'coasting' during controlled ovarian stimulation (COS) for IVF. Hum Reprod 2004; 19: 2561–8.

24. Camus M, Papanikolaou EG, Pozzobon C, et al. Ovarian hyperstimulation syndrome (OHSS) incidence in GnRH antagonist IVF cycles. Can estradiol levels or the number of follicles on the day of hCG administration predict the patients at risk of developing OHSS? Communication 176, 21st Annual Meeting of ESHRE, Copenhagen, 2005.

25. Blankstein J, Shalev J, Saadon T, et al. Ovarian hyperstimulation syndrome: prediction by number and size of preovulatory ovarian follicles. Fertil Steril 1987; 47: 597–602.

26. Tal J, Paz B, Samberg I, et al. Ultrasonographic and clinical correlates of menotropin versus sequential clomiphene citrate: menotropin for induction of ovulation. Fertil Steril 1985; 44: 342–5.

27. MacDougall MJ, Tan SL, Balen A, et al. A controlled study comparing patients with and without polycystic ovaries undergoing in-vitro fertilization. Hum Reprod 1993; 8: 233–7.

28. Lyons CA, Wheeler CA, Frishman GN, et al. Early and late presentation of the ovarian hyperstimulation syndrome: two distinct entities with different risk factors. Hum Reprod 1994; 9: 792–9.

29. Delvigne A, Dubois M, Battheu B, et al. The ovarian hyperstimulation syndrome in in-vitro fertilization: a Belgian multicentric study. II. Multiple discriminant analysis for risk prediction. Hum Reprod 1993; 8: 1361–6.

30. Oyesanya OA, Parsons JH, Collins WP, et al. Total ovarian volume before human chorionic gonadotrophin administration for ovulation induction may predict the hyperstimulation syndrome. Hum Reprod 1995; 10: 3211–12.

31. Danninger B, Brunner M, Obruca A, et al. Prediction of ovarian hyperstimulation syndrome by ultrasound volumetric assessment [corrected] of baseline ovarian volume prior to stimulation. Hum Reprod 1996; 11: 1597–9.

32. Moohan JM, Curcio K, Leoni M, et al. Low intraovarian vascular resistance: a marker for severe ovarian hyperstimulation syndrome. Fertil Steril 1997; 67: 728–32.

33. Agrawal R, Conway G, Sladkevicius P, et al. Serum vascular endothelial growth factor and Doppler blood flow velocities in in vitro fertilization: relevance to ovarian hyperstimulation syndrome and polycystic ovaries. Fertil Steril 1998; 70: 651–8.

34. Pan HA, Wu MH, Cheng YC, et al. Quantification of Doppler signal in polycystic ovarian syndrome using 3D power Doppler ultrasonography. Hum Reprod 2002; 17: 201–6.

35. Pinkas H, Mashiach R, Rabinerson D, et al. Doppler parameters of uterine and ovarian stromal blood flow in women with polycystic ovary syndrome and normally ovulating women undergoing controlled ovarian stimulation. Ultrasound Obstet Gynecol 1998; 12: 197–200.

36. Delvigne A, Rozenberg S. Preventive attitude of physicians to avoid OHSS in IVF patients. Hum Reprod 2001; 16: 2491–5.

37. Enskog A, Nilsson L, Brannström M. Peripheral blood concentrations of inhibin B are elevated during gonadotrophin stimulation in patients who later develop ovarian OHSS and inhibin A concentrations are elevated after OHSS onset. Hum Reprod 2000; 15: 532–8.

38. Abramov Y, Barak V, Nisman B, et al. Vascular endothelial growth factor plasma levels correlate to the clinical picture in severe ovarian hyperstimulation syndrome. Fertil Steril 1997; 67: 261–5.

39. McClure N, Healy DL, Rogers PA, et al. Vascular endothelial growth factor as capillary permeability agent in ovarian hyperstimulation syndrome. Lancet 1994; 344: 235–6.

40. Ludwig M, Jelkmann W, Bauer O, et al. Prediction of severe ovarian hyperstimulation syndrome by free serum vascular endothelial growth factor concentration on the day of human chorionic gonadotropin administration. Hum Reprod 1999; 14: 2437–41.

41. Agrawal R, Tan SL, Wild S, et al. Serum vascular endothelial growth factor concentrations in in vitro fertilization cycles predict the risk of ovarian hyperstimulation syndrome. Fertil Steril 1999; 71: 287–93.

42. Mizunuma H, Takagi T, Yamada K, et al. The role of endogenous gonadotropin release in the etiology of ovarian enlargement during purified urinary follicle-stimulating hormone therapy. Fertil Steril 1991; 55: 66–72.

43. Al-Shawaf T, Zosmer A, Tozer A, et al. Value of measuring serum FSH in addition to serum estradiol in a coasting programme to prevent severe OHSS. Hum Reprod 2002; 17: 1217–21.

44. Levin I, Gamzu R, Hasson Y, et al. Increased erythrocyte aggregation in ovarian hyperstimulation syndrome: a possible contributing factor in the pathophysiology of this disease. Hum Reprod 2004; 19: 1076–80.

45. Tateishi N, Suzuki Y, Shirai M, et al. Reduced oxygen release from erythrocytes by the acceleration-induced flow shift, observed in an oxygen-permeable narrow tube. J Biomech 2002; 35: 1241–51.

46. Bishop JJ, Nance PR, Popel AS, et al. Effect of erythrocyte aggregation on velocity profiles in venules. Am J Physiol 2001; 280: H222–36.

47. Froom P. Blood viscosity and the risk of death from coronary heart disease. Eur Heart J 2000; 21: 513–14.

48. Weng X, Cloutier G, Beaulieu R, et al. Influence of acute phase proteins on erythrocyte aggregation. Am J Physiol 1996; 271: H2346–52.

49. Gabay C, Kushner I. Acute-phase proteins and other systemic responses to inflammation. N Engl J Med 1999; 340: 448–54.

50. Ridker PM, Rifai N, Rose L, et al. Comparison of C-reactive protein and low-density lipoprotein cholesterol levels in the prediction of first cardiovascular events. N Engl J Med 2002; 347: 1557–65.

51. Meier Ewert HK, Ridker PM, Rifai N, et al. Absence of diurnal variation of C-reactive protein levels in healthy human subjects. Clin Chem 2001; 47: 426–30.

52. Orvieto R, Chen R, Ashkenazi J, et al. C-reactive protein levels in patients undergoing controlled ovarian hyperstimulation for IVF cycle. Hum Reprod 2004; 19: 357–9.

53. Kluft C, Leuven JA, Helmerhorst FM, et al. Proinflammatory effects of oestrogens during use of oral contraceptives and hormone replacement treatment. Vascul Pharmacol 2002; 39: 149–54.

CHAPTER 4

Clinical manifestations of ovarian hyperstimulation syndrome

Gamal Serour

Ovarian hyperstimulation syndrome (OHSS) is mostly an iatrogenic complication of ovarian stimulation. It has been observed over the past 60 years, since gonadotropins were first used to induce ovulation in infertile patients. OHSS is the consequence of an exaggerated response to ovulation induction therapy. Ideally, ovulation induction should stimulate the ovaries to obtain the desired level of ovulation, i.e. monofollicular development. However, the narrow range between no response at all and an exaggerated response to ovulation induction agents combined with the unpredictable patient response makes prevention of OHSS virtually impossible, and prediction unlikely[1]. Some degree of ovarian hyperstimulation occurs in all women who respond to ovulation induction, but this should be distinguished from the clinical entity of OHSS. OHSS may also be encountered in clinical practice in some rare conditions not related to the intake of ovulation-inducing drugs (Table 1).

OVARIAN HYPERSTIMULATION NOT RELATED TO INTAKE OF OVULATION-INDUCING DRUGS

OHSS may be encountered in patients not receiving ovulation-inducing drugs. Physicians should be aware of these conditions, to be able to diagnose them and avoid unnecessary harmful management because of misdiagnosis. These clinical entities include the following.

Ovarian hyperstimulation in intrauterine life

Fetal ovarian hyperstimulation in a pregnancy of 35 weeks was reported by Berezowski *et al.*[2]. Two large cystic septate ovaries without internal vegetations were observed in the fetal abdomen by ultrasonography. There was significant elevation of maternal serum β-human chorionic gonadotropin (hCG) levels. Spontaneous regression of fetal ovarian volume and of maternal serum β-hCG occurred after delivery. The failure to diagnose this condition may result in unnecessary termination of pregnancy and/or neonatal surgery which may lead to castration of the female child.

Ovarian hyperstimulation in preterm infants

Ovarian cysts are a relatively frequent finding in neonates. In preterm infants, the simultaneous occurrence of estradiol-producing ovarian cysts and edematous swelling of the vulva, the thighs and the lower abdominal wall has been described. Vochem reported four cases of

Table 1 Various forms of ovarian hyperstimulation (OHS) encountered in clinical practice

Form of OHS	*Diagnostic criteria*
Spontaneous OHS	
OHS in intrauterine life and in preterm infants	35–39 weeks of pregnancy, large cystic ovaries, stimulation of external and internal genitalia, elevated maternal β-hCG, fetal E_2
OHS with gonadotroph adenoma	Ovarian enlargement, headache, galactorrhea, elevated E_2, FSH and β-LH, CT scan and MRI
OHS in spontaneous pregnancy	Usually associated with hypothyroidism, PCO, MP or hydatidiform mole May be recurrent and familial Develops between 8 and 14 weeks of pregnancy Serial color and pulsed Doppler ultrasonography, elevated hCG, VEGF and TSH
Iatrogenic OHS	
OHS in IVF/ICSI cycles	Abdominal discomfort, nausea, vomiting, abdominal distension Large cystic ovaries, with > 25 small and intermediate-sized follicles E_2 > 4000 pg/ml (> 14 500 mol/l)
OHS in ovulation induction/ ovulation enhancement	History of intake of hMG, FSH or CC Large cystic ovaries and elevated E_2 level

IVF, *in vitro* fertilization; ICSI, intracytoplasmic sperm injection; hCG, human chorionic gonadotropin; E_2, estradiol; FSH, follicle stimulating hormone; LH, luteinizing hormone; CT, computerized tomography; MRI, magnetic resonance imaging; PCO, polycystic ovaries; MP, multiple pregnancy; VEGF, vascular endothelial growth factor; TSH, thyroid-stimulating hormone; hMG, human menopausal gonadropin; CC, clompiphene citrate

extremely low-birth-weight infants with ovarian cysts, and stimulation of the external and internal genitalia beginning at 35–39 weeks[3]. Serum estradiol was elevated. The findings receded during the first 5–9 weeks of neonatal life. The physiologically high concentration of gonadotropins in preterm infants stimulates the ovaries to produce ovarian cysts as well as to secrete high amounts of estradiol, which induce transient stimulation of the external and internal genitalia. The condition subsides spontaneously within a few weeks and does not need any surgical interference.

Spontaneous and severe ovarian hyperstimulation due to gonadotroph adenoma

Spontaneous and severe ovarian hyperstimulation due to gonadotroph adenoma has been reported[4,5]. Patients present with ovarian enlargement simulating hyperstimulation, headache, galactorrhea, a dramatic rise in plasma estradiol, elevated levels of follicle stimulating hormone (FSH) and marginally elevated levels of β-luteinizing hormone (LH). Computerized tomography and pituitary magnetic resonance imaging reveal a huge pituitary adenoma. Transvaginal ultrasound shows enlarged ovaries resembling a hyperstimulation-like pattern. Although the estradiol level is extremely high in these patients, they do not present with ascites, suggesting that chronically elevated estradiol does not play a crucial role in OHSS. The condition subsides after trans-sphenoidal surgery.

OHSS in spontaneous pregnancy

The rare condition of OHSS during spontaneous pregnancy has been reported. The overproduction of endogenous chorionic gonadotropin during pregnancy has been associated with spontaneous OHSS (also termed hyperreactio-luteinalis of the first trimester), as well as hyperemesis gravidarum and transient gestational thyrotoxicosis[6–10]. OHSS in spontaneous pregnancy is particularly associated with primary hypothyroidism, polycystic ovaries, multiple gestations or hydatidiform mole, known to be associated with abnormally high levels of hCG[6,11–16]. In OHSS associated with hypothyroidism it has been suggested that the high level of thyroid-stimulating hormone (TSH) could stimulate the ovaries[14]. Familial recurrent gestational spontaneous OHSS has also been reported[17–20]. The follicular recruitment occurs later through stimulation of the FSH receptor by pregnancy-derived hCG. Massive luteinization of enlarged stimulated ovaries induces the release of vasoactive mediators, resulting in the development of OHSS[21].

Severe spontaneous OHSS during pregnancy with normal levels of chorionic gonadotropin was explained by Smits *et al.* and by Vasseur *et al.* to be due to a chorionic gonadotropin-sensitive mutation in the follicle-stimulating hormone receptor[22,23]. This is treated in more detail in Chapter 13.

Spontaneous forms of OHSS have generally been reported to develop between 8 and 14 weeks of amenorrhea. The initial corpus luteum related to the pregnancy is not responsible for the development of OHSS. The formation of secondary multiple corpora lutea, or at least of a critical mass of luteinized granulosa cells, could induce a massive release of vasoactive substances resulting in the development of OHSS[21].

Spontaneous OHSS is often misdiagnosed as an ovarian carcinoma with consequent laparotomy and castration, or severe complications such as renal insufficiency may develop because the diagnosis and treatment of OHSS are delayed. Serial color and pulsed Doppler ultrasonographic imaging and hCG, vascular endothelial growth factor (VEGF), TSH, free triiodothyronine and free thyroxine levels estimation can help in the diagnosis of spontaneous OHSS and evaluation of the patient, and permit conservative therapy.

OVARIAN HYPERSTIMULATION RELATED TO INTAKE OF OVULATION-INDUCING DRUGS (IATROGENIC OHSS)

In iatrogenic OHSS, follicular recruitment and enlargement occur during ovarian stimulation with exogenous FSH, or rarely with clomiphene citrate followed by the administration of gonadotropin-releasing hormone (GnRH)[24].

OHSS in *in vitro* fertilization programs

With the currently widespread use of GnRH agonists (GnRHa) for pituitary desensitization in combination with exogenous gonadotropin administration in *in vitro* fertilization (IVF) programs, up to 10% of IVF cycles result in OHSS, with severe OHSS observed in 0.5–2% of IVF cycles[25]. Considering the large number of IVF cycles performed annually around the world, OHSS is not a rare clinical problem. In a center performing 1000 IVF and intracytoplasmic sperm injection (ICSI) cycles/year, between 5 and 20 patients will become seriously ill from

OHSS every year. Moreover, we are dealing here with a condition that can result in thromboembolism, requires hospitalization and may even cause the death of a young, healthy woman who may not have been the primary source of the infertility for which she had received treatment.

OHSS in ovulation induction/ovulation enhancement

It has been reported that OHSS occurs in < 4% of cycles of ovulation induction[1]. It is difficult to obtain an accurate incidence of OHSS attributable to ovulation induction/ovulation enhancement (OI/OE) procedures as there is no system for recording the use of ovulation-inducing drugs not in association with IVF programs. The syndrome is becoming more common as the number of women receiving ovulation induction with gonadotropins for OI/OE, apart from IVF, is increasing. It is rarely seen in conjunction with clomiphene citrate or GnRH usage[24]. However, there are a few reports in the literature concerning the occurrence of OHSS in patients receiving clomiphene citrate for OI/OE[26], especially with repeated use over 3 consecutive months[27]. The failure to recognize and diagnose the possibility of OHSS with clomiphene citrate could result in unnecessary oophorectomy.

Patients at risk of iatrogenic OHSS

Patients who are at risk of OHSS should be identified before scheduling them for ovarian stimulation, whether for IVF/ICSI cycles or OI/OE, during ovarian stimulation and after oocyte pick-up (Table 2). According to the European Society of Human Reproduction and Embryology (ESHRE) special interest group (SIG) on safety and quality, these include: polycystic ovarian syndrome (PCOS) patients, and those with incomplete forms of PCOS, a high number of resting follicles, i.e. ≥ 10 in each ovary, a LH/FSH ratio ≥ 2, hyperandrogenism and a previous history of OHSS[28]. Also, young age (< 35 years), lean bodily habitus, allergies and using

Table 2 Patients at risk of iatrogenic ovarian hyperstimulation syndrome (OHSS)

Before stimulation	*During stimulation*	*After stimulation*
PCOS patients	Patients requiring high dose of gonadotropin	OPU > 25 oocytes
Incomplete forms of PCOS	Rapidly rising E_2 level	Exogenous hCG for luteal phase support
≥ 10 resting follicles in each ovary	E_2 > 4000 pg/ml	Pregnancy particularly multiple pregnancy
LH/FSH ≥ 2	> 25 small and intermediate follicles	
Hyperandrogenism	Exogenous hCG for ovulation induction	
Previous OHSS		
Young age < 35 years		
Lean bodily habitus		
GnRHa down-regulation		

PCOS, polycystic ovarian syndrome; LH, luteinizing hormone; FSH, follicle stimulating hormone; GnRHa, gonadotropin-releasing hormone agonist; E_2, estradiol; hCG, human chorionic gonadotropin; OPU, oocyte pick-up

GnRHa for down-regulation are reported to be possible risk factors[28–33].

During stimulation, patients who are more likely to develop OHSS include those requiring higher doses of exogenous gonadotropins or those with a high absolute or rapidly rising serum estradiol level (> 4000 pg/ml; > 14 500 mol/l) (with no clear cut-off value); other factors are the occurrence of > 25 small and intermediate-sized follicles, and the use of exogenous hCG for ovulation induction and luteal phase support[34,35].

Women at increased risk of OHSS should be on the lowest possible dose of gonadotropins with the aim of reducing the granulosa/luteal cell mass[36]. Patients who yield a large number of oocytes (> 25 oocytes) and those who become pregnant, particularly with a multiple pregnancy, are more likely to develop OHSS. Pregnancy increases the likelihood, duration and severity of OHSS.

OHSS may occur early or late, with two different risk factors. Luteinization is mandatory for the manifestation of OHSS. An early form of OHSS presents 3–7 days following hCG administration, is usually severe and reflects the degree of ovarian stimulation. Late OHSS presents about 12–17 days after hCG administration, is due to a pregnancy-related rise in hCG, is usually mild and is more prolonged. It is related more to pregnancy and to the number of gestational sacs seen on ultrasound 4 weeks after ovulatory hCG injections. However, a prospective observational study by Mathur *et al.*[37] comparing patient and cycle characteristics among three study groups – early OHSS, late OHSS and non-OHSS – showed that late OHSS was more likely than early OHSS to be severe, and is only poorly related to preovulatory events.

Clinical manifestations of iatrogenic OHSS

OHSS has a broad spectrum of clinical manifestations, from mild illness, which is usually self-limiting and requires no active therapy apart from careful observation, to moderate and severe disease which is life-threatening, and requires hospitalization, intensive-care monitoring and expert management. OHSS has traditionally been classified into three categories: mild, moderate and severe, and into six grades of increasing severity. Probably the most commonly used classification is the Golan classification[38]. Mild OHSS occurs in 23–33% of gonadotropin-stimulated IVF treatment cycles, moderate OHSS in 3–6% and severe OHSS in 0.2–1.9%[32,35,39].

The clinical symptoms and signs of OHSS exhibit a continuum of scope and severity that defies attempts at specific classification or staging. Unless the treating physician is aware of and predicts OHSS from the beginning, the moderate form passes on easily to the severe form in a short period of time. The guidelines of the ESHRE SIG for quality and safety in assisted reproductive technologies (ART) describe clinical manifestations of OHSS collectively as clinical symptoms, paraclinical signs and biological findings[28]. The Practice Committee of the American Society for Reproductive Medicine have classified clinical manifestations of OHSS into mild and severe types[24].

Clinical manifestations of mild OHSS Clinical manifestations of mild OHSS include: transient lower abdominal discomfort, mild nausea, vomiting, diarrhea and abdominal distension, which is observed in up to a third of superovulation cycles. The onset of symptoms typically occurs soon after ovulation (in superovulation cycles) or after oocyte retrieval in ART cycles, but it may be delayed. Progression of illness is recognized when the symptoms persist, worsen or include ascites that may be demonstrated by increasing abdominal girth or ultrasound evaluation (Table 3).

Clinical manifestations of severe OHSS Severe illness exists when pain is accompanied by one or more of the following symptoms and signs: rapid weight gain, tense ascites, hemodynamic instability (orthostatic hypotension,

Table 3 Clinical manifestations of iatrogenic OHSS

Mild OHSS	*Progression of illness*	*Severe OHSS*
Observed in up to a third of superovulation cycles	Symptoms persist or worsen	Occurs in 0.5–2% of superovulation cycles
Transient lower abdominal discomfort	Ovarian enlargement	Lower abdominal pain
Mild nausea, vomiting and diarrhea	Ascites demonstrated clinically or by ultrasound evaluation	Intractable nausea and vomiting
Abdominal distension		Increased abdominal girth and ovarian enlargement
Normal blood tests		Dyspnea
		Hypovolemia
		Hemoconcentration
		Oliguria
		Rapid weight gain
		Ascites, plural effusion and pericardial effusion
		Hypercoagulability
		Abnormal blood tests

tachycardia), respiratory difficulty (tachypnea), progressive oliguria and laboratory abnormalities. The symptoms and signs of severe OHSS can be grouped under the following items depending on the severity of the condition and the time the diagnosis is made. Physicians should not wait until all these symptoms and signs appear before diagnosing severe OHSS. Any group of these symptoms and signs combined with ovarian enlargement, abdominal pain and distension would qualify for the diagnosis of severe OHSS in a patient receiving drugs for induction of ovulation:

(1) Intractable nausea and vomiting that prevent ingestion of food and adequate fluids;

(2) Hypovolemia and hemoconcentration as a result of extravasation of protein-rich fluid from the vascular compartment to the third space, which in turn results in contraction of the vascular volume and lowered blood pressure and central venous pressure;

(3) Oliguria or anuria because of reduced renal perfusion due to decreased vascular volume and/or tense ascites; when not corrected the decreased renal perfusion stimulates the renal tubules to increase salt and water resorption in the proximal tubules, producing oliguria and low urinary sodium excretion; with less sodium being delivered to the distal tubules there

is a decrease in exchange of hydrogen and potassium for sodium, resulting in hyperkalemic acidosis;

(4) Rapid weight gain, because of salt and water retention;

(5) Dyspnea due to pulmonary compromise from an elevated diaphragm and/or hydrothorax;

(6) Ascites, pleural effusion and pericardial effusion; pleural effusion is usually secondary to ascites and possibly similar in pathogenesis to Meig's syndrome[40]; as the ascitic fluid is an exudate and, therefore, protein-rich fluid, serum albumin levels decrease markedly, producing hypoalbuminemia;

(7) Hypercoagulability with thromboembolic sequelae; this results from hemoconcentration, immobilization due to abdominal distension and pain, mechanical compression of venous blood flow in the pelvic brim and lower limb, high estradiol levels and endothelial cell damage due to stress-induced leukocytosis[41]; Arterial and venous thromboses occur in various sites, including upper and lower limbs as well as intracerebrally[42];

(8) Adult respiratory distress syndrome (ARDS), due to pulmonary edema and restricted lung movement, may occur.

If OHSS is not quickly managed and hemodynamics restored, multiple organ dysfunction syndrome and death may occur. Brinsden *et al.* believe that death is rare following OHSS, and occurs in approximately 1:500 000 stimulated cycles[1]. This seems to be an underestimation of this complication. There have been few, isolated, published reports of women who died from OHSS. Serour *et al.* in a series of 3500 IVF/ICSI cycles reported one death due to hepatorenal failure that occurred in a patient with moderate OHSS, who was retrospectively found to have an unrevealed history of hepatitis C with impairment of liver function[39]. Semba *et al.* reported a patient who died suddenly of rapid respiratory insufficiency. Autopsy examination revealed massive pulmonary edema, intra-alveolar hemorrhage and pleural effusion without any evidence of pulmonary thromboembolism. Histopathology of the ovary showed a picture consistent with OHSS[43]. Death may also occur due to acute respiratory failure, lactic acidosis, shock, massive cerebral infarction, myocardial infarction, supraventricular tachycardia or massive thromboembolic manifestations. Mortality due to OHSS is underreported in the literature. The author is aware of many cases in different parts of the world which were never published. Many of these patients, when seriously ill, end up in emergency and intensive care or the neurosurgery unit, and may never report to the IVF center.

Laboratory findings

Laboratory findings in women with severe OHSS comprise: hemoconcentration (hematocrit > 45%) due to an increase in capillary permeability and leakage of protein-rich fluid from the intravascular space; leukocytosis (white blood cell count > 15 000) due to hemoconcentration and generalized stress reaction; electrolyte imbalances (hyponatremia: sodium < 135 mEq/l; hyperkalemia: potassium > 5.0 mEq/l); elevated liver enzymes; decreased creatinine clearance (serum creatinine > 1.2 mg/dl; creatinine clearance < 50 ml/min), and low serum albumin level < 30 g/l.

CLINICAL MANIFESTATIONS OF COMPLICATIONS OF OHSS

Not uncommonly, the reproductive medicine physician is not the one who is consulted when patients are admitted to hospital with complications of OHSS. Many of these patients end up in the surgical, vascular, neurosurgery, neurology, chest or critical-care units. Furthermore, a large number of publications on the complications of OHSS appear in the medical journals of vascular surgery, neurosurgery, neurology, chest medicine, intensive care units and others. Consequently, many reproductive medicine physicians are unfortunately not fully aware of the frequency of occurrence of these complications, or familiar with their clinical manifestations. Reciprocally, the attendant physicians in these different subspecialty units should be aware of clinical manifestations of the complications of OHSS. This is essential for early diagnosis and proper management of this potentially fatal syndrome. It necessitates a continuous dialog between reproductive medicine physicians and their colleagues in other subspecialties relating to this newly emerging set of complications due to the widespread use of ovulation-induction drugs for OI/OE or in IVF programs. A history of the recent intake of these drugs should be included in the admission sheets of all women of reproductive age admitted to these units.

The diagnosis of some complications of OHSS may be masked by the pain, distension and ascites associated with OHSS. Sometimes, one or another of these complications may be the first presenting manifestation of OHSS (Table 4). The complications of OHSS include the following.

Ovarian torsion

While the overall risk of ovarian torsion is about 1 per 5000 stimulations, it is greater in the presence of OHSS. Mashiach *et al.* noted torsion in 16% of pregnant patients with OHSS compared with 2.3% in non-pregnant patients[44]. The risk of torsion increases with an increase in ovarian size and with ligamentous softening, which explains the increased susceptibility in early pregnancy after ovarian hyperstimulation[40].

The characteristic symptoms include sudden, extreme abdominal pain accompanied by nausea. If undiagnosed and neglected this may result in ovarian necrosis. The risk of torsion may even persist beyond the treatment cycle, and it may be precipitated by exercise or strenuous activity if regression to normal ovarian size has not been achieved[45].

Ovarian hemorrhage

Ovarian hemorrhage may occur in OHSS due to ovarian rupture or, rarely, intraovarian hemorrhage. Ovarian rupture may be precipitated by abdominal trauma, strenuous activity or bimanual examination. It is manifested by severe abdominal pain, distension, hypotension, severe pallor and free fluid in the peritoneal cavity. Pain and ascites associated with severe OHSS can easily mask ovarian rupture.

Hemorrhage inside the ovarian follicles may also occur, and lead to a picture similar to internal hemorrhage. The ovaries become large, tense and edematous with multiple cystic structures filled with blood. Ultrasonography and repeat hemoglobin level assessment will help to diagnose these conditions.

Thromboembolism

This is a rare but extremely serious complication of OHSS. Most cases of thrombosis are late complications of OHSS, and may or may not be associated with hereditary hypercoagulability. It may occur in patients with mild, moderate or severe OHSS[39,42,46–60].

The clinical manifestations and mechanisms[61–64] underlying thromboembolic complications are treated in further detail in Chapter 5.

Venous compression due to enlarged ovaries and ascites, in addition to the immobility due to pain and distension, and all the above transient changes in coagulation factors, are the main etiological factors in the increased incidence of thromboembolic complications in OHSS. Thromboembolism of the internal jugular veins presents with pain and swelling in the neck and dyspnea, or it may present with pulmonary embolism. Thrombosis of the middle cerebral

Table 4 Diagnostic criteria of complications of iatrogenic OHSS

Complication	*Diagnostic criteria*
Torsion	Exercise or strenuous activity followed by extreme abdominal pain and nausea
Ovarian hemorrhage	Abdominal trauma or strenuous activity followed by severe abdominal pain, distension, hypotension, severe pallor, low Hb level and ultrasound scan
Thromboembolism which may be arterial or venous in various sites including upper and lower limbs, neck and intracerebral vessels	A possible positive family history of thrombosis and/or thrombophilias, signs depend upon site of thromboembolism Usually presents between 7 and 10 weeks' gestation. Positive specific tests for blood hypercoagulability MRI and MRA
Hepatocellular and cholestatic disorders	Usually in third trimester Mild to moderate increase in AST and ALT May persist for > 2 months
Impaired renal function and anuria	Oliguria or anuria Serum creatinine > 1.2 mg/dl Creatinine clearance < 50 ml/min Sodium < 135 mEq/l Potassium > 5.0 mEq/l Hyperkalemic acidosis
Temporary failure of transplanted kidney	Anuria
Bilateral or unilateral hydrothorax	Chest tightness, dry cough and dyspnea Chest ultrasonography or chest X-ray
ARDS	Rapid respiratory insufficiency Chest X-ray or ultrasonography Blood gases assessment Lung function tests MRI and MRA
Pulmonary embolism	Fever, dyspnea, wheeze and hemoptysis Chest X-ray, MRI and MRA
Pericardial effusion	Supraventricular arrhythmia Echocardiography

ARDS, adult respiratory distress syndrome; Hb, hemoglobin; MRI, magnetic resonance imaging; MRA, magnetic resonance angiography; AST, aspartate aminotransferase; ALT, alanine aminotransferase artery presents with a picture of cerebral infarct. Deep vein thrombosis presents with pain and swelling of the leg.

Duplex Doppler ultrasonographic examination and magnetic resonance angiography of suspected occluded vessels based on the clinical manifestations will help in the diagnosis and initiation of treatment before the onset of serious complications.

Liver dysfunction

Liver dysfunction is a rare complication of severe OHSS. More recently it has been reported even in moderate OHSS[39,65]. Both hepatocellular and cholestatic disorders were reported. Abnormal hepatic function has been increasingly recognized as a complication of severe OHSS that may persist for more than 2 months. Liver biopsy shows significant morphological abnormalities only at the ultrastructural level.

Midgley *et al.*[66] describe a case of recurrent cholestasis following OHSS during a twin pregnancy. On the first occasion cholestasis developed unusually in the first trimester, and on the second occasion it developed in the third trimester as usual. In a large prospective longitudinal study of 50 consecutive patients with ascites due to severe OHSS, Fabregues *et al.*[67] showed that 15 patients (30%) had abnormal liver tests characterized by a mild to moderate increase in aspartate aminotransferase (AST) (mean 103 ± 17.1 IU/l and alanine aminotransferase (ALT) (76 ± 8.3 IU/l), which was associated in some cases with an increase in γ-glutamyl transpeptidase or alkaline phosphatase. All abnormalities reverted to normal after resolution of the syndrome. The death of a patient, with an unrevealed history of hepatitis C, from hepatorenal failure following moderate OHSS has been reported by Serour *et al.*[39]. Davis *et al.*[68] describe a case of severe OHSS with

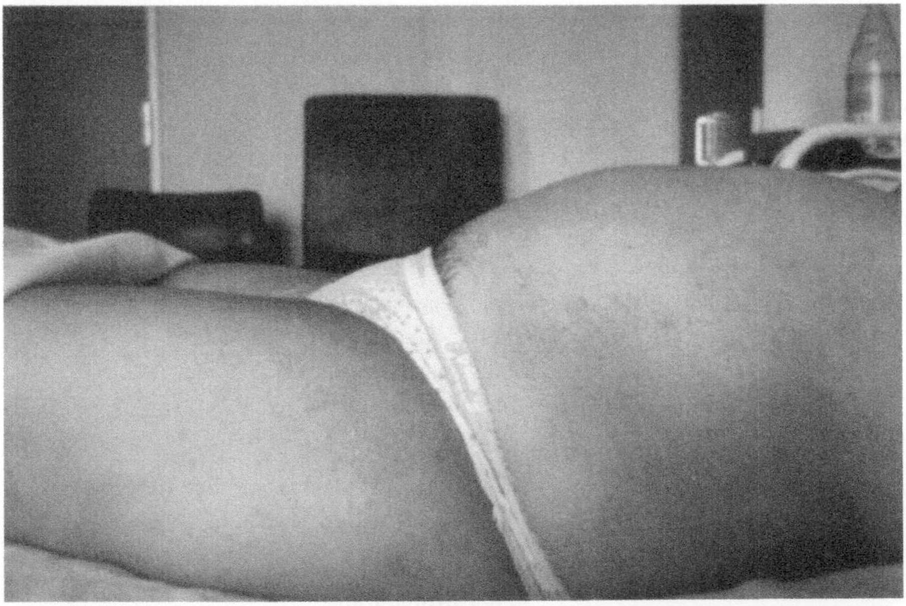

Figure 1 Severe abdominal distension in a patient with severe OHSS. Picture taken on day 16 after embryo transfer. The patient was pregnant with twins. Courtesy Dr J Gerris, Belgium

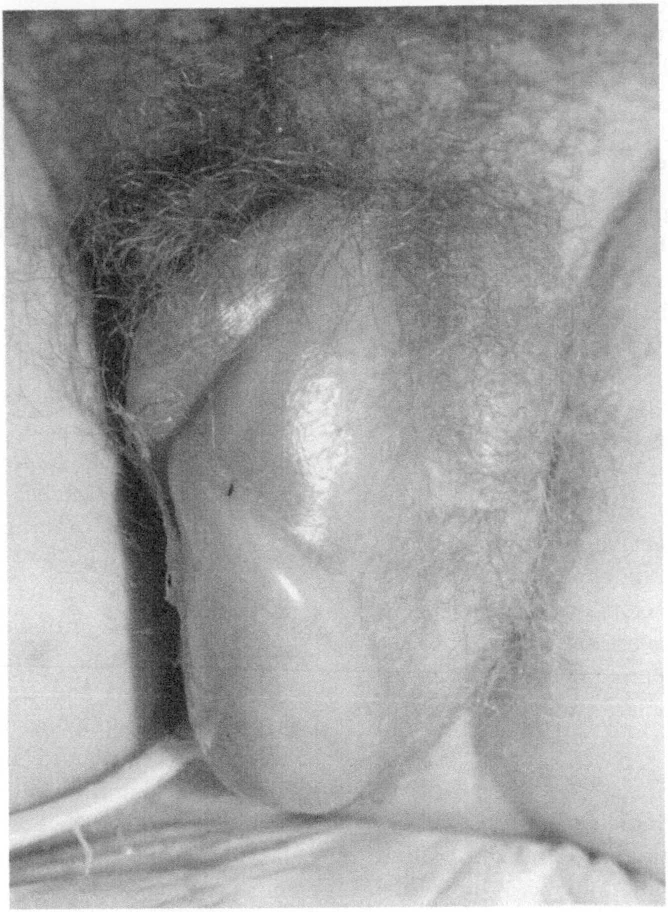

Figure 2 Vulvar edema in a patient with OHSS. Courtesy Dr J J Amy, Belgium

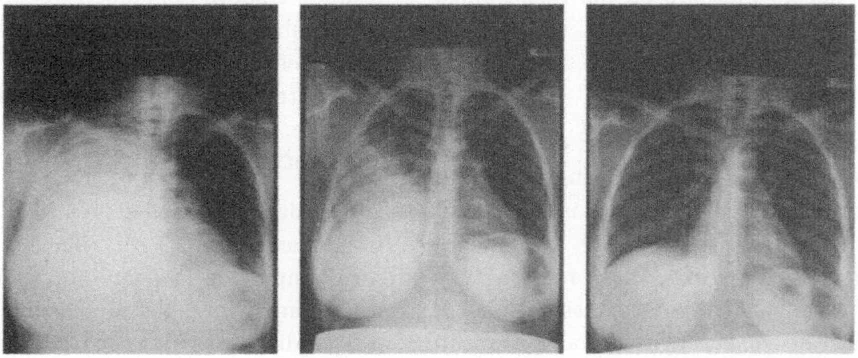

Figure 3 Three subsequent images of thorax X-ray in the same patient, showing severe resolving and resolved hydrothorax. Courtesy Dr J Gerris, Belgium

malnutrition, severe hypoalbuminemia with gross edema and progressively worsening liver function.

Gastrointestinal complications

Gastrointestinal symptoms such as nausea and vomiting may be initial presentations of OHSS. Failing to suspect such a condition may result in later presentation of these patients with cerebrovascular accidents. These symptoms are usually due to a high level of estradiol, ovarian enlargement and abdominal distension. Uhler *et al.*[69] reported a perforated posterior duodenal ulcer associated with OHSS. Stress associated with invasive monitoring, multiple medical therapies in the intensive-care unit and *Helicobacter pylori* infection appear to be the most probable causative factors of the ulcer. Prompt recognition of this complication and an emergency exploratory laparotomy will help to save the life of these patients.

Renal complications

Tension ascites can impair renal function, and in severely hypovolemic cases, prerenal failure will be heralded by oliguria, raised blood urea and creatinine, followed by anuria, hyperkalemia and uremia[30,40]. Temporary failure of a transplanted pelvic kidney has also been reported, due to pressure on the transplanted kidney by enlarged ovaries[70].

Respiratory complications

OHSS usually causes ascites and occasionally hydrothorax. When ascites is lacking an isolated pleural effusion in a pregnant or non-pregnant patient can be mistaken for pulmonary embolism. Several workers have reported this not so uncommon sole presentation of OHSS[71–74]. The isolated hydrothorax may result from a combination of positive intra-abdominal pressure, negative intrathoracic pressure and diaphragmatic defects that promote the transfer of intra-abdominal fluid into the pleural fluid, resulting in hydrothorax in the absence of abdominal fluid. The preferential location of hydrothorax on the right side in most cases might be explained by a capillary leak and exudation into the pleural space due to the decreased right lymphatic drainage as compared with the left side, in addition to the defect in the diaphragm being more common in its right portion. Clinically, hydrothorax manifests with chest tightness, dry cough and dyspnea. There is a negative history of fever, wheeze, hemoptysis or leg swelling. The diagnosis can be confirmed with chest ultrasonography or X-ray. Early recognition and diagnosis of the condition should allow for appropriate therapeutic management.

Bibasilar partial atelectasis or ARDS may occur. This may be attributable to lung movement restriction because of pain, tense ascites or large ovarian cysts and transudation of fluid from pulmonary capillaries into the alveoli. The condition can be diagnosed by chest X-ray, ultrasonography and assessment of blood gases and lung function. Other diagnostic procedures such as magnetic resonance imaging (MRI) and magnetic resonance angiography (MRA) can help to differentiate the condition from pulmonary embolism.

Pulmonary embolism may also occur as a result of a shower of emboli from different sites of thrombosis. The patient develops fever, dyspnea, wheeze and hemoptysis. The diagnosis can be confirmed with chest X-ray, MRI and MRA.

Cardiac complications

Pericardial effusion may present with supraventricular arrhythmia. Pericardial effusion and cardiac tamponade is a rare and potentially fatal event, and once the diagnosis is made by echocardiography, drainage of the fluid by a cardiologist is necessary. Massive myocardiac infarction may also occur, and results in sudden death.

Ventriculoperitoneal shunt failure

Ventriculoperitoneal shunt dysfunction has been reported by Lee *et al.*[75]. Shunt dysfunction is attributed to intra-abdominal hypertension as a consequence of ascites and enlarged ovaries. Neurosurgeons should be alerted to this possibility with the increasing number of patients developing OHSS.

ACKNOWLEDGMENT

I would like sincerely to thank my infertile patients at the Egyptian IVF center, Maadi Cairo, and at Al-Azhar University IVF unit, whose sufferings from OHSS over the past 19 years have contributed a great deal to my understanding of this potentially fatal complication. I sincerely hope that this chapter will play a role in the better understanding and early diagnosis of OHSS by those who manage to read this book, to reduce the risks of OHSS to their patients.

Many thanks are due to my secretarial staff, Mrs Azza El Tobgy and Mrs Gihan El Fiqy. Without their dedication this chapter would not have been completed before the deadline set by the Editors of the book.

REFERENCES

1. Brinsden PR, Wada I, Tan SL, et al. Diagnosis, prevention and management of ovarian hyperstimulation syndrome. Br J Obstet Gynaecol 1995; 102: 767–72.
2. Berezowski AT, Machado JC, Mendes MC, et al. Prenatal diagnosis of fetal ovarian hyperstimulation. Ultrasound Obstet Gynecol 2001; 3: 259–62.
3. Vochem M. Ovarian hyperstimulation syndrome in preterm infants. Z Geburtsh Neonatol 2002; 4: 156–60.
4. Christin-Maitre S, Rongieres-Bertrand C, Kottler ML, et al. A spontaneous and severe hyperstimulation of the ovaries revealing a gonadotroph adenoma. J Clin Endocrinol Metab 1999; 10: 3450–3.
5. Pentz-Vidovic I, Skoric T, Grubisic G, et al. Evolution of clinical symptoms in a young woman with a recurrent gonadotroph adenoma causing ovarian hyperstimulation. Eur J Endocrinol 2000; 5: 607–14.
6. Ludwig M, Gembruch U, Bauer O, et al. Ovarian hyperstimulation syndrome (OHSS) in a spontaneous pregnancy with fetal and placental triploidy: information about the general pathophysiology of OHSS. Hum Reprod 1998; 8: 2082–7.
7. Furneaux EC, Langley-Evans AJ, Langley-Evans SC. Nausea and vomiting of pregnancy: endocrine basis and contribution to pregnancy outcome. Obstet Gynecol Surv 2001; 56: 775–82.
8. Glinoer D. The regulation of thyroid function in pregnancy: pathways of endocrine adaptation from physiology to pathology. Endocr Rev 1997; 18: 404–33.
9. Coccia ME, Pasquini L, Comparetto C, et al. Hyperreactio luteinalis in a woman with high-risk factors. A case report. J Reprod Med 2003; 2: 127–9.
10. Wajda KJ, Lucas JG, Marsh WL Jr. Hyperreactio luteinalis: benign disorder masquerading as an ovarian neoplasm. Arch Pathol Lab Med 1989; 113: 921–5.
11. Olatunbosun OA, Gilliland B, Brydon LA, et al. Spontaneous ovarian hyperstimulation syndrome in four consecutive pregnancies. Clin Exp Obstet Gynecol 1996; 3: 127–32.
12. Rosen GF, Lew MW. Severe ovarian hyperstimulation in a spontaneous singleton pregnancy. Am J Obstet Gynecol 1991; 165: 1312–13.
13. Zalel Y, Katz Z and Capsi B. Spontaneous ovarian hyperstimulation syndrome concomitant with spontaneous pregnancy in a woman with polycystic ovarian disease. Am J Obstet Gynecol 1992; 167: 122–4.
14. Nappi RG, Di Nero E, D'Aries AP, et al. Natural pregnancy in hypothyroid woman complicated by spontaneous ovarian hyperstimulation syndrome. Am J Obstet Gynecol 1998; 187: 610–11.

15. Todros T, Carmazzi CM, Bontempo S, et al. Spontaneous ovarian hyperstimulation syndrome and deep vein thrombosis in pregnancy: case report. Hum Reprod 1999; 9: 2245–8.

16. He Dong C, Eun-Joo P, Sung-Hoon K, et al. Ovarian hyperstimulation syndrome complicating a spontaneous singleton pregnancy: a case report. J Assist Reprod Genet 2001; 2: 120–3.

17. Zalel Y, Orvieto R, Ben Rafael Z, et al. Recurrent spontaneous ovarian hyperstimulation syndrome associated with polycystic ovary syndrome. Gynecol Endocrinol 1995; 9: 313–15.

18. Olatunbosum OA, Gilliland B, Brydon LA, et al. Spontaneous ovarian hyperstimulation syndrome in four consecutive pregnancies. Clin Exp Obstet Gynaecol 1996; 23: 127–32.

19. Di Carlo C, Bruno PA, Cirillo D, et al. Increased concentration of renin, aldosterone and Ca^{125} in a case of spontaneous recurrent familial, severe ovarian hyperstimulation syndrome. Hum Reprod 1997; 12: 2115–17.

20. Edi-Osagie ECO, Hopkins RE. Recurrent idiopathic ovarian hyperstimulation syndrome in pregnancy. Br J Obstet Gynaecol 1997; 104: 952–4.

21. Delbaere A, Smits G, Olatunbosun O, et al. New insights into the pathophysiology of ovarian hyperstimulation syndrome. What makes the difference between spontaneous and iatrogenic syndrome? Hum Reprod 2004; 3: 486–9.

22. Smits GI, Olatunbosun O, Delbaere A, et al. Ovarian hyperstimulation syndrome due to a mutation in the follicle-stimulating hormone receptor. N Engl J Med 2003; 8: 760–6.

23. Vasseur C, Rodien P, Beau I, et al. A chorionic gonadotropin-sensitive mutation in the follicle-stimulating hormone receptor as a cause of familial gestational spontaneous ovarian hyperstimulation syndrome. N Engl J Med 2003; 8: 753–9.

24. The Practice Committee of the American Society for Reproductive Medicine. Ovarian hyperstimulation syndrome. Fertil Steril 2003; 5: 1309–14.

25. Egbase PE. Severe OHSS: how many cases are preventable? Hum Reprod 2000; 15: 8–10.

26. Mitchell SY, Fletcher HM, Williams E. Ovarian hyperstimulation syndrome associated with clomiphene citrate. West Indian Med J 2001; 3: 227–9.

27. Sills ES, Poiynor EA, Moomjy M. Ovarian hyperstimulation and oophorectomy following accidental daily clomiphene citrate use over three consecutive months. Reprod Toxicol 2000; 6: 541–3.

28. ESHRE. Special interest group (SIG) guidelines on ovarian hyperstimulation syndrome (OHSS) 2005. http//www.eshre.com/emc.

29. Navot D, Bergh PA, Laufer N. Ovarian hyperstimulation syndrome in novel reproductive technologies: prevention and treatment. Fertil Steril 1992; 58: 249–61.

30. Serour GI, Rhodes C, Sattar M, et al. Complications of assisted reproductive techniques: a review. Assist Reprod 1999; 4: 214–32.

31. Whelan JG III, Vlahos NF. The ovarian hyperstimulation syndrome. Fertil Steril 2000; 73: 883–96.

32. Ferraretti AP. The ovarian hyperstimulation syndrome (OHSS): definitions, clinical symptoms, classification and incidence. In Ferraretti AP, Gianaroli L, Tarlatzis BCC, eds. Ovarian Hyperstimulation Syndrome. Serono Fertility Series. Rome: Christengraf Press, 1997; 1: 1–10.

33. Ludwig M, Felderbaum RE, Devroey P, et al. Significant reduction of the incidence of ovarian hyperstimulation syndrome OHSS by using LHRH antagonist cetrorelix (Cetrotide) in controlled ovarian stimulation for assisted reproduction. Arch Gynecol Obstet 2000; 264: 29–32.

34. Aboulghar M, Mansour R, Serour GI, et al. Ovarian hyperstimulation syndrome: modern concepts in pathophysiology and management. Middle East Fertil Soc J 1996; 1: 3–16.

35. Schenker JG. Prevention and treatment of ovarian hyperstimulation syndrome. Hum Reprod 1993; 8: 653–9.

36. Al-Shawaf T, Grudzinskas JG. Prevention and treatment of ovarian hyperstimulation syndrome. Best Pract Res Clin Obstet Gynaecol 2003; 2: 249–61.

37. Mathur RS, Akande AV, Keay SD, et al. Distinction between early and late ovarian hyperstimulation syndrome. Fertil Steril 2000; 5: 901–7.

38. Golan A, Ron-el R, Herman A, et al. Ovarian hyperstimulation syndrome. An update review. Obstet Gynecol Surv 1989; 44: 430–40.

39. Serour GI, Aboulghar M, Mansour R, et al. Complications of medically assisted conception in 3500 cycles. Fertil Steril 1998; 70: 638–42.

40. McManus J, McClure N. Complications of assisted reproduction. The Obstetrician and Gynaecologist. Royal College of Obstetricians and Gynaecologists 2002; 3: 124–9.

41. Pinntucci G, Coviello L, Castelli MP, et al. Cathepsin G-induced release of PAI-1 in the culture medium of endothelial cells: a new thrombogenic role for polymorphonuclear leukocytes? J Lab Clin Med 1993; 122: 69–79.

42. Stewart JA, Hamilton PJ, Murdoch AP. Thromboembolic disease associated with ovarian stimulation and assisted conception techniques. Hum Reprod 1997; 12: 2167–73.

43. Semba S, Moriya T, Youssef EM, et al. An autopsy case of ovarian hyperstimulation syndrome with massive pulmonary edema and pleural effusion. Pathol Int 2000; 7: 549–52.

44. Mashiach S, Bider D, Morano, et al. Adnexal torsion of hyperstimulated ovaries in pregnancies after gonadotrophin therapy. Fertil Steril 1990; 53: 76–80.

45. Littman ED, Rydfors JR, Milki AA. Exercise-induced ovarian torsion in the cycle following gonadotrophin therapy: case report. Hum Reprod 2003; 8: 1641–2.

46. Aurosseau MH, Samama MM, Belhassen A, et al. Risk of thrombo-embolism in relation to an in-vitro fertilization programme: three case reports. Hum Reprod 1995; 10: 94–7.

47. Kligman I, Noyes N, Benadiva CA, et al. Massive deep vein thrombosis in a patient with antithrombin III deficiency undergoing ovarian stimulation for in vitro fertilization. Fertil Steril 1995; 63: 673–6.

48. Germond M, Wirthner D, Thorin D, et al. Aorto-subclavian thrombo-embolism: a rare complication associated with moderate ovarian hyperstimulation syndrome. Hum Reprod 1996; 11: 1173–6.

49. Aboulghar MA, Mansour RT, Serour GI, et al. Moderate ovarian hyperstimulation syndrome complicated by deep cerebrovascular thrombosis. Hum Reprod 1998; 13: 2088–91.

50. Elford K, Leader A, Wee R, et al. Stroke in ovarian hyper-stimulation syndrome in early pregnancy treated with intra-arterial recombinant tissue plasminogen activator (rt-PA). Neurology 2002; 8: 1270–2.

51. Hwang WJ, Lai ML, Hsu CC, et al. Ischemic stroke in a young woman with ovarian hyperstimulation syndrome. J Formos Med Assoc 1998; 7: 503–6.

52. Koo EJ, Rha JH, Lee B, et al. A case of cerebral infarct in combined antiphospholipid antibody and ovarian hyperstimulation syndrome. J Korean Med Sci 2002; 4: 574–6.

53. Tavmergen E, Ozcakir HT, Levi R, et al. Bilateral jugular venous thromboembolism and pulmonary emboli in a patient with severe ovarian hyperstimulation syndrome. J Obstet Gynaecol Res 2001; 4: 217–20.

54. Jesudason WV, Small M. Internal jugular vein thrombosis following ovarian hyperstimulation. J Laryngol Otol 2003; 3: 222–3.

55. Heinig J, Behre HM, Klockenbusch W. Occlusion of the ulnar artery in a patient with severe ovarian hyperstimulation syndrome. Eur J Obstet Gynecol Reprod Biol 2001; 1: 126–7.

56. Murrle GA, Wetzel V, Burck C, et al. Floating thrombus of the internal carotid artery as a rare complication in ovarian hyperstimulation syndrome after in vitro fertilization/embryo transfer. Chirurg 1998; 10: 1105–8.

57. Berker B, Demirel C, Satiroglu H. Internal jugular vein thrombosis as a late complication of ovarian hyperstimulation syndrome in an ICSI patient. Arch Gynecol Obstet 2004; 3: 197–8.

58. Ou YC, Kao YL, Lai SL, et al. Thromboembolism after ovarian stimulation: successful management of a woman with superior sagittal sinus thrombosis after IVF and embryo transfer: case report. Hum Reprod 2003; 11: 2375–81.

59. Arya R, Shehata HA, Patel RK, et al. Internal jugular vein thrombosis after assisted conception therapy. Br J Haematol 2001; 1: 153–5.

60. Tang OS, Ng EH, Wai Cheng P, et al. Cortical vein thrombosis misinterpreted as intracranial haemorrhage in severe ovarian hyperstimulation syndrome: case report. Hum Reprod 2000; 9: 913–16.

61. Aune B, Hoieke, Oian P, et al. Does ovarian stimulation for in vitro fertilization induce a hypercoagulable state? Hum Reprod 1991; 6: 925–7.

62. Kodama H, Fukuda J, Karube H, et al. Status of the coagulation and fibrinolytic systems in ovarian hyperstimulation syndrome. Fertil Steril 1996; 66: 417–24.

63. Balasch J, Reverter JC, Fabregues F, et al. Increased induced monocytes tissue factor expression by plasma from patients with severe ovarian hyperstimulation syndrome. Fertil Steril 1996; 66: 608–13.

64. Rogolino A, Coccia ME, Fedi S, et al. Hypercoagulability, high tissue factor and low tissue factor pathway inhibitor levels in severe ovarian hyperstimulation syndrome: possible association with clinical outcome. Blood Coagul Fibrinolysis 2003; 3: 277–82.

65. Elterk K, Scoccia B, Nelson LR. Hepatic dysfunction associated with moderate ovarian hyperstimulation syndrome. A case report. J Reprod 2001; 8: 765–8.

66. Midgley DY, Khalaf Y, Braude PR, et al. Recurrent cholestasis following ovarian hyperstimulation syndrome: case report. Hum Reprod 1999; 9: 2245–8.

67. Fabregues F, Balasch J, Gines, et al. Ascites and liver test abnormalities during severe ovarian hyperstimulation syndrome. Am J Gastroenterol 1999: 94; 994–9.

68. Davis AJ, Pandher GK, Masson GM, et al. A severe case of ovarian hyperstimulation syndrome with liver dysfunction and malnutrition. Eur J Gastroenterol 2002; 7: 779–82.

69. Uhler ML, Budinger GR, Gabram SG, et al. Perforated duodenal ulcer associated with ovarian hyperstimulation syndrome: case report. Hum Reprod 2001; 1: 174–6.

70. Khalaf Y, El Kington N, Anderson H, et al. Ovarian hyperstimulation syndrome and its effect on renal transplantation patients undergoing IVF. Hum Reprod 2000; 15: 1275–7.

71. Roden S, Juvin K, Homasson JP, et al. An uncommon etiology of isolated pleural effusion. The ovarian hyperstimulation syndrome. Chest J 2000; 1: 256–8.

72. Cordani S, Bancalari L, Maggiani R, et al. Massive unilateral hydrothorax as the only clinical manifestation of ovarian hyperstimulation syndrome. Monaldi Arch Chest Dis 2002; 5–6: 314–17.

73. Blandin S, Khouatra C, Geriniere L, et al. Isolated pleurisy revealing ovarian hyperstimulation syndrome. Rev Pneumol Clin 2002; 3: 151–3.

74. Murray A, Rombauts L. Unilateral pleural effusion as the main presentation of 'early onset severe' ovarian hyperstimulation syndrome. Fertil Steril 2004; 4: 1127–9.

75. Lee G, Daniel RT, Jones NR. Ventriculoperitoneal shunt failure as a secondary complication of ovarian hyperstimulation syndrome. Case report. J Neurosurg 2002; 4: 992–4.

CHAPTER 5

Thromboembolic complications of ovarian hyperstimulation syndrome

Jane Stewart

Ovarian hyperstimulation syndrome (OHSS) is a complex phenomenon which has not yet been fully elucidated. Whilst rare cases of spontaneous OHSS can occur for example in molar pregnancy[1] or as a result of gonadotropin receptor abnormalities[2], it is primarily an iatrogenic condition. It is incumbent therefore upon the practitioner supervising the risk-causing treatment to ensure that the recipient is fully informed of those risks and that they are kept to a minimum.

Mild cases of OHSS may be uncomfortable, inconvenient and time-consuming; however, it should not be forgotten that serious complications can arise and may result in significant morbidity both acutely and in the longer term. There is a risk of mortality if severe or unrecognized, and there are implications for future health and well-being even if appropriate treatment is given. One such complication is thromboembolism. The aim of this chapter is to discuss the nature of thromboembolic disease and put it in the context of the woman of reproductive age and indeed of women undergoing assisted reproductive treatment. OHSS is considered as a specific risk factor. The prevention, diagnosis and treatment of thromboembolism in relation to ovarian stimulation and OHSS are discussed.

THROMBOEMBOLISM IN WOMEN OF REPRODUCTIVE AGE

Venous thromboembolic disease (VTE) is widely experienced and much highlighted in the public forum. It is a significant cause of peroperative morbidity[3], and is still a feared risk in the use of the combined oral contraceptive pill (COCP)[4] and hormone replacement treatment (HRT)[5]. It has been drawn again and most recently to public attention as a silent risk of long-haul air travel[6]. It is broadly understood, therefore, in the lay population that it results from some form of intervention and is preventable. Increasing awareness has led to a drive to consider more formally the risk of venous thromboembolism (VTE) in hospital in-patients other than the postoperative population.

Whilst there is an increased risk of VTE in the elderly population, and hence the concerns regarding medical in-patients and long-haul flights in this group in particular, in a woman of reproductive age the risk of VTE occurring is said to be 5–21/100 000 women/year[7]. This risk increases to 15–25/100 000 women/year in users of the combined oral contraceptive pill (COCP) and increases to 60/100 000 women/year during pregnancy[8]. Despite this awareness, the risk associated with an otherwise uncomplicated pregnancy is probably unknown to most women and may not be generally discussed as part of normal antenatal care unless there are other associated risk factors, and even then not always appropriately: 30 cases of direct maternal death from thromboembolic disease were reported in the UK from 2000 to 2002, representing an incidence of 1.5/100 000 maternities, over half of which were considered to have received suboptimal care[9].

There are numerous additional risk factors that play a role in the incidence of this disorder in an otherwise healthy population (Table 1).

THROMBOEMBOLISM

Intravascular thrombosis is the inappropriate formation of clots within vessels, and embolism results from the movement of these clots or portions of them, to lodge downstream in smaller vessels. The result of these episodes is development of symptoms related to poor blood flow in the affected, occluded vessels and also in downstream organs or tissues. Thrombosis can occur in both arteries and veins, and, peculiarly, arterial thromboembolism is associated with ovarian stimulation and OHSS[10].

Virchow's triad describes the combination of features which allows clots to form: stasis, endothelial damage and hypercoagulability (Figure 1). The natural process of clot formation works to reduce bleeding at the site of injury and promote the healing process. Intravascular thrombosis results from the inappropriate triggering of this process by one of a number of factors. If Virchow's triad is considered, then numerous mechanisms can be derived (Table 2). These various factors may be invoked as a basis for considering the nature of thrombosis and in particular for the etiology when associated with OHSS.

PREGNANCY AND THROMBOSIS

The effects of pregnancy on the hemostatic mechanism are well known and take effect from early on in the process. Pregnancy induces a hypercoagulable state by virtue of changes in numerous clotting and thrombolytic factors. An increase in the von Willebrand factor (VIIIR.vWf), factor VIII, factor V and fibrinogen, an acquired resistance to activated protein C and a reduction of protein S with associated increases in plasminogen activator inhibitors 1

Table 1 General risk of thromboembolism in women of reproductive age

Background risk factors	*Additional risk factors*
Age > 35 years	COCP, HRT
Obesity	Pregnancy
Mobility problems	Cancer
Significant family history of thrombosis	Surgery
Thrombophilia – inherited or acquired	Immobility including bedrest and long-haul travel
Previous thrombosis	
Varicose veins	

COCP, combined oral contraceptive pill; HRT, hormone replacement treatment

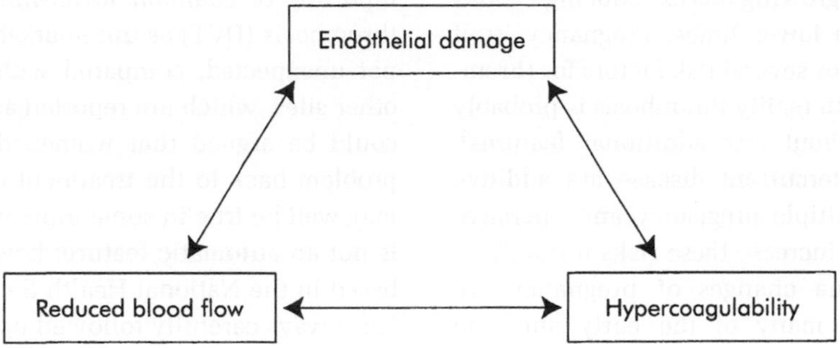

Figure 1 Virchow's triad

Table 2 Virchow's triad and venous thromboembolism

Stasis	*Endothelial damage*	*Hypercoagulation*
Immobility fracture debilitating illness long-haul travel postoperative	Local injury trauma intravascular cannulation childbirth	Increased coagulability hyperestrogenemia, e.g. pregnancy, ovarian stimulation, COCP, HRT, cancer diagnosis
Occlusion intravascular long-line obstructive mass, e.g. tumor, pregnancy	Generalized injury postoperative burns	Reduced thrombolysis inherited thrombophilias hyperestrogenemia
Reduced intravascular volume severe dehydration, e.g. burns	Platelet disorders	Platelet disorders thrombocythemia
Increased intravascular viscosity	Cancer diagnosis	
Hematological disorders, e.g. polycythemia		
Atrial fibrillation		

COCP, combined oral contraceptive pill; HRT, hormone replacement treatment

and 2 induce a relative thrombophilia[11]. The process of placental invasion results in significant local vascular changes, and it is possible that such local changes are reflected in the endothelium throughout the vasculature, adding to hypercoagulability. As pregnancy progresses, generalized venous stasis occurs as a result of reduced vascular resistance and also the effect of the growing uterus reducing venous return from the lower limbs. Pregnancy itself thus encompasses several risk factors for thrombosis, although in reality thrombosis is probably uncommon without any additional features[9]. Obesity and intercurrent disease are additive factors, and multiple pregnancy and operative delivery simply increase these risks further[9].

The hormone changes of pregnancy are responsible for many of the early and late changes that occur, and both estrogen and progesterone are implicated in development of the hypercoagulable state.

OHSS AND THROMBOSIS

In OHSS, as in pregnancy, there are physical features that make the increased risk of thrombosis entirely explicable. The physical presence of greatly enlarged ovaries and potentially tense ascites will result in a degree of obstruction to venous drainage from the lower limbs, resulting in reduced blood flow. Women experiencing OHSS are nearly always nauseated and may have recurrent vomiting, and are therefore potentially dehydrated as well as being laid up in bed with general malaise, both being further contributors to their risk of thromboembolism at least in the lower limbs. There are features of this phenomenon in association with OHSS, however, which are less easy to understand.

In 1997 we summarized the worldwide reports available at that time of thromboembolic disease associated with a variety of fertility treatments, all but one involving ovarian stimulation[10]. Fifty-four cases had been reported then since 1964[12–47]. Most interesting about these reports, however, was that they were not all the lower-limb venous thromboses that might have been expected. The 54 cases comprised 25% arterial thrombosis, and, of the venous thromboses reported, 60% were sited in the upper limb or neck. It is possible that this idiosyncratic distribution is the result of under-reporting of *common* lower-limb deep venous thrombosis (DVT) as unremarkable and perhaps not unexpected, compared with thrombosis at other sites, which are reported as novel cases. It could be argued that women do not report a problem back to the treatment center, and this may well be true in some units where follow-up is not an automatic feature; however, this unit, based in the National Health Service in the UK, has always carefully followed up cases of OHSS and sees virtually every couple treated, back for review 6–8 weeks after completion of that treatment. In addition, there is a telephone advice service for first-line contact by couples in the event of acute problems, and open access to the unit is encouraged. Finally, since most couples live in the region, admission with complications and/or delivery if pregnant, if not to the unit's parent hospital, would be to one of the local district general hospitals. It is unlikely that a significant complication, therefore, would go unreported at base. In our experience, however, in over 15 years, although a number of women have undergone tests to exclude the possibility, where five cases of thromboembolism have occurred, we have never seen a *traditional* DVT following assisted conception treatment[47].

Since 1997 there have been a further 30 cases of thromboembolic disease reported in association with OHSS, the majority reviewed by Delvigne and Rozenberg[48]: two cases of pulmonary embolism[49]; ten cases of internal jugular venous and/or subclavian vein thrombosis (two bilateral and one including the superior vena cava)[50–58]; one superior sagittal sinus thrombosis[59] and one cortical vein thrombosis (with second site inferior vena cava extending to both iliac veins)[60]; two carotid artery thromboses, one resulting in a stroke[61,62]; a brainstem infarction from intracranial thrombosis[63] and seven further intracranial arterial complications[49,64–69], including one central retinal artery thrombosis[69]; two upper-limb arterial thromboses[70,71]; and, finally, coronary artery and intracardiac thromboses[72,73]. A single iliofemoral thrombosis has been reported[74], but there have been no reports of series of lower-limb DVT otherwise. There are at least two further reports of thrombosis associated with ovarian stimulation where OHSS was not implicated[75,76].

Whilst these cases do not represent a huge number in relation to the number of cases of ovarian stimulation performed internationally per year, they do represent important morbidity and occasional mortality, and it is clear that reported cases will not represent the full picture. Reporting bias results in skewing towards more 'interesting' and less 'routine' cases, and in addition some cases may indeed remain unnoted simply because the woman reports elsewhere than the fertility clinic and the link may not be made.

OHSS is not always the key factor, although present in the majority of these cases. The interpretation of this association remains problematic, however, due to the enormous differences both across international boundaries and over time in making the diagnosis.

Upper-limb thrombosis is a relative rarity, representing about 4% of all VTE in the general population[77]. Specific risk factors include long-line intravenous catheterization and obstructive lesions in the chest, whether tumors or bony abnormalities[78]. Arterial thrombosis is also rare in young healthy adults, occurring as a result of specific trauma, including arterial canalization, or in the elderly in the form of strokes. There are no specific features of assisted conception treatment which can account for this peculiar distribution of cases except the generation of a hypercoagulable state.

Importantly, in around 80% of the OHSS-associated cases, pregnancy was also a feature. Since severe OHSS is associated with high pregnancy rates it is not unreasonable that these factors should go hand in hand, but it is of interest to note that the timing of occurrence of the reported thrombosis does not generally coincide with the probable peak of OHSS severity. The mean period from treatment to diagnosis of venous thrombosis was about 34 days (upper limb, head and neck; range 14–50) and 20 days (lower limb and pulmonary embolism; range 11–24). That of arterial thrombosis was shorter at 13 (range 1–36 days)[10]. It is likely that there is a cumulative effect of the two conditions on risk, and whilst the hypercoagulability induced by pregnancy has been discussed above in general terms, the fact that thrombosis can occur with OHSS unaffected by pregnancy means that this must represent an independent risk factor, and numerous hypotheses have been put forward to explain this phenomenon.

THE HYPERCOAGULABLE STATE IN OHSS

As described above, there are a number of features of OHSS which contribute to the generalized increased risk of thrombosis. It is likely that the influence of hyperestrogenemia has a role to play in its pathogenesis. Working on the hypothesis that women undergoing ovarian stimulation may behave like pregnant women, Wramsby *et al.*[79] have considered acquired activated protein C (APC) resistance. They assessed 20 women undergoing *in vitro* fertilization (IVF) treatment, all of whom were confirmed non-carriers of the factor V Leiden mutation, and compared these with women tested during their normal menstrual cycles. They showed that, unlike pregnant women, there was no change in APC resistance during stimulation, and that it did not differ from that of unstimulated women who similarly showed no cyclical differences. Although a dose-dependent role has been confirmed in exogenous estrogen administration[80], the same effect of endogenous estrogen is less clear, although Kodama *et al.*[81] were able to show sequential changes, in particular thrombophilic features (D-dimer, plasmin–α^2-antiplasmin complex and thrombin–antithrombin III (ATIII) complex), which were more marked in women who generated high rather than low endogenous serum estradiol concentrations during treatment, and more so again where significant OHSS intervened. Of these changes, the thrombin–ATIII complex denotes activation of the coagulation pathway, and the plasmin–α^2-antiplasmin complex and D-dimer are associated with activation of the fibrinolytic pathway. The changes rapidly returned to normal if no pregnancy ensued, but persisted for several weeks when pregnancy occurred, a finding that fits with the observations regarding the combination of OHSS, pregnancy and the different timings of thrombosis. They were also able to show that changes in D-dimer and plasmin–α^2-antiplasmin were more marked and preceded the development of thrombosis in the one woman of age 22 with OHSS who developed the condition[43].

Kim *et al.*[82] described an increase in fibrinogen concentration in the blood of women undergoing ovulation induction which correlated with estrogen concentration. They also showed an increase in VIIIR.vWF and a reduction in ATIII. However, no difference in prothrombin time (PT) or activated partial thromboplastin time (APTT) was demonstrated. Other studies have suggested increased fibrinogen and reduced ATIII concentrations in association with an increase in clot lysis time[83], a thromboprotective reduction in factor VII and an increase in free protein C concentrations[84] and significant changes in PT and APTT, but within the normal ranges, thus negating the importance of the change[85]. Although these changes were related to ovarian stimulation, they were not studied in the context of OHSS.

Other studies specifically examining hematological changes in cycles affected by OHSS have been of limited use because they have not provided follow-up data of sufficient duration to include the period of risk, which appears to be some weeks after human chorionic gonadotropin (hCG) administration[10]. Philips *et al.*[86] reported increased concentrations of factor V, fibrinogen, profibrinolysin, fibrinolytic inhibitors and platelets in two women experiencing severe OHSS, and both Kaaja *et al.*[87] and Todorow *et al.*[88] suggested that changes in von Willebrand factor behavior could predict the onset of OHSS. Delvigne *et al.*[89] examined a number of clotting parameters in women suffering from OHSS, and showed no abnormality in PTR, APTT, ATIII or APC resistance. There was a slightly higher fibrinogen concentration in women with OHSS. Unfortunately, sampling was not done until after resolution of the OHSS symptoms and was done only once, so that any dynamics of these parameters throughout stimulation, OHSS and its resolution would not be seen.

It does, however, seem likely that there are changes in various factors associated with the thrombolytic and fibrinolytic pathways which may promote a thrombophilic state, but the combined studies are inconclusive, and whilst estrogen concentrations are implicated, the mechanism is uncertain.

Hemoconcentration is a cardinal feature of significant OHSS, and increases the risk of thrombosis because of increased blood viscosity and, potentially, also an increased concentration of circulating coagulation factors. Levin *et al.* suggested that increased erythrocyte aggregation detected in OHSS compared with unaffected controls may have a role in its pathogenesis[90]. It is not clear how this finding relates to the expected hemoconcentration, however. Hemoconcentration may also allow more prolonged exposure of circulating factors to the endothelial surface, thus increasing the effect of any local damage. There is evidence, for instance, that tissue factor in the coagulation pathway is increased and tissue factor pathway inhibitor decreased in severe OHSS[91]. Circulating factors may in themselves have effects on the endothelial surface, making it more prone to stimulate thrombus formation. Balasch *et al.*[92] suggested a role in thrombogenesis of tissue factors produced by monocytes in women with severe OHSS, and endothelial damage by stress-induced leukocytes has also been hypothesized[44]. Finally, Foong *et al.*[93] have hypothesized that a change in arteriolar reactivity observed in women with OHSS may predispose to its pathogenesis, but by changes in local blood flow this may also have a role in promotion of the prothrombotic state in these women.

There has been some discussion that predisposition to subfertility, the need for treatment and OHSS may be secondary to an associated thrombophilia. Dulitsky *et al.*[49] found that 17 out of 20 women experiencing severe OHSS compared with 11 of 41 controls had at least one thrombophilic marker, albeit that some were acquired. Of these women, three had some form of thromboembolic disorder. Each of these had a combination of at least two thrombophilic markers. Importantly, Grandone *et al.*[94] examined 305 women undertaking a total of 747 cycles of IVF. They were able to show that the risk of thromboembolic disease corresponded to 1.6/100 000 cycles/woman (4/747 cycles were thus complicated), and that age over 39 years was a specific risk factor. Following testing for both inherited and acquired thrombophilias they also showed that mild hyperhomocysteinemia was strongly associated with the thromboembolic disorders that occurred. Whilst admitting that the study was not powered to do so, Delvigne *et al.*[89] showed no increased incidence in a full range of thrombophilias (including antiphospholipid syndrome) in women who developed OHSS, compared with matched controls. Similarly, Fabregues *et al.*[95] considered the prevalence of thrombophilias, both inherited and acquired, in women with severe OHSS and found no excess compared with unaffected controls.

These most recent papers are significant in that they highlight a change in knowledge that has occurred over recent years, with the recognition of thrombophilias and their clinical importance[7] (Table 3). When many of the cases of ovarian stimulation-associated thromboembolic disease were being reported, few considered these disorders, and many of the women whose problems were reported were not screened either before, in the case of known risk factors, or necessarily afterwards to make the diagnosis. It is likely, therefore, that in a number of those cases where this possibility was not considered mainly for historical reasons, there would have been an underlying thrombophilia. It is also likely, however, that thrombophilia represents an additional risk factor rather than a cause to explain fully the phenomenon of thrombosis in OHSS.

Table 3 The thrombophilias

Inherited thrombophilia	*Acquired thrombophilia*
Factor V Leiden	Antiphospholipid syndrome
Antithrombin III deficiency	Acquired hyperhomocysteinemia
Protein S deficiency	
Protein C deficiency	
Inherited hyperhomocysteinemia	
Raised factor VIII	
Prothrombin gene G20210A variant	

It is clear on reviewing the literature that there is as yet no firm pathogenetic link between the development of OHSS and its associated complication of thromboembolism. In the rest of this chapter a more pragmatic view is taken with regard to prophylaxis, diagnosis and treatment of thromboembolism in association with fertility treatment and OHSS.

PREVENTION OF THROMBOEMBOLIC DISEASE IN WOMEN UNDERGOING OVARIAN STIMULATION

The basis for prevention of thrombosis is first and foremost to recognize the risk. It is common in peroperative patients or hospital in-patients to assess formally that risk on the basis of age, weight, mobility, underlying disorder (including operation to be undergone), previous personal history or family history of thromboembolism and other intercurrent risk factors. A scoring system is often employed to determine the type of thromboprophylaxis relevant to their situation, whether it be simply early mobilization, the use of graduated stockings, prophylactic doses of heparin or full anticoagulation[3]. Most women undergoing assisted conception treatment are healthy individuals where the calculated risk is low, and no specific measures need to be taken. Regarding operative risk, oocyte retrieval under sedation does not constitute a high risk, although a lengthy procedure performed under general anesthesia probably warrants antiembolism stockings at least. There is, however, a need to maintain awareness of the changing nature of that risk as treatment progresses, particularly where there are other factors such as obesity to take into account. The development of OHSS requires reassessment of that risk. One such scoring system for ovarian stimulation is proposed in Table 4.

ADDITIONAL RISK FACTORS

It is of course true that if the process of ovarian stimulation increases the risk of thromboembolism then, as with pregnancy, this will be significantly enhanced by any other coincidental thrombophilic disorder or a previous history of thromboembolic disease, and in several of the case reports discussed above a thrombophilia was implicated along with other risk factors[19,42,45,50,73,75]. These must be taken into account when considering the appropriateness of fertility treatment and the type of treatment considered. Discussion of these risks must come into the process of information counseling of the couple undergoing treatment, and serious consideration given to thromboprophylaxis, not just for the ensuing treatment but also for any consequent pregnancy. This includes a consideration of multiple pregnancy and potential mode of delivery.

Table 4 Risk of thromboembolism in association with ovarian stimulation: proposed scoring system

Risk factor	*Score**
Age > 35 years	1
Obesity	1
Poor mobility	1
Family history of thromboembolism	1
Known thrombophilia	1–2
Previous VTE	3
Pregnancy	1
OHSS	1
Admission with OHSS or 3 or more days in absence of OHSS	2

*Score of 3 or more warrants thromboprophylaxis; VTE, venous thromboembolism

SCREENING

Screening for thrombophilia would allow for further risk assessment; however, thrombophilias are relatively rare: up to 1 in 20 are carriers for the commonest – factor V Leiden[96] – but homozygosity is much rarer. The clinical and cost-effectiveness of screening is therefore debatable. Fabregues *et al.*[95] concluded that even screening for the commonest inherited thrombophilias (factor V Leiden and prothrombin G20210A variant) is not cost-effective in this population, with a cost of nearly $500 000 estimated to prevent one thrombotic episode associated with factor V Leiden. The screening issue was thoroughly discussed in the debate around factor V Leiden and oral contraceptive use. The conclusion was, in that setting, where the risk was not high, that screening for thrombophilia was not worthwhile[97]. In addition, it was not clear how significant heterozygosity was, and it was possible that many women would be denied the use of the COCP spuriously as a result of testing. The relative risk of thromboembolism associated with fertility treatment, although difficult to assess in absolute terms, appears to be significantly lower than that with use of the COCP and certainly lower than that with pregnancy. Long duration of prophylactic doses of anticoagulants can in themselves be harmful (Table 5). It seems unreasonable to presume, therefore, that the benefits of screening may outweigh the risks in an otherwise low-risk population. Where there is a history suggestive of thrombophilia, however, such screening is almost certainly warranted, since for example a significant family history and positive screen combined constitutes a higher risk.

Table 5 Risks of anticoagulant treatment

	Warfarin	*Unfractionated heparin*	*Low-molecular-weight heparin*
Short term	Exacerbation of protein C deficiency Drug interactions Bleeding	Bleeding	Low risk
Long term	Drug interactions Bleeding	Thrombocytopenia Osteoporosis	Low risk
Pregnancy[100]			
maternal	Bleeding	Bleeding Thrombocytopenia Osteoporosis	Bleeding
fetal	Nasal hypoplasia Bony abnormalities CNS malformations Neonatal bleeding	Safe	Safe
Breast-feeding	Safe	Safe	Safe
Monitoring required	Yes	Yes	In pregnancy

CNS, central nervous system

ANTIPHOSPHOLIPID SYNDROME

Antiphospholipid syndrome is a condition characterized by both arterial and venous thrombosis. Whilst in this severe form it is rare, it can be manifest in young women by recurrent poor obstetric outcome, and is the only treatable cause of recurrent miscarriage[98]. Whilst the role of otherwise asymptomatic antiphospholipid syndrome in subfertility is more controversial, there may be an association. Women with the syndrome who have had successive pregnancy problems are treated in subsequent pregnancy with low-dose aspirin and heparin[99], which can have a significant impact on the outcome of pregnancy. It is not clear what, if any role, asymptomatic and unrecognized antiphospholipid syndrome may have on the risk of thrombosis in fertility treatment. It is possible that such a condition could be responsible for the arterial thromboses experienced in this population. Thus, consideration of antiphospholipid syndrome constitutes part of standard thrombophilia screening when this is warranted, as well as in screening for recurrent pregnancy loss.

PROPHYLAXIS

Whilst short-term thromboprophylaxis is used to cover a particular risk period, as a general rule, if thromboprophylaxis for the period of fertility treatment is considered, then extension into subsequent pregnancy is likely to be required. Similarly, if prophylaxis is required for pregnancy, then its commencement as early as possible is warranted, and that is likely to include preceding ovarian stimulation treatment.

Low-risk prophylaxis

Aside from the above, OHSS and pregnancy combined appear to constitute the greatest risk of thromboembolism to women undergoing assisted conception treatment. Pregnancy alone does not require intervention, but the development of OHSS necessitates further assessment. Our practice is to manage OHSS on an outpatient basis as far as possible, admitting women to hospital if intravenous therapy is required, if there is significant ascites warranting paracentesis or if the woman simply is not coping. In these situations, women are probably spending large periods of time resting, and are therefore accumulating significant risk factors for thrombosis. All women with a diagnosis of OHSS who require admission to hospital therefore receive a prophylactic dose of subcutaneous heparin throughout their admission, and treatment is discontinued usually on discharge. If they are clinically improved but retain a significant degree of abdominal distension by fluid and are pregnant then this may be continued after discharge until the OHSS, prolonged by pregnancy, has resolved.

Prophylaxis for high risk

Where a woman has a personal history of venous thrombosis, then it is incumbent upon the practitioner to ensure that appropriate measures are taken to avoid recurrence. In this situation, unless there was an obvious provocative and temporary risk factor, the decision is probably clear-cut, and for any woman undergoing superovulation, prophylactic doses of heparin should be considered for the duration of treatment and into pregnancy[100,101]. Where there has been a specific episode contributing to the previous thrombosis, prophylaxis for pregnancy may be withheld and thus is probably not necessary preceding fertility treatment unless there are other risk factors. The development of OHSS during such treatment warrants review of that decision.

Prophylaxis for thrombophilia

The consideration of thromboprophylaxis is more complicated when there is a known thrombophilia, since, as has been discussed, screening for the condition is not advocated in otherwise asymptomatic women without a personal or significant family history. It is difficult, therefore, in this situation to recommend prophylaxis for all women who incidentally test positive but have no other risk factors except planned fertility treatment and anticipated pregnancy[102]. The need for pretreatment prophylaxis then depends on the type of thrombophilia, and, if inherited, the zygosity, as it would in pregnancy.

The risk of thrombosis is greatest in women who are homozygous for an inherited disorder, are heterozygous for more than one thrombophilia or have ATIII deficiency[11]. In these situations thromboprophylaxis would usually be offered for pregnancy, and should probably therefore also be offered for ovarian stimulation. In lower-risk situations, for example heterozygosity for factor V Leiden, thromboprophylaxis would perhaps be offered only in the presence of other significant risk factors such as a family history, and considered in older or obese women[100–102].

Other measures

Whilst the value of graduated stockings in thromboprophylaxis is uncertain, it is our practice to provide these to women admitted to hospital with OHSS.

DIAGNOSIS OF THROMBOEMBOLISM

Thromboembolism may of course present as a cause of sudden death. A large pulmonary embolus or significant intracranial arterial thrombosis may be the first sign of the condition. A high index of suspicion should be maintained in any sudden collapse of a young woman undergoing fertility treatment, since only by prompt treatment in that situation in an intensive-care setting may the outcome be improved. Where the presentation is less sudden, a suspicion of thromboembolism is raised initially by unusual symptoms in such women. The woman may complain of unilateral limb pain or swelling, or, in the case of neck thrombosis, neck stiffness. In arterial thrombosis there may be symptoms associated with ischemia, although if intra-abdominal this may be difficult to elucidate. In the case of intracranial thrombosis neurological sequelae may be present. Where there is a suspicion of venous thrombosis, examination may reveal swelling, skin discoloration and limb warmth and tenderness. Some form of imaging is generally necessary to confirm and assess the thrombosis. First-line for venous thrombosis is ultrasonography, including occlusion ultrasound and Doppler studies. The interpretation of negative results depends upon the history and considered likelihood of DVT[103] (Table 6). If the likelihood of thrombosis is high, further imaging may be of benefit – venography remains the gold standard for diagnosis of venous thrombosis – and ventilation with or without perfusion scan is used for confirmation of pulmonary embolism, but may not be considered necessary in a woman with positive ultrasound results and chest symptoms. Computerized tomography (CT) scanning and magnetic resonance imaging (MRI) have a role in evaluating more complex situations, for example to confirm vena cava involvement, or arteriography for arterial thromboses. Where ultrasonography is negative and suspicion of thrombosis is low, no further action need necessarily be taken; however, if symptoms persist, a repeat assessment is of value a few days later[100]. This strategy is recommended for pregnant women with a suspicion for thrombosis, and is easily transferable to the fertility patient[100]. The assessment of blood D-dimer (fibrinogen breakdown product) concentration has been lauded as a useful adjunct to initial ultrasound assessment and even as a screening test prior to undertaking imaging procedures[104]. The concentration of D-dimer rises physiologically in pregnancy, however, and this appears to be paralleled in

Table 6 Clinical probability of diagnosis of venous thrombosis based on reference 103

Risk factor	*Score**
Prior history of DVT	1
OHSS and/or pregnancy	1
Paralysis, paresis (recent plaster or immobilization of lower limb)	1
Localized tenderness	1
Entire limb swollen	1
Calf swelling > 3 cm compared with contralateral limb	1
Pitting edema	1
Collateral superficial veins	1
Alternative diagnosis as likely or greater than DVT	–2

*Score of –2 to 1 = low risk, 2 or more = high risk; DVT, deep venous thrombosis

OHSS[81]. A raised concentration, whilst otherwise indicative of pathology, cannot therefore be interpreted as such in these situations. D-dimer in the normal range, however, effectively rules out significant thrombus formation even in pregnancy[11].

TREATMENT

As has been discussed, the occurrence of thromboembolism in fertility treatment is rare. When diagnosed, however, it requires rapid and expert intervention. The mainstay of treatment is of course anticoagulation to prevent extension of the primary clot, reduce the risk of embolism and facilitate its organization such that recanalization of the affected vessel can occur. With appropriate imaging techniques the extent of the thrombus can be assessed, which allows for symptoms to be accounted for, and the possible risks and effects of embolism to be considered. Where this risk is significant, operative intervention may be considered by means of thrombectomy, as may be necessary in arterial thrombosis, or insertion of an upstream 'umbrella' in the case of inferior vena cava thrombosis[105]. Thus, the diagnosis and treatment of thromboembolism requires a multidisciplinary decision-making approach including the radiologist and potentially also the vascular surgeon.

In the case of otherwise uncomplicated venous thrombosis, standard treatment would involve anticoagulation with heparin, initially intravenously and followed by subcutaneous administration of a maintenance dose of either unfractionated heparin monitored using APTT or, more conveniently, an appropriate therapeutic dose of one of the low-molecular-weight (LMW) heparins. Conversion to a therapeutic dose of warfarin, monitored by International Normalized Ratio (INR) assessment, is an alternative suitable for women where there is no associated pregnancy. A therapeutic dose is continued for 6 months and consideration then given to its cessation[105].

In the event of pregnancy heparin is used, since there are significant potential adverse effects of warfarin to the fetus[100]. LMW heparin is the preferred choice for maintenance therapy in pregnancy, and is considered to be as safe as unfractionated heparin in this setting. The advantage of LMW heparin is that it can be given as a standard dose in relation to the woman's weight, and does not require such rigorous monitoring. As with heparin the therapeutic dose is continued for about 6 months, but should be extended into the postpartum period. It can be readily reduced for delivery and reinstated immediately after delivery. Conversion to warfarin maintenance may be considered following delivery, and either drug is considered safe to the breast-feeding infant[100].

Graduated compression stockings should be worn by all women undergoing treatment for DVT, as there is evidence that they may reduce the risk of prolonged symptoms[106]. The effect of some form of similar compression on the long-term symptomatology associated with upper-limb thrombosis is unknown[107].

LONG-TERM OUTLOOK

The morbidity associated with thromboembolism depends on its site, severity and treatment. In the case of intracerebral arterial thrombosis, whilst in the long term recovery may be good, the process of rehabilitation may be prolonged, and the woman may well be left with some form of disability or weakness as a result of the stroke. Successful treatment of venous thrombosis does not necessarily exclude the possibility of long-term problems. Post-thrombotic syndrome refers to the residual effects of vascular occlusion, and includes altered sensation, heaviness and reduced mobility in the limb. It occurs in both lower- and to a lesser extent upper-limb venous thromboses[107] and can be progressive (at least in the first 2 years), prolonged and debilitating, culminating, for example, in some cases in venous ulceration.

Finally, of course, upon completion of therapeutic treatment for thrombosis, consideration needs to be given to the risk of recurrence and long-term prophylaxis. Whilst it may be considered that OHSS with or without pregnancy is explanation enough for thrombosis occurring, it is necessary to assess the woman's risk in more detail. However, if there are other obvious factors such as obesity these should be addressed in this situation. Whilst it will not affect management of the primary thrombosis, it is necessary to ensure that such women have had thrombophilia screening performed. A positive result not only allows a fuller assessment of her ongoing risk, but will affect the recommendations made regarding prophylactic treatment in either similar or different circumstances in the future. A significant result (for example confirmation of homozygosity where the risk is high) may also have an effect on her decision to pursue further fertility treatment and indeed pregnancy. A positive result for inherited thrombophilia also has implications for other members of her family, which needs to be discussed.

CONCLUSION

There is a small but important risk of venous or arterial thrombosis in women undergoing ovarian stimulation for fertility treatment, which is heightened by both OHSS and pregnancy. Whilst most women are at low risk of thromboembolic disease at the outset of treatment, this risk needs to be considered and reviewed as clinical conditions change. Women who have known risk factors for thromboembolism should be assessed for thromboprophylaxis, and, if considered appropriate, it should be instituted at the start of treatment and probably maintained throughout the subsequent pregnancy. OHSS brings with it a number of factors which increase the likelihood of thromboembolism, and whilst the pathogenetic links have yet to be fully determined, when women are hospitalized with this condition consideration should be given to appropriate thromboprophylaxis even in the absence of other risk factors.

REFERENCES

1. Ludwig M, Genbruch U, Bauer O, et al. Ovarian hyperstimulation syndrome (OHSS) in a spontaneous pregnancy with fetal and placental triploidy: information about the general pathophysiology of OHSS. Hum Reprod 1998; 13: 2082–7.
2. Delbaere A, Smits G, Olatunbosun O, et al. New insights into the pathophysiology of ovarian hyperstimulation syndrome. What makes the difference between spontaneous and iatrogenic syndrome? Hum Reprod 2004; 19: 486–9.
3. Scottish Intercollegiate Guidelines Network (SIGN). Section 2: Risk factors for venous thromboembolism. In Prophylaxis of Venous Thromboembolism. SIGN, 2002. www.sign.ac.uk/guidelines/fulltext/62.
4. McPherson K. Third generation oral contraception and venous thromboembolism. Br Med J 1996; 312: 68–9.
5. Rymer J, Wilson R, Ballard K. Making decisions about hormone replacement therapy. Br Med J 2003; 326: 322–6.
6. Kelman CW, Kortt MA, Becker NG, et al. Deep venous thrombosis and air travel: record linkage study. Br Med J 2003; 327: 1072–3.
7. Rosendaal FR. Venous thrombosis: a multicausal disease. Lancet 1993; 353: 1167–73.
8. Committee on Safety of Medicines (CSM) and Medicines and Healthcare Products Regulatory Agency (MHRA). Combined oral contraceptives containing desogestrel or gestodene and the risk of venous thromboembolism. Curr Prob Pharmacovigilance 1999; 25: 11–12.
9. Confidential Enquiry into Maternal and Child Health. Why mothers die 2000–2002. London: RCOG Press, 2004.
10. Stewart JA, Hamilton PJ, Murdoch AP. Thromboembolic disease associated with ovarian stimulation and assisted conception techniques. Hum Reprod 1997; 12: 2167–73.
11. Greer IA. Thrombosis in pregnancy. Lancet 1999; 353: 1258–65.
12. Mozes M, Bogokowsky H, Anteri E, et al. Thromboembolic phenomena after ovarian stimulation with human gonadotrophins. Lancet 1965; 2: 1213–15.
13. Humbert G, Delauney P, Leroy J, et al. Accident vasculaire cérébrale au cours d'un traitement par les gonadotrophines. Nouv Presse Med 1973; 2: 28–30.
14. Nwosu UC, Corson SL, Bolognese RJ. Hyperstimulation and multiple side-effects of menotropin therapy: a case report. J Reprod Med 1974; 12: 117–20.
15. Schenker JG, Weinstein D. Ovarian hyperstimulation syndrome: a current survey. Fertil Steril 1978; 30: 255–68.
16. Dumont M, Combet A, Domenichini Y. Thrombose artérielle cérébrale à la suite d'une hyperstimulation ovarienne, grossesse sextuple. Avortement thérapeutique. Nouv Presse Med 1980; 9: 3628–31.
17. Dalrymple JC, Smith DH, Sinosich MJ, et al. Venous thrombosis with high estradiol levels following gonadotrophin therapy. Infertility 1982–3; 5:239–45.
18. Salat-Baroux J, Cornet D, Antoine JM, et al. Un cas de stimulation grave au cours d'une fécondation in vitro suivie de grossesse. Gynécologie 1987; 38: 69–72.
19. Boulieu D, Ninet J, Pinede L, et al. Thrombose veineuse précoce de siege inhabituel, en début de grossesse après hyperstimulation ovarienne. Contracept Fertil Sex 1989; 17: 725–7.
20. Kaaja R, Siegberg R, Tiitinen A, et al. Severe ovarian hyperstimulation syndrome and deep venous thrombosis. Lancet 1989; 2: 1043.
21. Neau J-P, Maréchaud M, Guitton P, et al. Occlusion de l'artère cérébrale moyenne lors d'une induction de l'ovulation par les gonadotrophines. Rev Neurol (Paris) 1989; 145: 859–61.
22. Rizk B, Meagher S, Fisher AM. Severe ovarian hyperstimulation syndrome and cerebrovascular accidents. Hum Reprod 1990; 5: 697–8.

23. Fournet N, Surrey E, Kerin J. Internal jugular vein thrombosis after ovulation induction with gonadotrophins. Fertil Steril 1991; 56: 354–6.

24. Ong ACM, Elsen V, Rennie DP, et al. The pathogenesis of ovarian hyperstimulation syndrome (OHS): a possible role for ovarian renin. Clin Endocrinol 1991: 34: 43–9.

25. Rajah R, Boothroyd A, Lees WR. Case of the month. A pain in the neck! Br J Radiol 1991; 64: 867–8.

26. Mills MS, Eddowes HA, Fox R, et al. Subclavian vein thrombosis: a late complication of ovarian hyperstimulation syndrome. Hum Reprod 1992; 7: 370–1.

27. Waterstone JJ, Summers BA, Hoskins MC, et al. Ovarian hyperstimulation syndrome and deep cerebral venous thrombosis. Br Med Obstet Gynaecol 1992; 99: 439–40.

28. Ayhan A, Urman B, Gürgen T, et al. Thrombosis of the internal jugular vein associated with severe ovarian hyperstimulation syndrome. Aust NZ J Obstet Gynecol 1993; 33: 436.

29. Kermode AG, Churchyard A, Carroll WM. Stroke complicating severe ovarian hyperstimulation syndrome. Aust NZ J Med 1993; 23: 219.

30. Vauthier-Brouzes D, Lefebvre G, Seebacher J, et al. Thrombose voineuse jugulaire interne en cours de grossesse après hyperstimulation ovarienne pour FIV. Contracept Fertil Sex 1993; 21: 33–5.

31. Bachmeyer C, Grateau G, Bruel D, et al. Thrombose de la veine jugulaire interne au cours d'un syndrome d'hyperstimulation ovarienne. Rev Méd Interne 1994; 15: 52–4.

32. Bénifla J-L, Conard J, Naouri M, et al. Syndrome d'hyperstimulation ovarienne et thrombose. J Gynecol Obstet Biol Reprod 1994; 23: 778–83.

33. Inbar OJ, Levran D, Shlomo M, et al. Ischaemic stroke due to induction of ovulation with clomiphene citrate and menotropins without evidence of ovarian hyperstimulation syndrome. Fertil Steril 1994; 62: 1075–6.

34. Thill B, Rathat C, Akula A, et al. Accidents thrombo-emboliques lors des fécondations in vitro. Ann Fr Anesth Réanim 1994; 13: 726–9.

35. Aurousseau MH, Samama MM, Belhassen A, et al. Risk of thromboembolism in relation to an in-vitro fertilization programme: three case reports. Hum Reprod 1995; 10: 94–7.

36. Benshushan A, Shushan A, Paltiel O et al. Ovulation induction with clomiphene citrate complicated by deep venous thrombosis. Eur J Obstet Gynecol Reprod Biol 1995; 62: 261–2.

37. Choktanasiri W, Rojanasakul A. Acute arterial thrombosis after gamete intrafallopian transfer: A case report. J Assist Reprod Genet 1995; 12: 335–7.

38. el Kouri D, Bani-Sadr F, De Faucal P, et al. Thrombose jugulaire après hyperstimulation ovarienne: une complication evitable? Presse Med 1995; 24: 547.

39. Hignett M, Spence JEH, Claman P. Internal jugular vein thrombosis: a late complication of ovarian hyperstimulation syndrome despite minidose heparin prophylaxis. Hum Reprod 1995; 10: 3121–3.

40. Hocke C, Guyon F, Dulucq MC, et al. Accidents thromboemboliques et hyperstimulation ovariennes. J Gynecol Obstet Biol Reprod 1995; 24: 691–6.

41. Hulinsky I, Smith HC. External jugular vein thrombosis: a complication of the ovarian hyperstimulation syndrome. Med J Aust 1995; 162: 335–6.

42. Kligman I, Noyes N, Benadiva CA, et al. Massive deep vein thrombosis in a patient with antithrombin III deficiency undergoing ovarian stimulation for in vitro fertilisation. Fertil Steril 1995; 63: 673–6.

43. Kodama H, Matsui T, Fukuda J, et al. Characteristics of blood hemostatic markers in a patient with ovarian hyperstimulation syndrome who actually developed thromboembolism. Fertil Steril 1995; 64: 1207–9.

44. Germond M, Wirthner D, Thorin D, et al. Aorto-subclavian thromboembolism: a rare complication associated with moderate ovarian hyperstimulation syndrome. Hum Reprod 1996; 11: 1173–6.

45. Horstkamp B, Lübke M, Kentenich H, et al. Internal jugular vein thrombosis caused by resistance to activated protein C as a complica-

tion of ovarian hyperstimulation after in-vitro fertilization. Hum Reprod 1996; 11: 280–2.

46. Huong DLT, Wechsler B, Piette J-C, et al. Risks of ovulation induction therapy in systemic lupus erythematosus. Br J Rheumatol 1996; 35: 1184–6.

47. Stewart JA, Hamilton PJ, Murdoch AP. Upper limb thrombosis associated with assisted conception treatment. Hum Reprod 1997; 12: 2174–5.

48. Delvigne A, Rozenberg S. Review of clinical course and treatment of ovarian hyperstimulation syndrome (OHSS). Hum Reprod Update 2003; 9: 77–96.

49. Dulitsky M, Cohen SB, Inbal A, et al. Increased prevalence of thrombophilia among women with severe ovarian hyperstimulation syndrome. Fertil Steril 2002; 77: 463–7.

50. Hollemaert S, Wautrecht JC, Capel P, et al. Thrombosis associated with ovarian hyperstimulation syndrome in a carrier of the factor V Leiden mutation. Thromb Haemost 1996; 76: 275–7.

51. Moutos DM, Miller MM, Mahadevan MM. Bilateral internal jugular venous thrombosis complicating severe ovarian hyperstimulation syndrome after prophylactic albumin administration. Fertil Steril 1997; 68: 174–6.

52. Ellis MH, Nun IB, Rathaus V, et al. Internal jugular vein thrombosis in patients with ovarian hyperstimulation syndrome. Fertil Steril 1998; 69: 140–2.

53. Jacob S, Byrne P, Harrison RF. Symptomatic cystic swelling at the root of the neck with left sided pleural effusion as a presentation of ovarian hyperstimulation syndrome. Br J Obstet Gynaecol 1999; 106: 986–8.

54. Todros T, Carmazzi CM, Bontempo S et al. Spontaneous ovarian hyperstimulation syndrome and deep venous thrombosis in pregnancy: case report. Hum Reprod 1999; 14: 2245–8.

55. Lamon D, Chang CK, Hruska L, et al. Superior vena cava thrombosis after in vitro fertilization: case report and review of the literature. Ann Vasc Surg 2000; 14: 283–5.

56. Loret de Mola JR, Kiwi R, Austin C, et al. Subclavian deep vein thrombosis associated with the use of recombinant follicle-stimulating hormone (Gonal F) complicating mild ovarian hyperstimulation syndrome. Fertil Steril 2002; 73: 1253–6.

57. Schanzer A, Rockman CB, Jacobowitz GR, et al. Internal jugular venous thrombosis in association with the ovarian hyperstimulation syndrome. J Vasc Surg 2000; 31: 815–18.

58. Belaen B, Geerinckx K, Vergauwe P, et al. Internal jugular vein thrombosis after ovarian stimulation. Hum Reprod 2001; 16: 510–12.

59. Ou YC, Kao YL, Lai SL, et al. Thromboembolism after ovarian stimulation: successful management of a woman with superior sagittal sinus thrombosis after IVF and embryo transfer: case report. Hum Reprod 2003; 18: 2375–81.

60. Shan Tang O, Ng E, Wai Cheng P, et al. Cortical vein thrombosis misinterpreted as intracranial haemorrhage in severe ovarian hyperstimulation syndrome. Hum Reprod 2000; 15: 1913–16.

61. Yoshii F, Ooki N, Shinohara Y, et al. Multiple cerebral infarctions associated with ovarian hyperstimulation syndrome. Neurology 1999; 53: 225–7.

62. Di Micco P, D'Uva M, Romano M, et al. Stroke due to left carotid thrombosis in moderate ovarian hyperstimulation syndrome. Thromb Haemost 2003; 90: 957–60.

63. Morris RS, Paulson RJ. Increased angiotensin-converting enzyme activity in a patient with severe ovarian hyperstimulation syndrome. Fertil Steril 1999; 72: 749–50.

64. Hwang WJ, Lai ML, Hsu CC, et al. Ischemic stroke in a young woman with ovarian hyperstimulation syndrome. J Formos Med Assoc 1998; 97: 503–6.

65. Aboulghar MA, Mansour RT, Serour GI, et al. Moderate ovarian hyperstimulation syndrome complicated by deep cerebrovascular thrombosis. Hum Reprod 1998; 13: 2088–91.

66. El Sadek MM, Amer MK, Fahmy M. Acute cerebrovascular accidents with severe ovarian hyperstimulation syndrome. Hum Reprod 1998; 13: 1793–5.

67. Davies AJ, Patel B. Hyperstimulation – brain attack! Br J Radiol 1999; 72: 923–4.

68. Elford K, Leader A, Wee R, et al. Stroke in ovarian hyperstimulation syndrome in early pregnancy treated with intra-arterial rt-PA. Neurology 2002; 59: 1270–2.

69. Turkistani IM, Ghourab SA, Al-Sheikh OH, et al. Central retinal artery occlusion associated with severe ovarian hyperstimulation syndrome. Eur J Ophthalmol 2001; 11: 313–15.

70. Mancini A, Milardi D, Di Pietro ML, et al. A case of forearm amputation after ovarian hyperstimulation for in vitro fertilisation–embryo transfer. Fertil Steril 2001; 76: 198–200.

71. Heinig J, Behre HM, Klockenbusch W. Occlusion of the ulnar artery in a patient with severe ovarian hyperstimulation syndrome. Eur J Obstet Gynecol Reprod Biol 2001; 96: 126–7.

72. Ludwig M, Tolg R, Richardt G, et al. Myocardial infarction associated with ovarian hyperstimulation syndrome. JAMA 1999; 282: 632–3.

73. Andrejevic S, Bonaci-Nikolic B, Bukilica M, et al. Intracardiac thrombosis and fever possibly triggered by ovulation induction in a patient with antiphospholipid antibodies. Scand J Rheumatol 2002; 31: 249–51.

74. Cil T, Tummon IS, House AA et al. A tale of two syndromes: ovarian hyperstimulation and abdominal compartment. Hum Reprod 2000; 15: 1058–60.

75. McGowan BM, Kay LA, Perry DJ. Deep vein thrombosis followed by internal jugular vein thrombosis as a complication of in vitro fertilisation in a woman heterozygous for the prothrombin 3' UTR and factor V Leiden mutations. Am J Haematol 2003; 73: 276–8.

76. Ulug U, Aksoy E, Erden H, et al. Bilateral internal jugular vein thrombosis following successful assisted conception in the absence of ovarian hyperstimulation syndrome. Eur J Obstet Gynecol Reprod Biol 2003; 109: 231–3.

77. Horattas MC, Wright DJ, Fenton AH, et al. Changing concepts of deep venous thrombosis of the upper extremity – report of a series and review of the literature. Surgery 1988; 104: 561–7.

78. Burihan E, de Figueiredo LF, Francisco J Jr, et al. Upper extremity deep venous thrombosis: analysis of 52 cases. Cardiovasc Surg 1993; 1: 19–22.

79. Wramsby ML, Bokanewa MI, Blombäek M, et al. Response to activated protein C during normal menstrual cycles and ovarian hyperstimulation. Hum Reprod 2000; 15: 795–7.

80. Inman WHW, Vessey MP, Westerholm B, et al. Thromboembolic disease and the steroidal content of oral contraceptives. A report to the Committee on Safety of Drugs. Br Med J 1970; 2: 203–9.

81. Kodama H, Matsui T, Fukuda J, et al. Status of the coagulation and fibrinolytic systems in ovarian hyperstimulation syndrome. Fertil Steril 1996; 66: 417–24.

82. Kim HC, Kemmann E, Shelden R, et al. Response of blood coagulation parameters to elevated endogenous 17β-estradiol levels induced by human menopausal gonadotrophins. Am J Obstet Gynecol 1981; 140: 807–10.

83. Aune B, Høie KE, Øian P, et al. Does ovarian stimulation for in vitro fertilisation induce a hypercoagulable state? Hum Reprod 1991; 6: 925–7.

84. Bremme K, Wramsby H, Andersson O, et al. Do lowered factor VII levels at extremely high endogenous oestradiol levels protect against thrombin production? Blood Coagul Fibrinol 1994; 5: 205–10.

85. Lox C, Dorsett J, Cañez M, et al. Hyperoestrogenism induced by menotropins alone or in conjunction with luprolide acetate in in vitro fertilisation cycles: the impact on haemostasis. Fertil Steril 1995; 63: 566–70.

86. Philips LL, Gladstone W, van de Wiele R. Studies of the coagulation and fibrinolytic systems in hyperstimulation syndrome after administration of human gonadotrophins. J Reprod Med 1975; 14: 138–43.

87. Kaaja R, Siegberg R, Titinen A, et al. Severe ovarian hyperstimulation syndrome and deep venous thrombosis. Lancet 1989; 2: 1043.

88. Todorow S, Schricker ST, Siebzenreubl ER, et al. Von Willebrand factor: an endothelial marker to

monitor in vitro fertilisation patients with ovarian hyperstimulation syndrome. Hum Reprod 1993; 8: 2039–49.

89. Delvigne A, Kostyla K, De Leener A, et al. Metabolic characteristics of women who developed ovarian hyperstimulation syndrome. Hum Reprod 2002; 17: 1994–6.

90. Levin I, Gamzu R, Hasson Y, et al. Increased erythrocyte aggregation in ovarian hyperstimulation syndrome: a possible contributing factor in the pathophysiology of this disease. Hum Reprod 2004; 19: 1076–80.

91. Rogolino A, Coccia ME, Fedi S, et al. Hypercoagulability, high tissue factor and low tissue factor pathway inhibitor levels in severe ovarian hyperstimulation syndrome: possible associate on with clinical outcome. Blood Coag Fibrinolysis 2003; 14: 227–82.

92. Balasch J, Tàssies D, Reverter JC, et al. Increased induced monocyte tissue factor expression by plasma from patients with severe ovarian hyperstimulation syndrome. Fertil Steril 1996; 66: 608–13.

93. Foong L-C, Bhagavath B, Kumar J, et al. Ovarian hyperstimulation syndrome is associated with reversible impairment of vascular reactivity. Fertil Steril 2002; 78: 1159–63.

94. Grandone E, Colaizzo D, Vegura P, et al. Age and homocysteine plasma levels are risk factors for thrombotic complications after ovarian stimulation. Hum Reprod 2004; 18: 1796–9.

95. Fabregues F, Tassies D, Reverter JC, et al. Prevalence of thrombophilia in women with severe ovarian hyperstimulation syndrome and cost-effectiveness of screening. Fertil Steril 2004; 81: 989–95.

96. Vandenbroucke JP, Koster T, Briet E, et al. Increased risk of venous thrombosis in oral contraceptive users who are carriers of factor V Leiden mutation. Lancet 1994; 344: 1453–7.

97. Vandenbroucke JP, van der Meer FJM, Helmerhorst FM, et al. Factor V Leiden: should we screen oral contraceptive users and pregnant women. Br Med J 1996; 313: 1127–30.

98. Royal College of Obstetricians and Gynaecologists The investigation and treatment of couples with recurrent miscarriage. RCOG Guideline No. 17. London: RCOG Press, 2003.

99. Empson M, Lassere M, Craig JC, et al. Recurrent pregnancy loss with anti-phospholipid antibody: a systematic review of therapeutic trials. Obstet Gynecol 2002; 99: 135–44.

100. Jilma B, Kamath S, Yip GYH. Antithrombotic therapy in special circumstances. I – Pregnancy and cancer. Br Med J 2003; 326: 37–40.

101. Royal College of Obstetricians and Gynaecologists Thromboprophylaxis during pregnancy, labour and after vaginal delivery. Green Top Guidelines. RCOG Guideline No. 37. London: RCOG Press, 2004.

102. Jilma B, Kamath S, Yip GYH. Antithrombotic therapy in special circumstances. II – In children, thrombophilia and miscellaneous conditions. Br Med J 2003; 326: 93–6.

103. Wells PS, Anderson DR, Rodger M, et al. Evaluation of D-dimer in the diagnosis of suspected deep venous thrombosis. N Engl J Med 2003; 349: 1227–35.

104. Fancher TL, White RH, Krawitz RL. Combined use of rapid D-dimer testing and estimation of clinical probability in the diagnosis of deep venous thrombosis: systematic review. Br Med J 2004; 329: 821–4.

105. Tovey C, Wyatt S. Diagnosis, investigation and management of deep venous thrombosis. Br Med J 2003; 326: 1180–4.

106. Brandjes DP, Buller HR, Heijboer H, et al. Randomised trial of effect of compression stockings in patients with symptomatic proximal vein thrombosis. Lancet 1997; 349: 759–62.

107. Prandoni P, Bernardi E, Marchiori A, et al. The long term clinical course of acute deep vein thrombosis of the arm: prospective cohort study. Br Med J 2004; 329: 484–5.

CHAPTER 6

Anonymous reports of lethal cases of ovarian hyperstimulation syndrome

Didi Braat, Rob Bernardus and Jan Gerris

INTRODUCTION

Severe ovarian hyperstimulation syndrome (OHSS) in patients undergoing hormonal treatment for multiple follicular recruitment prior to *in vitro* fertilization (IVF) has been discussed extensively in the literature. Iatrogenic lethal outcome of these elective treatment modalities, however, is sparsely found: is this due to the very low incidence or due to (for obvious reasons) unwillingness to report it? It goes without saying that the impact of this most serious complication is devastating to the partners and families, as well as to the medical professionals concerned. Should we not learn from each other? Do we have to wait a generation before long-term observational studies may become available, and should we, medical professionals, remain blind and/or deaf to reports that appear meanwhile in the lay literature?

When trying to write this chapter, the aim was to identify lethal cases for which as many objective data as possible could be collected. This has proved difficult. Questionnaires were sent to Dutch and Flemish gynecologists asking for anonymous information regarding lethal cases of OHSS. A letter asking for information was published in *Human Reproduction*[1]. The primary aim was to obtain information as to what had been the primary cause of death in these cases, and whether some intervention could have prevented the patient from dying. Reactions to these requests were scant and mostly negative.

In total, 11 published cases could be identified, three in The Netherlands, two in Belgium and six cases in other countries, published over recent decades; four more cases have been published in the lay literature.

Between 1992 and 1997, three lethal cases occurred in IVF treatments in The Netherlands that can be attributed to the stimulatory phase. In an effort to initiate transparency by sharing these shocking experiences, as well as possible measures to prevent recurrence, we report these lethal cases. The same holds for the two cases in Belgium and for the six previously published cases.

LETHAL CASES ORIGINATING IN THE NETHERLANDS

Patient 1 (1992)

The patient was 28 years old and had primary infertility because of polycystic ovarian syndrome (PCOS). Eventually, IVF was initiated owing to the extreme difficulty in obtaining mono-ovulatory induction of ovulation. The patient was treated with a combination of gonadotropin-releasing hormone (GnRH) analogs and gonadotropins. There was a discrepancy between the number of follicles and the number of oocytes retrieved. Two days after egg collection the patient was admitted to hospital because of dyspnea, nausea and general malaise. Because of the risk of OHSS all embryos were frozen. One day later she was transferred to the intensive-care unit because of adult respiratory distress syndrome (ARDS), oliguria and hydrothorax. Unfortunately, she developed multiorgan failure and died 29 days after oocyte pick-up (OPU).

Patient 2 (1994)

This was a 35-year-old patient who had been suffering from primary infertility for 9 years. She had PCOS. She had undergone ovulation induction for many cycles, some of which had been ovulatory and some anovulatory. After 12 ovulatory cycles, of which the last 6 cycles were combined with intrauterine insemination (IUI), IVF was initiated. The woman had a normal body mass index (BMI) (24.2).

Ovarian hyperstimulation was combined with GnRH analogs. She started with 225 IU of gonadotropins for 7 days. This dosage was changed to 150 IU from day 8 onwards, because of the growth of many follicles. Four days later the dominant follicle reached 19 mm, and the next day 10 000 IU of human chorionic gonadotropin (hCG) was administered. No serum estrogen levels were measured. Follicular aspiration was technically difficult because of many small follicles. Seventeen oocytes were obtained. The day following egg collection the patient complained of abdominal pain. Ultrasonography revealed multicystic ovaries (6 cm in diameter) and a small amount of fluid. The next day she was admitted to hospital because of an aggravation of complaints and symptoms. The ovaries were 7 cm in diameter and there was a large amount of ascites. She became dyspneic and was transferred to the intensive-care unit. No embryo transfer was performed, and all (16) embryos were frozen. She developed ARDS and artificial respiration was applied. Two days later electrolytes and kidney function tests were normal; antibiotics were started because of suspicion of a lung infection. One day later, however, kidney function deteriorated and the patient was transferred to a tertiary center, where she died because of multiple organ failure. Her decease was 25 days after egg collection. Autopsy revealed 1 l of ascitic fluid, no pleural effusion and ovaries of size less than 10 cm in diameter.

Patient 3 (1997)

This patient was 40 years of age. She had had primary infertility for 3 years due to a tubal factor, for which IVF was indicated. She started her first IVF cycle with a short GnRH analog protocol combined with gonadotropins. She was given 200 IU for 7 days from cycle day 3 onwards, followed by 150 IU for 4 days, and subsequently 50 IU for 1 day. That same evening, 5000 IU hCG was administered. At oocyte collection, 29 follicles (of which 17 were > 16 mm) were aspirated, resulting in 11 oocytes. Serum estradiol levels were 2.1, 7.7 and 21.9 nmol/ml (656, 2406 and 6844 pg/ml) on cycle days 10, 12 and 14, respectively.

One day later the patient complained of abdominal pain. Ultrasonography revealed multicystic ovaries (8.8 × 8 × 7 cm and 8 × 7 × 5 cm in diameter) and a small amount of peritoneal fluid. Because of threatening OHSS, daily visits were arranged. However, the next morning she was admitted to hospital because she felt worse. According to her husband, she sometimes acted confused. There were no complaints of headache, nor of an increase of abdominal pain. Blood pressure was 130/90 mmHg, pulse rate 100, temperature 36.7°C. No signs of an acute abdomen were found. Prophylactic heparin treatment was started. Three hours later the patient lapsed into a coma. Angiography revealed occlusion of the A. vertebralis dextra, A. basilaris and Aa. cerebri posteriores. Selective streptokinase was administered, but although this resulted in passage of the A. basilaris, the Aa. cerebri posteriores remained obstructed. The patient died on the third day after OPU. Autopsy was refused. A family history of thromboembolic disease was negative; retrospective analysis of thrombophilia factors turned out negative for factor V (Leiden), proteins C and S and antithrombin III.

LETHAL CASES ORIGINATING IN BELGIUM

Patient 1 (1995)

The report regarding this patient is constructed on the basis of personal remembrance of one of the physicians who was working in the treating center, called here center B. The patient died in another hospital in another city (called here center A), and the reporting physician learnt of the patient's death by pure accident a long time after the events took place. Notwithstanding, several efforts at obtaining a written report of what went wrong, and direct telephone contact with the physicians who treated the patient after she was admitted to their hospital, did not until now result in any manner of formal report. The patient was a Caucasian G_1P_1 who was 41 years of age at the time she consulted center A for secondary infertility. She had been trying to conceive since 1992 (3 years). She had already been treated by ovulation hyperstimulation and with one IVF cycle, in which no fertilization had occurred. Routine sperm characteristics were within normal values. In center B, intracytoplasmic sperm injection (ICSI) was proposed, accepted and performed, and led to a pregnancy ending in clinical miscarriage at 8 weeks of amenorrhea and the patient's demise. The fatal cycle was her second treatment cycle. It was carried out with the classical long protocol, using buserelin for 3 weeks followed by stimulation with 300 IU of human menopausal gonadotropin (hMG). On the day of hCG administration, serum estradiol was 3921 pg/ml, and the day after hCG it rose to 7200 pg/ml. On the subsequent day of oocyte collection, serum estradiol dropped to 2331 pg/ml and a total of 26 oocytes were collected, of which 20 were in metaphase II. Fourteen of these were normally fertilized after ICSI; four embryos were transferred and another eight could be cryopreserved. Eight days after transfer, serum hCG was 13 mIU/ml with an estradiol level of 3115 pg/ml. Nothing more was heard from the patient, and it was not until much later that the physicians at center B learned that the patient had died. According to indirect and anonymous information obtained at center A, the patient had been admitted at 6 weeks of pregnancy with severe OHSS. The ovaries both had a diameter of > 10 cm and there was much ascites. She was treated by doctors from the department of internal medicine who administered diuretics. Transabdominal ascites puncture was performed by a gynecologist. During the puncture, the patient developed hypovolemic shock, from which she did not recover. Via another source of information, we learned that as much as 4 l of ascitic fluid had been collected over a short period of time (1 h).

Patient 2

The same center B has in its records one other lethal case of which, however, nothing is known apart from the fact that the patient died. She was a foreign patient who died in her country of origin. Taken together, and for what it is worth, two patients from this center died in a cohort of > 55 000 IVF/ICSI cycles spanning an activity period of 22 years (incidence 1 : 27 500).

CASE REPORTS FROM THE LITERATURE

To our knowledge, in the literature only six other cases of lethal OHSS are reported, with four additional case reports available in the lay literature.

The first mortal case was published by Gotzsche in 1951 (cited by Esteban-Altirriba[2]). The patient was a 28-year-old woman with secondary amenorrhea who was treated with urinary menopausal gonadotropins and human chorionic gonadotropins according to the then prevailing scheme proposed by Rydberg, who was also the first, in 1942, to attract attention to the existence of what was the called *massive hyperluteinization of the ovaries* (cited by Esteban-Altirriba[2]). Six days after administration of hCG, the now well-known acute abdominal distension syndrome developed and became so pronounced that a surgical intervention was performed. Both ovaries were enlarged to the size of the fist of a man and appeared necrotic. There was a large quantity of serosanguinolent fluid in the abdominal cavity. Colic adhesions had formed around several large blood clots. The 'cysts' were *partially* removed but the patient died soon afterwards.

The second mortal case was published by Figueroa-Casas in 1958[3]. This was a patient who, after three failed treatment cycles, received huge doses of hMG (a total dose of 15 000 IU) and hCG (45 000 IU). She developed the typical OHSS syndrome, showing abdominal distension compatible with a pregnancy of 20 weeks' amenorrhea. Put to rest with antispasmodic and antibiotic treatment, the patient remained stable. Further stimulation was conducted during another 11 days, when the situation quickly became critical (nausea, tachycardia, biliary vomiting, severe oliguria). It was decided to operate on the patient (under local anesthesia): 3.5 l of a foul fluid were removed, as well as two hugely cystically enlarged ovaries; the uterus was left in place. The patient died the next day of anuria.

A third dramatic case with death in the end was published by Mozes *et al.*[4]. This patient died as the result of thrombosis of the carotid arteries leading to a deep coma.

Much later, another case of lethal OHSS was published relating to a 39-year-old woman who initially developed moderate OHSS[5]. After OPU she was drowsy, and she never regained full consciousness. She deteriorated quickly over a 10-day period and died of hepatorenal failure. Retrospective review of her medical records revealed a history of hepatitis C with residual impairment of liver function.

Another recent case relates to a patient who died 11 days after OPU because of severe OHSS with cerebral infarction[6].

The last published case report describes a 28-year-old Japanese woman with PCOS[7]. Because of primary infertility she had undergone ovulation induction with 150 IU hMG for 6 days, followed by 5000 IU hCG. No evidence of ovulation was detected. Twelve days after the start of treatment she was admitted because of abdominal pain, possibly due to the enlargement of her ovaries. On ultrasound scan the right ovary measured 8.5 cm and the left ovary 8.1 cm in diameter. Her blood analysis suggested moderate OHSS (hemoglobin 15.0 g/dl, hematocrit 43.9%). She was treated with dopamine, after which her condition improved. However, 16 days after the start of hMG she suddenly developed respiratory arrest and she died of respiratory failure. On autopsy, 500 ml ascites and 550 ml (right) and 320 ml (left) pleural effusion was found. There was massive pulmonary edema and intra-alveolar hemorrhage, without any evidence of pulmonary thromboembolism.

Four other unpublished cases are mentioned on the Internet on a commercial website called LifeSite, describing itself as 'a web portal dedicated to issues of culture, life, and family.' It has Catholic inspiration. At http://www.lifesite.net/ldn/2005/apr/05041408.html, the four cases are mentioned to the lay public. A professional report on these cases could not be tracked.

They include one woman who died in 1996 in the USA and whose death was reported by the Centers for Disease Control (CDC). She died from intracranial hemorrhage supposedly due to IVF-induced OHSS. Another woman seems to have died in 1995 in New Zealand as the result of an OHSS-triggered cerebral embolism. Another 32-year-old Irish woman died in 2004 as the result of adult respiratory distress syndrome arising as a complication of OHSS. Most recently, a 33-year-old UK woman collapsed at a bus-stop, and was disconnected from life support 5 days later after reportedly suffering a massive heart attack. Although it is difficult to see how this could have been typical OHSS, the woman's death seems nevertheless related to thrombophilic complications elicited by hormonal treatment.

For the sake of completeness, it should be mentioned that in an Australian survey of mortality in a cohort of IVF patients, Venn *et al.* concluded that there were no more deaths than among women not treated with IVF[8]. In particular, no death in the cohort studied could be linked to OHSS.

WHAT CAN WE LEARN FROM THESE CASE REPORTS?

Dutch cases and the literature

All three Dutch women were hyperstimulated in an IVF setting, and they all had an early (3–7 days after hCG) onset of OHSS, with rapid aggravation of symptoms. Two of the three patients in our report suffered from PCOS, as well as the Japanese woman from the literature. This is also probably true for the very early cases published in the 1950s. In both PCOS women there was a discrepancy between the number of follicles and the amount of oocytes. This may indicate that the real number of small (and intermediate) follicles was higher than measured, and/or that not all follicles had been aspirated. It is known that especially the number of intermediate (10–14 mm in diameter) follicles is important for the prediction of OHSS[9]. Monitoring of estradiol is lacking in our first two cases. Although monitoring with ultrasound is sufficient in most IVF patients, it may be helpful to predict OHSS in the case of high-risk women. Young (< 35 years), lean women and women with polycystic ovaries, as well as women who have had previous OHSS, are prone to develop OHSS. At the Capri European Society of Human Reproduction and Embryology (ESHRE) consensus meeting it was concluded that individuals at high risk for developing the syndrome have estradiol levels > 12.8 nmol/l (4000 pg/ml) and/or > 35 follicles at the time of induced ovulation[10]. The woman in case 3 did not have PCOS. Furthermore, she was 40 years old. However, the level of estradiol in case 3 had strongly increased from cycle day 12 to cycle day 14.

Based on the existing literature on severe OHSS, primary measures should involve knowledge of risk factors in the individual patient, before treatment starts. In those PCOS patients who are difficult to stimulate with gonadotropins, other treatment modalities such as laparoscopic electrocautery of the ovaries[11] or metformin as a (co)treatment should be considered, before converting to IVF. If there is an indication for IVF, the unpredictive nature of the ovarian response in PCOS patients must warrant an individually tailored, slow step-up (or even step-down) protocol of gonadotropin stimulation. Monitoring of estradiol production on a routine basis is debatable, but may be advantageous as an early warning sign. As there is no advantage of a higher dose of hCG for final follicular maturation, a standard dose of 5000 IU should be administered. In the case of threatening OHSS, discontinuation of the cycle should be considered by not providing hCG. Embryo transfer can be postponed in cases at risk, by freezing all embryos. A 7/7 days and 24/24 h availability of the clinic does not guarantee a good outcome, but will prevent further delay in diagnosing patients at risk.

Further to the recognition of risk factors associated with the OHSS, an awareness of the change in hyperstimulated patients into a hypercoagulable state[12,13], most probably due to the hyperestrogenic condition, should always be present. Extreme vigilance for signs and symptoms of developing thromboembolism (venous or arterial) may change the course of events, when dealt with timely and properly. Patient number 3 acted confused; in retrospect, this phenomenon could have served as an early warning sign, which could have led to more diagnostic measures. A quest for familial thromboembolism in the patient's history and for thrombophilia factors, when indicated, can lead to prophylactic measures.

Severe OHSS, if managed well, is 'a self-limiting' disease. However, the course of events in the presented cases detiorated rapidly and resulted in (multiple) organ failure, most probably due to the hypercoagulable state. Until the underlying pathophysiology in OHSS and thromboembolism is found and leads eventually to possibilities to identify women at risk, extreme suspicion of possible complications is mandatory in patients who undergo assisted reproductive treatments.

The reported cases have been discussed extensively by the Dutch Society of Obstetrics and Gynecology (NVOG). Although there is yet no reliable national complication register, it is agreed by all IVF specialists that all serious complications are to be reported to the IVF working party of the NVOG. Since 1998 there has been a national guideline, 'OHSS'[12].

Today, we are more aware of the risks of ovarian hyperstimulation, especially in women with PCOS. To our best knowledge, since 1997, no lethal cases of OHSS have occurred in The Netherlands.

Belgian cases

If anything can be learned, it is that other doctors apart from those working in an IVF unit should be aware of the existence and the potential severity of OHSS. It is the conviction of the authors of this chapter that in severe cases, it is mandatory to refer the patient to the center where the patient was primarily treated for her infertility, or at least to a hospital where such a center and the expertise with OHSS exist. Perhaps it can also be underlined that ascitic fluid should not be evacuated too quickly. Patients usually experience a marked subjective relief even after the removal of a small quantity of fluid, and there is no need for quickly losing large volumes.

Recently, a guideline on OHSS was issued by the Reproductive Working Group of Flanders. It can be surmised that, in most countries, such guidelines exist and can often be found on the Internet. The short form of the planned OHSS guideline of the ESHRE is given in the Appendix to this chapter.

THE IMPORTANCE OF REGISTRIES

It is understandable but remains to be deplored that lethal cases of OHSS are almost never reported. It is impossible that the 11 cases which have been (summarily) identified should be the only ones that have occurred in recent decades. If three cases occur over a 10-year period in The Netherlands, i.e. over an estimated 100 000 cycles, the incidence can be estimated at 0.003%. Given an annual number of IVF/ICSI cycles worldwide of ~500 000, i.e. over a period of 10 years a total number of cycles of ~5 000 000, this would mean ~150 lethal cases in the world over the past 10 years. This is only a very rough estimate, because the number of annual cycles has been rising steadily. This would come to one case in 33 333 cycles. Brinsden *et al.*[14] estimate the incidence to be 1/500 000. In reality, the true incidence could be significantly higher.

The only way to obtain a better idea of the true incidence is to strive towards prospective registration of all fertility treatments (ovulation induction, IUI, IVF/ICSI), as well as of their most important complications. This chapter aspires no more than to create the awareness that, in the long term, such registries are unavoidable. It is unacceptable that young women should die while being treated for a problem that, in one case out of two, is not theirs.

For the issue of multiple pregnancy, centers worldwide have come a long way in registering the incidence of this most frequent complication. Expressing the efficacy of a center by an indicator called CUSIDERA (cumulative singleton delivery rate) and its safety by another indicator called CUTWIDERA (cumulative twin delivery rate) could be one way of reporting multiples, as suggested by Germond *et al.*[15].

In contrast, few countries ask their centers to report the incidence of OHSS, and if they do, lethal cases are not reported. Such reports could help in understanding the direct mechanisms of death as well as help in suggesting measures to prevent the death of these patients.

Moreover, before such a register of complications could have any usefulness (apart from creating unwanted reactions from an incompletely informed public), there must be unity of definition of OHSS, when it is mild, moderate and serious, and a guarantee of anonymity to avoid under-reporting. National and supranational registries, such as the American Society for Reproductive Medicine (ASRM), the European IVF Monitoring (EIM) program and the World Registry on assisted reproductive technologies (ART) should ask their accredited members to report all cases of severe OHSS and all cases of maternal mortality, whatever the cause of death.

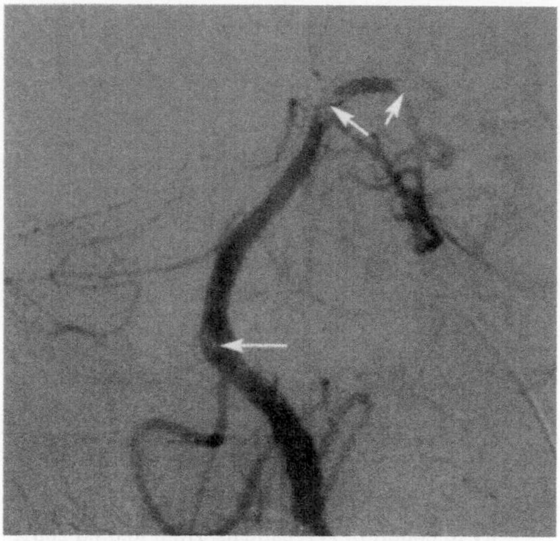

Figure 1 Thrombi (arrowheads) in right arteria basilaris of patient who died of thromboembolic complications of OHSS. Courtesy of Dr R Bernardus, The Netherlands

ACKNOWLEDGMENTS

The authors thank Dr A Th Alberda, Sint Franciscus Gasthuis, Rotterdam; Dr D A Gietelink, Amphia Ziekenhuis, Breda, The Netherlands; and Dr M Camus, Center for Reproductive Medicine of the VUB, Brussels, for their contribution to the manuscript.

REFERENCES

1. Delvigne A. Request for information on unreported cases of severe ovarian hyperstimulation syndrome (OHSS) [Letter]. Hum Reprod 2005; 20: 2033.
2. Esteban-Altirriba J. Le syndrome d'hyperstimulation massive des ovaries. Rev Fr Gynecol Obstet 1961; 56: 555.
3. Figueroa-Casas P. Reaccion ovarica monstruosa a las gonadotrofinas a proposito de un caso fatal. Ann Cirug 1958; 23: 116.

4. Moses M, Bogowsky H, Anteby E, et al. Thromboembolic phenomena after ovarian stimulation with menopausal gonadotrophins. Lancet 1965; 2: 1213.

5. Serour GI, Aboulgar M, Mansour R, et al. Complications of medically assisted conception in 3,500 cycles. Fertil Steril 1998; 70: 638–42.

6. Cluroe AD, Synek BJ. A fatal case of ovarian hyperstimulation syndrome with cerebral infarction. Pathology 1995; 27: 344–6.

7. Semba S, Moriya T, Youssef EM, et al. An autopsy case of ovarian hyperstimulation syndrome with massive pulmonary edema and pleural effusion. Pathol Int 2000; 50: 549–52.

8. Venn A, Hemminski E, Watson L, et al. Mortality in cohort of IVF patients. Hum Reprod 2001; 16: 2691–6.

9. Beerendonk CC, Van Dop PA, Braat DD, et al. Ovarium hyperstimulation syndrome: facts and fallacies. Obstet Gynecol Surv 1998; 53: 439–49.

10. ESHRE Capri Workshop. Infertility revisited: the state of the art today and tomorrow. Hum Reprod 1996; 11: 1779–806.

11. Bayram N, van Wely M, Kaaijk EM, et al. Using an electrocautery strategy or recombinant follicle stimulating hormone to induce ovulation in polycystic ovary syndrome: randomised controlled trial. Br Med J 2004; 328: 192–7.

12. Het ovarieel hyperstimulatiesyndroom. Utrecht: NVOG, richtlijn no. 11, 1998. www.nvog/nl.

13. Stewart JA, Hamilton PJ, Murdoch AP. Thromboembolic disease associated with ovarian stimulation and assisted conception technique. Hum Reprod 1997; 10: 2167–73.

14. Brinsden PR, Wada I, Tan SL, et al. Diagnosis, prevention and management of ovarian hyperstimulation syndrome. Br J Obstet Gynaecol 1995; 102: 767–72.

15. Germond M, Urner F, Chanson A, et al. What is the most relevant standard of success in assisted reproduction? The cumulated singleton/twin delivery rates per oocyte pick-up: the CUSIDERA and CUTWIDERA. Hum Reprod 2004; 19: 2442–4.

APPENDIX

OVARIAN HYPERSTIMULATION SYNDROME

Short management guidelines

F Olivennes, J Gerris, A Delvigne and K Nygren

Primary risk factors before treatment

- Polycystic ovarian syndrome;
- Incomplete forms of PCOS:
  - High number of resting follicles: ≥ 10 follicles of 4–10 mm in each ovary;
  - Luteinizing hormone/follicle stimulating hormone (LH/FSH) ratio > 2;
  - Hyperandrogenism;
- Previous history of OHSS;
- Young age*;

- Low body weight*;
- Allergies*.

*Scientific evidence to confirm these factors is weak.

Criteria for defining a patient as being at risk of OHSS during stimulation for IVF

- Serum estradiol value > 3000/4000 pg/ml:
  - No clear cut-off value;
  - Poor predictive value (8–73%);
  - Not a mediator as OHSS possible with low estradiol;
  - The slope of the estradiol rise is the main risk factor and of more importance than the maximum estradiol value;
- Follicle numbers > 20–25 in both ovaries:
  - No clear cut-off value (10–35);
  - Variation due to operator and technique;
- Other predictors not used as routine:
  - Vascular endothelial growth factor (VEGF) > 200 pg/ml.

Clinical diagnosis and staging

Most common symptoms and signs.

Clinical symptoms

- Lower abdominal discomfort;
- Progressive increase in umbilical circumference;
- Nausea, vomiting;
- Dyspnea;
- Diarrhea;
- Respiratory distress;
- Rapid weight gain;
- Oliguria, anuria.

Para-clinical signs

- Enlarged ovaries;
- Ascites;
- Pleural effusion (right > left);
- Thromboembolism (especially from upper-body veins);
- Pericardiac effusion.

Biological findings

- Electrolyte imbalance;
- Hypovolemia;
- Hemoconcentration (increased hematocrit);
- Leukocytose (related to hemoconcentration);
- Low creatinine clearance;
- Low blood pressure;
- High liver enzymes;
- Hypercoagulability;
- Hypoalbuminemia.

Forms and classification

Early forms:

3–7 days after hCG;

Related to the intensity of ovarian response;

More severe form.

Late forms:

12–17 days after hCG;

Related to fetal hCG secretion;

Milder but more prolonged.

Clinical classification:

Mild OHSS
Abdominal distension and discomfort (grade 1);
Grade 1 plus nausea, vomiting and/or diarrhea, ovaries 5–12 cm.
Moderate OHSS
Grade 2 and ultrasonic evidence of ascites (grade 3).
Severe OHSS
Moderate OHSS plus clinical evidence of ascites and/or hydrothorax or dyspnea (grade 4);
All above plus hemoconcentration, coagulation abnormalities, diminished renal perfusion (grade 5).

Management

Criteria for hospitalization:
Hemoconcentration > 45%;
Any sign of severe OHSS.

Out-patient management:

Fluid chart;
Weight gain;
Follow-up of abdominal circumference;
Instruction to consult at any sign of complication;
Out-patient follow-up every 48 h with blood tests and sonographic examination.

Management in hospital:

Pulse;
Blood pressure;
Fluid balance charts;
Sonographic examination: ascites volume, ovarian size;
Thorax X-ray (if dyspnea);
ECG (to exclude pericardiac effusion);
Red and white blood cell count, electrolytes, renal function tests, liver function tests (mainly albumin and total protein), coagulation tests.

Treatment

Maintain diuresis.

Fluid management

Intravenous administration of Ringer's lactate solution;
First 24 h: 1500–3000 ml;
Subsequent days: amount of fluid amount depending on fluid balance;
Combination of Ringer's lactate + dextrose 5% solution or sodium chloride 0.9% (saline) + dextrose 5% (standard) solution.

Plasma expanders

HES: hydroxyethyl starch 6% solution in isotonic sodium chloride solution;
Maximum daily dose: 33 ml/kg in 250–500 ml per day, dropwise, slow administration to avoid lung congestion.

Albumin administration

Should be kept for a later stage, once hypoalbuminemia is proven, because of risk of hepatitis, excessive albumin overload, renal function impairment and potential vial contamination. Administration is mainly important during drainage of ascites.
Daily dose: 25–75 g (100–300 ml) per day according to the severity of hypoalbuminemia and the total volume of ascitic fluid drained.

Anticoagulants

Should be given only when clinical evidence exists for:

Thromboembolic phenomena;

Thrombophilia;

Hypercoagulability or thromboembolic history;

Uncorrected hemoconcentration after 48 h of the usual intravenous treatment.

Low-dose aspirin

For prevention of thromboembolic complication;
Patients who are immobilized because of obesity (not recommended if ascites drainage).

Ascites drainage

Abdominally or vaginally;
Proposed if patient discomfort is important, or systematically, or when biological anomalies are not corrected by the usual intravenous treatment (persistent hemoconcentration and/or renal failure).
Gradual manner: 4 l within 12 h;
Ultrasound guidance recommended.

CHAPTER 7

Modern classification of the ovarian hyperstimulation syndrome

Zalman Levine and Daniel Navot

INTRODUCTION

Ovarian hyperstimulation syndrome (OHSS) is the gravest complication of so-called controlled (far too often uncontrolled) ovarian hyperstimulation (COH)[1]. From a perspective of priorities in reproductive medicine in general, and assisted reproductive technologies in particular, OHSS is second only to high-order multiple birth on the list of adverse outcomes which need to be minimized or completely eliminated.

NEED FOR CLASSIFICATION

Like many other diseases, OHSS exists in a clinical spectrum. Some patients, at one end of the spectrum, exhibit only mild signs and symptoms of the disease; others, at the other extreme, require intensive management and may even be at risk for death from the disease[2–6]. Diseases that can manifest in a range of severity need classification systems for two reasons. First, if clinicians are to evaluate and treat patients with the disease, parameters must exist which can be applied to each patient to assess the extent of disease and to plan an appropriate management strategy. Just as congestive heart failure is classified based on the level of functional ability to help clinicians determine whether the patient can be managed medically or should be placed on a heart-transplant list, so must OHSS be classified to help clinicians determine whether the patient should be managed supportively or intensively, medically or surgically, at home or in hospital.

Second, if clinical researchers are to study disease epidemiology and investigate various strategies for treatment and prevention, a uniform classification scheme will ensure consistency by allowing researchers to speak in a common language about the disease and by enabling clinicians to apply the results of these studies to individual patients. Just as the revised American Fertility Society classification system for endometriosis enables standardized research into the disease and ensures the relevance of clinical trials for clinical practice, so must OHSS be classified to ensure uniform definitions in clinical research and to maximize application of the research to everyday clinical care.

CLASSIFICATION SCHEMES BY DISEASE SEVERITY

Over the past 25 years, several classification systems have been suggested to categorize OHSS better and disseminate uniform guidelines for prevention and treatment. Most of these classification systems are based on the severity of the disease, which is in turn based on a combination of the severity of the patient's symptoms as well as severity of the physical, laboratory and radiological signs of the disease (Table 1). Five major schemes have been suggested to classify OHSS.

Rabau (1967)

Although pregnant mare serum gonadotropin was used clinically as early as the 1930s to induce ovulation, the results of these early trials were disappointing. Gonadotropin treatments began to enter the clinical armamentarium in 1958, when a combination of follicle stimulating hormone derived from cadaveric human pituitary glands and human chorionic gonadotropin (hCG) successfully induced ovulation and pregnancy[7]. With the use of these agents, and with the later introduction of clomiphene citrate[8] and human menopausal gonadotropins[9], experience with the spectrum of ovarian hyperstimulation syndrome unfortunately grew.

The original classification, suggested by Rabau *et al.* in 1967[10], categorizes the syndrome into six grades by levels of increasing severity. Grade 1 disease is defined by the presence of supraphysiological levels of estradiol and pregnanediol, as measured by 24-h urinary excretion greater than 150 μg and 10 μg, respectively.

Table 1 Classification of OHSS

Mild	*Moderate*	*Severe*	*Critical*
Bloating	Vomiting	Massive ascites	Tense ascites
Nausea	Abdominal pain	Hydrothorax	Hypoxemia
Abdominal distension	US evidence of ascites	Hct > 45%	Pericardial effusion
Ovaries ≤ 5 cm	Hct > 41%	WBC > 15 000/mm^3	Hct > 55%
	WBC > 10 000/mm^3	Oliguria	WBC > 25 000/mm^3
	Ovaries > 5 cm	Creatinine 1–1.5 mg/dl	Oliguria or anuria
		Creatinine clearance ≥ 50 ml/min	Creatinine > 1.5 mg/dl
		Hepatic dysfunction	Creatinine clearance < 50 ml/min
		Anasarca	Renal failure
		Ovaries variably enlarged	Thromboembolic phenomena
			ARDS
			Ovaries variably enlarged

US, ultrasound; Hct, hematocrit; WBC, white blood cell count; ARDS, adult respiratory distress syndrome

Grade 2 adds to these laboratory measurements the presence of enlarged ovaries and, questionably, palpable cysts. Interestingly, Rabau did not define grades 1 and 2 as OHSS at all, and felt that these grades were expected by-products of ovarian stimulation and required no attention or treatment.

In the Rabau classification system, grade 3 disease adds the presence of abdominal distension and definitively palpable ovarian cysts, and grade 4 includes vomiting and possibly diarrhea. To Rabau, patients with grades 3 and 4 OHSS are at possible risk for future worsening and complications, and require observation but no intervention. Grades 5 and 6, in this system, require hospitalization with aggressive observation and intervention. Grade 5 is defined by fluid shifts and third spacing leading to ascites and hydrothorax, and grade 6 is defined by hematological changes in blood volume, blood viscosity and coagulation time.

Schenker (1978)

Schenker and Weinstein[11] modified the Rabau classification system to group the grades into a less cumbersome mild/moderate/severe terminology, but maintained the grading system as well. In the Schenker scheme, grades 1 and 2 are termed mild OHSS, and include the same definitions: urinary excretion of estradiol and pregnanediol for grade 1, and enlarged ovaries with small cysts for grade 2. Grades 3 and 4 are termed moderate OHSS, and include abdominal distension for grade 3, and nausea, vomiting and/or diarrhea for grade 4. Grades 5 and 6 are defined as severe disease, including large ovarian cysts and ascites and/or hydrothorax for grade 5, and hemoconcentration, increased blood viscosity and coagulation changes for grade 6.

Golan (1989)

While the Rabau and Schenker classification systems seemed at the time to be comprehensive, they suffer from several drawbacks. First, they focus more on ovarian response, particularly in the lower grades of the disease, than on the clinical syndrome. Second, they are difficult to incorporate into the clinical setting, as 24-h urinary hormones are not routinely measured. Third, they incorporate unnecessarily cumbersome subdivisions; simple classification as mild, moderate and severe OHSS would be adequately descriptive and more clinically useful. Finally, these schemes were developed through observation of women undergoing ovulation induction. More recently, with the evolution of assisted reproductive technologies (ART) and routine use of controlled ovarian hyperstimulation (COH) in ART patients, the laboratory and clinical findings in the lower grades of the Rabau and Schenker classifications are routinely observed and may reflect not a syndrome but an acknowledgment that COH has indeed been achieved. Therefore, there was a need for a simpler, more clinically useful and more relevant system.

Golan *et al.* in 1989[12] attempted such a revision of these older systems by classifying OHSS into mild, moderate and severe, eliminating hormone measurements from the system, and including in the mild category clinical symptoms previously classified as moderate disease prior to the days of routine COH for ART. Golan maintains a grading scheme, defining grades 1 and 2 as mild OHSS, grade 3 as moderate OHSS and grades 4 and 5 as severe OHSS. In the mild category, grade 1 includes abdominal discomfort and distension, and grade 2 adds enlarged ovaries to 5–12 cm and nausea, vomiting and/or diarrhea. For moderate OHSS, Golan introduces the use of ultrasound, defining ultrasound evidence of ascites as grade 3, even if the degree of ascites is not detectable clinically. Severe OHSS features respiratory symptoms such as dyspnea and tachypnea and clinical evidence of ascites and/or hydrothorax as grade 4, and hemoconcentration, oliguria, increased blood viscosity, coagulation abnormalities, hypotension and renal hypoperfusion as grade 5. Perhaps one of the most important innovations of the Golan system is the introduction of ultrasound as a tool in classifying OHSS, encouraging the use of this technology, already in widespread use in the monitoring of ovarian response, for the evaluation and monitoring of OHSS as well. The moderate form of OHSS includes significant ovarian enlargement (5–12 cm), and accompanying symptoms such as abdominal pain, significant bloating, nausea and diarrhea.

Navot (1992)

The major deficiency of the Golan classification scheme is the absence of a distinction between forms of the disease that are severe but not life-threatening, and forms that are critical and potentially fatal. If one of the major purposes of the classification scheme is to aid the clinician in appropriately managing the patient with OHSS, such a distinction would be of great clinical import. Additionally, clinicians routinely assess the severity and course of OHSS with laboratory measurements of hematological parameters, electrolytes and renal function, yet the classification system does not address these widely used measurements in a quantitative way.

To correct these deficiencies, Navot *et al.*[13] subdivided the 'severe' category into 'severe OHSS' and 'critical OHSS'. According to the Navot scheme, patients with severe OHSS have variably enlarged ovaries, massive ascites with or without hydrothorax, a hematocrit greater than 45%, a leukocyte count greater than 15 000, clinically measured oliguria, serum creatinine 1.0–1.5, creatinine clearance at least 50 ml/min, laboratory evidence of hepatic dysfunction and anasarca. Patients with critical, life-threatening OHSS have a critically contracted blood volume and multiorgan failure. They exhibit more extreme forms of the same parameters, including a hematocrit greater than 55%, a leukocyte count greater than 25 000, serum creatinine at least 1.6, creatinine clearance 50 ml/min or less, prerenal azotemia, thromboembolic phenomena and adult respiratory distress syndrome (ARDS).

Of note, unlike the earlier schema, the Navot system minimizes the significance of ovarian enlargement. In the past, ovulation induction was the primary cause of OHSS, and ovarian size may have been an important parameter in assessing the disease. However, now that much OHSS results from COH for ART, follicular aspiration and iatrogenic follicular trauma during oocyte retrieval may minimize ovarian size even in the face of severe OHSS. With COH, anasarca can frequently coexist with relatively minor ovarian enlargement. Therefore, the Navot scheme downplays ovarian enlargement, relying more on the general clinical picture and on common laboratory parameters.

Rizk (1999)

In an attempt to subdivide further Golan's severe category, Rizk and Aboulghar[14] defined three grades of severe OHSS. Grade A severe OHSS features dyspnea, oliguria, nausea, vomiting, diarrhea, abdominal pain, clinical or ultrasound evidence of ascites, hydrothorax and enlarged ovaries on ultrasound. Patients with grade A disease have a normal biochemical profile. Grade B severe OHSS adds massive ascites, markedly enlarged ovaries, severe dyspnea, severe oliguria, increased hematocrit, hepatic dysfunction and elevated serum creatinine. Grade C OHSS, which features complications that Rizk feels can also occur in the setting of moderate disease, resembles Navot's 'critical' category, with end-organ complications such as renal failure, venous thrombosis and ARDS.

Over the past decade, this Navot modification of the prior classification systems has become the most widely used scheme in clinical practice and in research settings. It is comprehensive and logical, and we advocate it to be universally adopted for clinical evaluation as well as for academic investigation.

CLASSIFICATION BY DISEASE ONSET: EARLY AND LATE OHSS

Since 1994, investigators[15–17] have recognized that what is commonly called OHSS actually includes two distinct disease entities: OHSS that occurs 3–7 days after hCG triggering, and OHSS that occurs more than 10 days after hCG triggering. As a disease, OHSS seems to include these two distinct forms based on the timing of its onset, and can consequently be classified into early OHSS and late OHSS. Both forms of OHSS share a common pathophysiology; in both, hCG triggers granulosa cells to produce vasoactive substances which induce the capillary permeability that yields the clinical sequelae of OHSS. What distinguishes the early and late forms of the disease is the source of the hCG. In early OHSS, the exogenously injected hCG drives the granulosa directly to secrete sufficient vasoactive substances to produce the syndrome within 3–7 days, while in late OHSS, early pregnancy is responsible for the granulosa cell activity, as the implanting trophoblast produces increasing levels of endogenous hCG.

Clinically, these two entities ought to be distinguished, because they are distinct. Early OHSS, but not late OHSS, is dependent on ovarian stimulation; higher peak estradiol levels and greater gonadotropin doses are correlated with an increased incidence of early OHSS, but not of late OHSS. Therefore, criteria related to ovarian response can be used to predict early OHSS, but not late OHSS. Early OHSS can occur in any stimulated cycle, while late OHSS occurs only in the setting of a pregnancy. Late OHSS is more likely to be severe; in fact, late OHSS may account for almost 70% of all cases of severe OHSS. Late OHSS can occur with either a singleton or multiple pregnancy. While some authors have suggested that multiple pregnancy has a stronger association with late OHSS than singleton pregnancy by virtue of higher trophoblastic hCG production, a recent report found an equal association of singleton and multiple pregnancies with late OHSS[18].

Of interest, OHSS has recently been reported in several women with spontaneous pregnancies[19–21], and the cause of this OHSS seems to be a familial mutation in the follicle stimulating hormone (FSH) receptor, increasing its sensitivity to trophoblastic hCG. The mutation allows for constitutive stimulation of the FSH receptor by hCG, triggering the ovarian cascade responsible for OHSS. This form of OHSS clearly illustrates the distinction between early and late OHSS; these women did not have stimulated ovaries and did not have hCG triggering, yet developed OHSS due to endogenous production of hCG by the developing pregnancy. This spontaneous late OHSS in at least one report was severe, requiring hospitalization and intensive management. Whether FSH receptor mutations, or polymorphisms, play a role in the onset or severity of iatrogenic OHSS will require further research (see also Chapter 13).

SUMMARY

OHSS can be classified in various ways based on its severity and based on the timing of its onset. Any and all of these systems can be of both clinical and academic utility, helping to establish uniform standards for clinical research into the epidemiology, prevention and management of OHSS and for the clinical care of a patient with OHSS.

REFERENCES

1. Abramov Y, Elchalal U, Schenker JG. An epidemic of severe OHSS; a price we have to pay? Hum Reprod 1999; 14: 2181–3.

2. Moses M, Bogowsky H, Anteby E, et al. Thromboembolic phenomena after ovarian stimulation with menopausal gonadotrophins. Lancet 1965; 2: 1213.

3. Esteban-Altirriba J. Le syndrome d'hyperstimulation massive des ovaries. Rev Fr Gynecol Obstet 1961; 56: 555.

4. Figueroa-Casas P. Reaccion ovarica monstruosa a las gonadotrofinas a proposito de un caso fatal. Ann Cir 1958; 23: 116.

5. Cluroe AD, Synek BJ. A fatal case of ovarian hyperstimulation syndrome with cerebral infarction. Pathology 1995; 27: 344–6.

6. Semba S, Moriya T, Youssef EM, et al. An autopsy case of ovarian hyperstimulation syndrome with massive pulmonary edema and pleural effusion. Pathol Int 2000; 50: 549–52.

7. Gemzel CA, Diczfalusy E, Tillinger G. Clinical effect of human pituitary follicle-stimulating hormone. J Clin Endocrinol Metab 1958; 18: 1333.

8. Greenblatt RB, Barfield WE. Induction of ovulation with MRL/41. JAMA 1961; 178: 101.

9. Lunenfeld B. Treatment of anovulation by human gonadotropins. J Int Fed Gynecol Obstet 1963; 1: 153.

10. Rabau E, David A, Serr DM, et al. Human menopausal gonadotrophin for anovulation and sterility. Am J Obstet Gynecol 1967; 98: 92–8.

11. Schenker JG, Weinstein D. Ovarian hyperstimulation syndrome: a current survey. Fertil Steril 1978; 30: 255–68.

12. Golan A, Ron-El R, Herman A, et al. Ovarian hyperstimulation syndrome: an update review. Obstet Gynecol Surv 1989; 44: 430–40.

13. Navot D, Bergh PA, Laufer N. Ovarian hyperstimulation syndrome in novel reproductive technologies: prevention and treatment. Fertil Steril 1992; 58: 249–61.

14. Rizk B, Aboulghar MA. Classification, pathophysiology, and management of ovarian hyperstimulation syndrome. In Brinsden P, ed. A Textbook of In Vitro Fertilization and Assisted Reproduction. Carnforth, UK: Parthenon Publishing, 1999: 131–55.

15. Dahl Lyons CA, Wheeler CA, Frishman GN, et al. Early and late presentation of the ovarian hyperstimulation syndrome: two distinct entities with different risk factors. Hum Reprod 1994; 9: 792–9.

16. Mathur RS, Akande VA, Keay SD, et al. Distinction between early and late ovarian hyperstimulation syndrome. Fertil Steril 2000; 73: 901–7.

17. Papanikolaou EG, Tournaye H, Verpoest W, et al. Early and late ovarian hyperstimulation syndrome: early pregnancy outcome and profile. Hum Reprod 2005; 20: 636–41.

18. De Neubourg D, Mangelschots K, Van Royen E, et al. Singleton pregnancies are as affected by ovarian hyperstimulation syndrome as twin pregnancies. Fertil Steril 2004; 82: 1691–3.

19. Smits G, Olatunbosun O, Delbaere A, et al. Ovarian hyperstimulation syndrome due to a mutation in the follicle-stimulating hormone receptor. N Engl J Med 2003; 349: 760–6.

20. Vasseur C, Rodien P, Beau I, et al. A chorionic gonadotropin-sensitive mutation in the follicle-stimulating hormone receptor as a cause of familial gestational spontaneous ovarian hyperstimulation syndrome. N Engl J Med 2003; 349: 753–9.

21. Montanelli L, Delbaere A, Di Carlo C, et al. A mutation in the follicle-stimulating hormone receptor as a cause of familial spontaneous ovarian hyperstimulation syndrome. J Clin Endocrinol Metab 2004; 89: 1255–8.

CHAPTER 8

Ovarian hyperstimulation syndrome in singleton and twin pregnancies

Diane De Neubourg and Jan Gerris

INTRODUCTION

The most important adverse effect of *in vitro* fertilization/intracytoplasmic sperm injection (IVF/ICSI) is the occurrence of multiple pregnancies. Due to the scale of this problem and the seriousness of the obstetric and neonatal complications, multiple pregnancies remain the number-one complication of assisted reproductive technologies (ART). Although ovarian hyperstimulation syndrome (OHSS) is less frequent, it is a potentially life-threatening condition for a young woman undergoing ART.

Ovarian hyperstimulation syndrome is an iatrogenic complication of the use of gonadotropins. The pathophysiology of the disease is poorly understood, but the condition and disease are related to estrogens, vascular endothelial growth factor (VEGF) and the luteal phase induced by luteinizing hormone (LH) or human chorionic gonadotropin (hCG). The syndrome is caused by a change in vascular permeability by factors such as VEGF. This leads to a shift of fluid from the intravascular compartment to the third space, causing ascites and pleural effusion. The consequences of this shift are hypovolemia, hypoproteinemia and hemoconcentration leading to hypercoagulability, increased liver enzymes, elevated leukocytes, disturbance of electrolytes and renal failure.

It is well known that the development of ovarian hyperstimulation syndrome is related to the presence of hCG. The administration of hCG for ovulation induction in IVF/ICSI procedures can trigger 'early-onset' OHSS, whereas hCG from a developing pregnancy causes 'late-onset' OHSS. This was first described by Lyons *et al.*[1]. These authors also suggested that in the case of late-onset OHSS, the risk of developing OHSS and the severity of the syndrome were related to the occurrence of multiple pregnancy[1]. The profile and early pregnancy outcome of early and late OHSS have most recently been described by Papanikolaou *et al.*[2]. They describe a higher risk of preclinical miscarriage in the early OHSS pattern, and a close association of late OHSS with conception cycles, especially multiple pregnancies, when compared with non-OHSS cycles. However, it should be stressed that a median of two embryos were transferred in all analyzed subgroups.

The question of whether the transfer of only one embryo in a larger number of cycles might decrease the incidence of OHSS cases, through avoiding a number of twins, has never been investigated. Some authors have supposed that this would be the case, but data to show this to be effectively true are lacking. We actually investigated whether the introduction of single embryo transfer (SET) with its subsequent decline in twin pregnancies would result in a lower incidence of OHSS. It is helpful to realize that the population at risk for OHSS we are thus considering remains the same, i.e. the young woman with a good or even exaggerated ovarian response who previously received double embryo transfer and conceived with a high chance of twin pregnancy and who is now advised to have single embryo transfer.

DOES SINGLE EMBRYO TRANSFER RESULT IN LESS OHSS THAN DOUBLE EMBRYO TRANSFER?

Clinical research data with respect to the occurrence of OHSS in singleton and twin pregnancies in a program introducing elective SET

We analyzed the incidence of OHSS over a 7-year period (January 1998 until December 2004), during which we gradually introduced SET into our IVF/ICSI program. The percentage of single embryo transfer increased from 13% in 1998 to 63% in 2004; coincidentally, the mean number of embryos per transfer declined from 2.26 to 1.41. The overall pregnancy rate remained stable at a mean of 31.3%, while the multiple pregnancy rate declined from 33.6 to 9.2% (11.9% when monozygous pregnancies are included)[3,4].

Patients were treated with the long gonadotropin-releasing hormone (GnRH) agonist desensitization protocol, starting in the mid-luteal phase, with 6 × 100 μg of buserelin (Suprefact®; Aventis, Frankfurt, Germany) given intranasally for a period of 3 weeks. Ovarian stimulation was initiated using 150 IU of Metrodin HP® (Serono, Geneva, Switzerland), Menopur® (Ferring, Copenhagen, Denmark), Gonal-F® (Serono) or Puregon® (Organon, Oss, The Netherlands) given subcutaneously, except in patients with known poor response, where the starting dose was augmented to 225 IU. The criterion for hCG administration was the presence of at least three mature follicles with a diameter of 18 mm. Ten thousand IU of hCG (Profasi®, Serono, or Pregnyl®, Organon) were given intramuscularly exactly 37 h prior to oocyte pick-up. The IVF/ICSI procedure, embryo quality assessment and embryo transfer technique were performed as previously described[5].

In brief, oocyte pick-up was performed vaginally under ultrasound guidance. Approximately 16–19 h after insemination/injection, normal fertilization was checked. On day 2, every embryo was scored for the total number of cells, the presence of anuclear fragments and multinucleated blastomeres. On day 3, embryo quality was again evaluated. Selection for embryo replacement was made according to embryo characteristics as elaborated previously by our team[6]. All transfers were performed on an out-patient basis using a Wallace embryo transfer catheter (Sims Portex Ltd, Hythe, Kent, UK), consisting of an inner catheter and an outer catheter.

In all cycles, the luteal phase was supported by vaginally administered micronized natural progesterone (200 mg three times a day, Utrogestan®; Besins, Belgium). When pregnant, the patient continued the treatment until the first ultrasound scan. hCG was never administered in the luteal phase. When a patient was identified as being at risk for OHSS, in general two types of preventive measures were taken. When the serum estradiol level was ≥ 4000 pg/ml on the day of hCG administration, a reduced amount of 5000 IU hCG was administered rather than the usual 10 000 IU. On the other hand, coasting was performed when serum estradiol levels were rapidly increasing and reaching a level of ≥ 5000 pg/ml before a sufficient number of dominant follicles (≥ 18 mm) were present. Gonadotropin injections were withdrawn until serum estradiol levels dropped to ≤3000 pg/ml and follicles with a diameter ≥18 mm were present[7,8].

We used the criteria of Golan *et al.* to classify OHSS[9]. According to these criteria, patients with moderate to severe OHSS requiring bedrest or admission to hospital were marked in our database.

Student's *t* test was used to evaluate statistical differences between continuous variables. A p value ≤ 0.05 was considered significant. Confidence interval analysis was performed to compare the incidence of OHSS in singleton versus twin conception cycles.

Evolution of pregnancy rate, multiple pregnancy rate and incidence of OHSS

Over this 7-year period, 44 cases of OHSS occurred in 2882 cycles (1.52%). The incidence of ovarian hyperstimulation syndrome was fairly stable over this period, varying between 0.5 and 2.4% with an average of 1.52% per cycle. The effect of the evolution of implementation of SET on the ongoing pregnancy rate, the multiple pregnancy rate and the incidence of OHSS is shown in Figure 1. Of the 44 cases of OHSS, eight cases occurred in a non-conception cycle during the first week after oocyte retrieval. Thirty-six cases of OHSS occurred in 906 conception cycles (4.0%). There were 30 cases in 727 singleton conception cycles (4.1%) and six cases in 157 twin pregnancy cycles (3.8%) (odds ratio 1.08, 95% confidence interval 0.44–2.64).

Analysis of cycle-related variables

We analyzed cycle-related variables in non-conception cycles (early OHSS) and conception cycles (late OHSS). In the latter group a comparison was made between singleton and twin pregnancies. A total of 48 cases were analyzed (four cases from 2005 were also included).

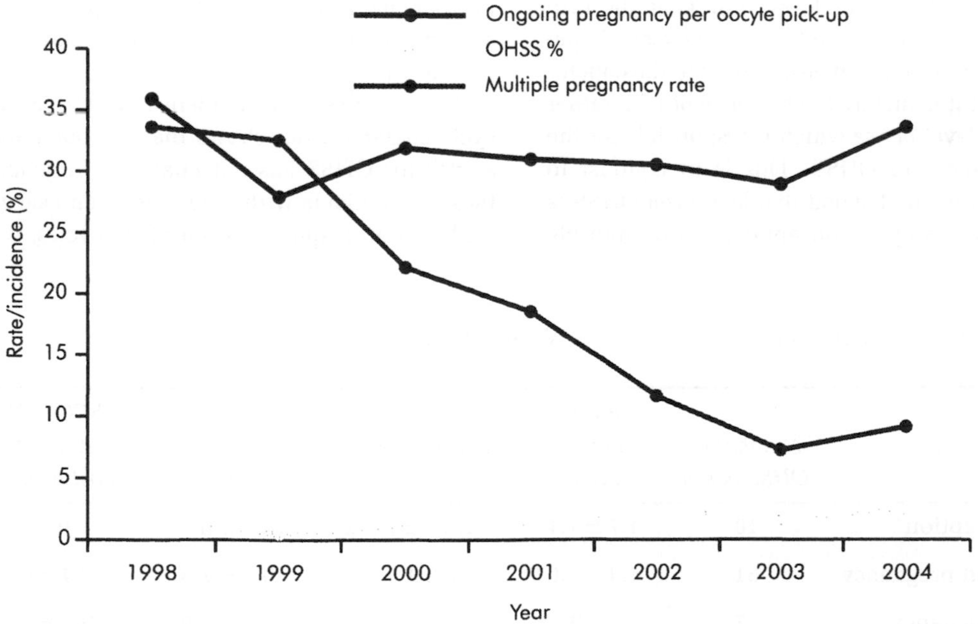

Figure 1 Evolution of pregnancy rate, multiple pregnancy rate and incidence of OHSS

These data showed no significant difference between the number of oocytes retrieved and the level of serum estradiol at the day of hCG administration (Table 1). However, the rank of the cycle in which OHSS occurred in twin pregnancies was significantly higher (cycle 3) than in singleton pregnancies (cycle 1.45) ($p = 0.001$). Also, the level of hCG on day 12 after day-3 embryo transfer was significantly higher in conception cycles leading to a twin pregnancy (247 ± 51 IU/l) compared with cycles resulting in a singleton pregnancy (154 ± 68 IU/l) ($p = 0.002$).

DISCUSSION

Over the 7-year period during which we registered the occurrence of OHSS, we did not detect any change in its incidence. The overall incidence of OHSS is 1.5% per cycle with egg retrieval and 4% in conception cycles. We did not find a significant difference in the incidence of OHSS between singleton and twin pregnancies. However, a significant difference could be detected in the serum levels of hCG on the 12th day after day-3 embryo transfer between singleton and twin pregnancies, leading to the conclusion that it is merely the presence of hCG rather than its level *per se* which is responsible for the development of OHSS. This is in contrast to publications that stated that late-onset OHSS is related not only to conceptions but to multiple pregnancies[1,2]. Therefore, one cannot conclude that prevention of multiple pregnancies is an adequate measure to prevent OHSS, as suggested by Orvieto[10], nor that single embryo transfer can, at present, be considered a prevention of OHSS. Cases of OHSS are, perhaps unfortunately, as frequent in pregnancies resulting from single embryo transfer as from two-embryo transfer.

There are no differences in cycle characteristics for number of oocytes and serum estradiol levels between conception and non-conception cycles, either between singleton and twin pregnancies.

However, the rank of the cycle in which OHSS occurred was higher for twin than for singleton pregnancies, reflecting the change in embryo transfer policy where double embryo transfer with a risk for twin pregnancies occurs in cycles with a higher rank. This observation stands in line with the transfer policy in Belgium, where a large proportion of first and second IVF/ICSI cycles are single embryo transfer cycles, resulting in a predictable 'shift' of twin pregnancies from first cycles a couple of years ago towards third and higher-rank cycles at the present time.

This analysis of incidence of OHSS and cycle characteristics shows that the population at risk for OHSS has not changed. In general, these are patients with a good to even exaggerated ovarian response in their first cycles, with

Table 1 Characteristics of cycles with OHSS. Values are expressed as mean ± SD

	Number of OHSS cases	*Rank of the cycle*	*Level of serum estradiol* (pg/ml)	*Number of oocytes*	*hCG* (IU/l) *at day 12 post-transfer*
No conception	10	1.7 ± 1.1	4771 ± 2432	18.0 ± 6.7	0
Singleton pregnancy	31	1.4 ± 0.9**	3592 ± 1769	15.3 ± 7.3	154 ± 68*
Twin pregnancy	7	3 ± 1.7**	3519 ± 1790	14.1 ± 6.6	247 ± 51*

*$p = 0.002$, **$p = 0.001$, singleton vs. twin pregnancy; hCG, human chorionic gonadotropin

a high chance of conception. These patients are offered single embryo transfer and, as previously shown by our group, the chance of conception is not affected through this embryo transfer policy[3,4]. Therefore, it could be anticipated that the incidence of OHSS will not be affected if the occurrence of OHSS is not related to the development of multiple pregnancy.

As it is clear that the late form of OHSS is induced by the presence of hCG originating from the early pregnancy, it appears that merely the presence of hCG rather than its level is responsible for the occurrence of late OHSS[11]. Therefore, to reduce the incidence of OHSS, measures other than those mentioned here should be considered. Embryo transfer can be postponed until the blastocyst stage, to evaluate the symptoms in a patient with early presentation of OHSS[12]. Another possibility is to proceed with hCG administration and oocyte retrieval but to cancel the embryo transfer and freeze all the embryos[13]. The success of this policy largely depends on the results of the cryopreservation program of the center.[14] Recently, the introduction of GnRH antagonists seems to offer a good perspective for prevention of OHSS[15]. An important advantage of the use of GnRH antagonists is the possibility of using GnRH agonists for ovulation induction in the prevention of OHSS[16].

This inevitably brings us to the consideration of 'friendly IVF', providing that lower numbers of oocytes and embryos do not decrease the chance to present an embryo with a high implantation potential, thus maintaining the high pregnancy rates for SET. Some of the investigated protocols appear to be very promising[17,18].

REFERENCES

1. Lyons CA, Wheeler CA, Frishman GN, et al. Early and late presentation of ovarian hyperstimulation syndrome. Hum Reprod 1994; 9: 792–9.
2. Papanikolaou E, Tournaye H, Verpoest W, et al. Early and late ovarian hyperstimulation syndrome: early pregnancy outcome and profile. Hum Reprod 2005; 20: 636–41.
3. De Neubourg D, Gerris J. SET – state of the ART. Reprod BioMed Online 2003; 7: 615–22.
4. Gerris J, De Neubourg D, Mangelschots K, et al. Elective single day-3 embryo transfer halves the twinning rate without decrease in the ongoing pregnancy rate of an IVF/ICSI programme. Hum Reprod 2002; 17: 2621–6.
5. De Neubourg D, Mangelschots K, Van Royen E, et al. Impact of patients' choice for single embryo transfer of a top quality embryo versus double embryo transfer in the first IVF/ICSI cycle. Hum Reprod 2002; 17: 1621–5.
6. Van Royen E, Mangelschots K, De Neubourg D, et al. Characterization of a top quality embryo, a step towards single-embryo transfer. Hum Reprod 1999; 14: 2345–9.
7. Urman, B, Pride SM, Ho Yuen B. Management of overstimulated gonadotrophin cycles with a controlled drift period. Hum Reprod 1992; 7: 213–17.
8. Waldenstrom U, Kahn J, Marsk L, et al. High pregnancy rates and successful prevention of severe ovarian hyperstimulation syndrome by 'prolonged coasting' of very hyperstimulated patients: a multicentre study. Hum Reprod 1999; 14: 294–7.
9. Golan A, Ron-El R, Herman A, et al. Ovarian hyperstimulation syndrome: an update review. Obstet Gynecol Surv 1989; 44: 430–40.
10. Orvieto R. Can we eliminate severe ovarian hyperstimulation syndrome? Hum Reprod 2005; 20: 320–2.
11. De Neubourg D, Mangelschots K, Van Royen E, et al. Singleton pregnancies are equally affected by ovarian hyperstimulation syndrome as twin pregnancies. Fertil Steril 2004; 82: 1691–3.
12. Trout SW, Bohrer MK, Seifer DB. Single blastocyst transfer in woman at risk of ovarian hyperstimulation syndrome. Fertil Steril 2001; 76: 1066–7.

13. Wada I, Matson PL, Troup SA, et al. Does elective cryo-preservation of all embryos of women at risk of ovarian hyperstimulation syndrome reduce the incidence of the condition? Br J Obstet Gynaecol 1993; 10: 265–9.

14. Queenan JT Jr, Veek LL, Toner JP, et al. Cryopreservation of all prezygotes in patients at risk of severe hyperstimulation syndrome does not eliminate the syndrome, but chances of pregnancy are excellent with subsequent frozen–thaw transfers. Hum Reprod 1997; 12: 573–6.

15. Olivennes F. GnRH antagonists: do they open new pathways to safer treatment in assisted reproductive techniques? Reprod Biomed Online 2002; 5: 20–5.

16. Itskovic J, Kol S, Mannaerts B. Use of a single bolus of GnRH agonist triptorelin to trigger ovulation after GnRH antagonist ganirelix treatment in women undergoing ovarian stimulation for assisted reproduction, with special reference to the prevention of ovarian hyperstimulation syndrome: preliminary report. Hum Reprod 2000; 15: 1965–8.

17. Olivennes F. Patient-friendly ovarian stimulation. Reprod Biomed Online 2003; 7: 30–4.

18. Hohmann FP, Macklon NS, Fauser BC. A randomized comparison of two ovarian stimulation protocols with gonadotropin-releasing hormone (GnRH) antagonist cotreatment for in vitro fertilization commencing recombinant follicle-stimulating hormone on cycle day 2 or 5 with the standard long GnRH agonist protocol. J Clin Endocrinol Metab 2003; 88: 166–73.

CHAPTER 9

Pathophysiology of the ovarian hyperstimulation syndrome

Annick Delvigne

INTRODUCTION

The ovarian hyperstimulation syndrome (OHSS) is characterized by an increase in size of the ovaries, with the appearance of multiple cysts, and by an increase in the vascular permeability of ovarian vessels causing ascites, pleural effusion and sometimes pericardiac effusion. The severe form is also accompanied by electrolyte disturbances, as well as by cardiopulmonary, hepatic, renal and hemodynamic disturbances, leading to an increased thromboembolic risk. The dominant finding is bilateral multicystic enlargement of the ovaries. Morphological examination of these ovaries reveals multiple corpora lutea, follicle cysts and massive edema of the ovarian stroma. It has been suggested that formation of the cysts is a direct reaction to stimulation with gonadotropins, since similar ovarian observations exist in other conditions associated with high levels of endogenous gonadotropins such as hydatidiform mole, choriocarcinoma and multiple pregnancy.

Animal experiments have shown that the main pathological feature of OHSS is an increase in capillary permeability, as demonstrated in a rabbit experimental model using intravenous dyes[1]. Furthermore, angiogenesis is also enhanced in OHSS. It has been demonstrated in animals that the amount of fluid shifting from the intravascular space into the abdominal cavity depends on the presence of the ovaries. The latter, however, do not have to be in the peritoneal cavity[2]. Neither estrogen nor a progestin in excessive amounts caused ascites in female rabbits[1]. Moreover, OHSS cannot be induced in male animals or in men treated with large doses of gonadotropins.

Consequently, the following principles can be considered as established: first, the presence of an ovary is a compulsory condition for OHSS; second, a vasoactive mediator secreted by the ovaries plays a major role in the development of OHSS, after ovarian stimulation. This factor is probably secreted into the peritoneal cavity and liberated in the systemic circulation where it can exert its action.

Some investigators have hypothesized that ascites in women with OHSS contains this chemical ovarian product responsible for OHSS. This hypothesis has been confirmed by *in vitro* permeability experiments, using follicular fluid and ascites of patients suffering from OHSS[3].

Subsequently, much research has been directed toward identifying this mediator either in the blood or in the ascites of patients with

OHSS, and these studies are presented in this review[4].

POTENTIAL BIOCHEMICAL MEDIATORS

Estrogens, prolactin and prostaglandins

Estrogen is a marker of ovarian response but is not the causative agent of OHSS, since the administration of estradiol does not induce OHSS. Some authors have suggested other causal candidates such as prolactin and prostaglandins, but no evidence of a directly causative role of these substances has been demonstrated so far[4].

Activation of the ovarian prorenin–renin–angiotensin system

There is a proven contribution of the prorenin–renin–angiotensin system (RAS) to the process of OHSS. It has been established that some factors of the RAS are secreted by the ovary, and that the RAS process can be influenced by some well-known risk factors associated with OHSS such as human chorionic gonadotropin (hCG). The systemic activation of the RAS during hemodynamic perturbations related to OHSS has also been documented. What remains to be established is whether an imbalance in the RAS is a 'primum movens' in the pathogenesis of OHSS or whether it is a catalyst of the hemodynamic degradation that occurs in OHSS. Alternatively, the activation of RAS may be a homeostatic response to hypovolemia during OHSS.

Cytokines

Studies of cytokines produce contradictory results, even in apparently similar populations, affected by OHSS for different reasons.

These low-molecular-weight proteins are active in extremely low concentrations, and can exert their influence in an autocrine, paracrine or endocrine fashion. Cytokine activity is influenced by the functional status of cytokine receptors, and the presence of cytokine inhibitors, soluble receptors and binding proteins. Nevertheless, most data converge to show that positive modulators of the early phase of inflammation (interleukins (IL) IL-1, IL-2, IL-6, IL-8, IL-18, tumor necrosis factor (TNF) and vascular endothelial growth factor (VEGF) are increased during the early stage of OHSS, and that immunosuppressive and anti-inflammatory cytokines (IL-10) tend to be lower in OHSS patients before treatment. One may hypothesize that patients with OHSS suffer from an intrinsic deficiency in their immune response, and that this differentiates them from those at high risk for OHSS who do not develop the condition.

Allergy cytokines and histamine

Because the pathophysiological changes during OHSS resemble an excessive inflammatory response, the possibility of hyperreactivity of ovarian mast cells in patients suffering from OHSS has been suggested. With regard to allergy, histamine and histamine blockade have been studied: histamine blocking has been shown to prevent the occurrence of OHSS in the rabbit model. However, OHSS in these rabbits did not involve antigen–antibody complexes, suggesting that antihistamine blocking of OHSS could take place directly at the ovarian level. Another rabbit study showed no difference in either histamine levels or ovarian mast-cell contents between OHSS and controls. Conflicting results were obtained for the inhibition of ascitic fluid formation and ovarian enlargement using H-1 receptor blockers[4].

Vascular endothelial growth factor

Vascular permeability and the subsequent development of ascitic fluid are thought to be induced by follicular fluid. The ovarian production of VEGF is demonstrated by the fact that, in most studies, higher concentrations are found in the follicular fluid than in the serum. Most, but not all, observations report an increase in plasma or serum VEGF concentrations in OHSS patients at the time of ovulation. In addition, hCG administration enhances the mRNA expression of VEGF by luteinized granulosa cells in a dose-dependent manner, explaining why the use of hCG in *in vitro* fertilization (IVF) protocols is often a critical step in the development of OHSS. The increased expression of VEGF mRNA has been described in women with polycystic ovarian syndrome (PCOS) who are at high risk of developing OHSS.

Nevertheless, many questions about the ovarian production and action of VEGF remain unanswered, and certain observations are contradictory. These conflicting results can be at least partially attributed to the method of VEGF assessment:

(1) VEGF can be measured in plasma or in serum, but the clotting process increases VEGF levels in serum 8–10-fold, and degranulation or hemoconcentration occurring in OHSS may entail misinterpretation of true levels of free active VEGF;

(2) OHSS ovarian-derived VEGF could be trapped in ascitic fluid or large cystic corpora lutea;

(3) Immunoassays cannot differentiate the four isoforms of VEGF;

(4) The biologically active isoform of VEGF in the circulation has not been determined;

(5) The relationship between soluble VEGF receptors and VEGF in the follicular fluid may influence the biological activity of VEGF, and different biological affinities of VEGF for receptors may exist[4].

The studied populations are heterogeneous, and the control group may influence the results; in particular, whether OHSS and control patients are matched for number of follicles is of paramount importance.

VEGF is thus certainly a mediator of the OHSS cascade, but it remains unknown whether disruption of the normal controlled follicular expression of VEGF constitutes a 'primum movens' of OHSS.

Miscellaneous substances that may play a role in OHSS[4]

Angiogenin has been found at significantly higher levels in the blood and ascitic fluid of OHSS patients, suggesting that angiogenin may be associated with neovascularization in OHSS.

The *kinin–kallikrein* system has been studied in the rat model. The results suggest that the kinin–kallikrein system plays an intermediate role in capillary permeability during OHSS.

Soluble vascular cell adhesion molecule-1 (sVCAM-1) and *soluble intercellular adhesion molecule-1 (sICAM-1)*, which belong to the immunoglobulin superfamily, are major mediators of white blood cell adhesion, interaction and extravasation during inflammatory and immune reactions. A case–control study of peritoneal fluid and plasma levels of sVCAM-1 and sICAM-1 suggested that soluble cell adhesion molecules may play a role in the pathogenesis and evolution of OHSS[5].

The serum and ascites concentrations of sICAM-1 and of *soluble E-selectin*, another endothelial cell adhesion molecule, were followed in a controlled study[6]. Higher levels of sICAM-1 and lower levels of E-selectin were observed in serum and ascitic fluid. More studies are needed to understand the kinetics and the cause–effect relationship between OHSS and these adhesion molecules. However, they seem to be implicated in the pathophysiological process leading to capillary hyperpermeability in severe OHSS.

The von Willebrand factor (vWF) is considered to be a marker of endothelial cell activation, and excessive endothelial cell VEGF production enhances vWF concentrations. The increased vWF on the day of embryo transfer has been shown to be related to the severity of OHSS, and an elevation of vWF precedes the clinical manifestations in severe OHSS[7]. This increase has not been observed in follicular fluid, suggesting that vWF is not produced by the ovary. vWF may be of endothelial origin and influenced by vasoactive ovarian factors. Higher plasma levels of vWF in OHSS patients compared with high responders on the day preceding oocyte retrieval lasted until after embryo transfer and were maintained well into the late luteal phase[8]. In high responders without OHSS, the levels of vWF also increased during the pre-ovulatory phase, but decreased from the day of oocyte retrieval onward. Subsiding levels of vWF in patients with severe OHSS indicate improvement of the disease. This test might become clinically useful as an additional 'discriminating parameter' or 'prognostic marker'. It is likely that vWF plays a role in the cascade that leads to OHSS, but rather as a consequence of the activation of endothelial cells by a factor of ovarian origin than as its causal factor.

Endothelin-1, another vasoconstrictor that increases capillary permeability, was found to be 100–300-fold higher in follicular fluid than in plasma. In OHSS patients, serum endothelin-1 level is elevated but in parallel with other neurohormonal vasoactive factors, and without correlation with the OHSS grading, suggesting a homeostatic response rather than an initiating role in OHSS[9].

Contribution of neurohormonal and hemodynamic changes to arteriolar vasodilatation

Balasch *et al.* evaluated systemic, endogenous vasoactive neurohormonal factors in severe OHSS during the appearance of the syndrome for a period of 4–5 weeks[9]. The authors recorded increased hematocrit, decreased mean arterial pressure, increased cardiac output and reduced peripheral vascular resistance. This was accompanied by marked increases in plasma renin, norepinephrine, antidiuretic hormone (ADH) and atrial natriuretic peptide levels. The authors compared previous results in women with and without hemoconcentration: similar values were observed except for renin, norepinephrine and ADH, which were found to be higher in OHSS patients. These observations suggest that OHSS is associated with arteriolar vasodilatation. Indeed, if circulatory dysfunction were to be due solely to an extravascular shift, contraction of the circulating blood volume should induce a reduction in cardiac output, an increase in peripheral vascular resistance and a decrease in atrial natriuretic peptide. In contrast, cardiac output and atrial natriuretic peptide are increased and peripheral vascular resistance is markedly reduced, indicating a marked peripheral arteriolar vasodilatation. The simultaneous occurrence of these disorders leads to hyperdynamic circulatory dysfunction, with marked stimulation of the sympathetic nervous system, renin–angiotensin system and ADH.

Evbuomwan *et al.* observed an alteration of osmoregulation during OHSS, with an osmotic threshold for arginine vasopressin secretion that is reset to lower plasma osmolality during superovulation[10]. This new, lower, body tonicity is maintained in OHSS patients until at least 10 days after the administration of hCG. These authors suggest that a decrease in plasma osmolality and plasma sodium levels is due to altered osmoregulation rather than to electrolyte losses.

CONCLUSION (Figure 1)

The main hypothesis concerning the development of OHSS is that regulation of the inflammation-like ovulation process is disturbed. This leads to overproduction of local proinflammatory factors in the ovary. In turn, this results in secondarily increased capillary leakage and transmission of inflammatory mediators to other

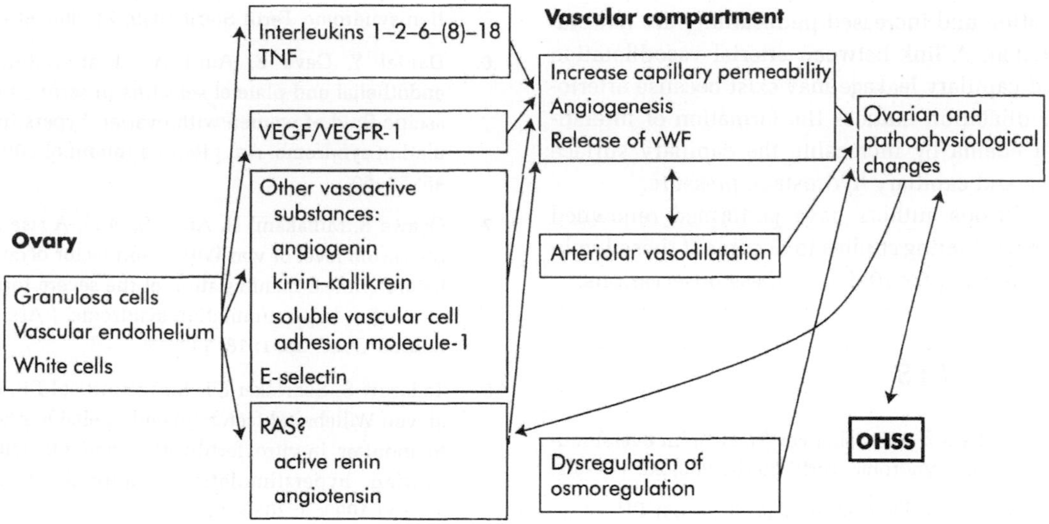

Figure 1 Pathophysiology of OHSS. TNF, tumor necrosis factor; VEGF, vascular endothelial growth factor; VEGFR-1, VEGF receptor-1; RAS, prorenin–renin–angiotensin system; vWF, von Willebrand factor

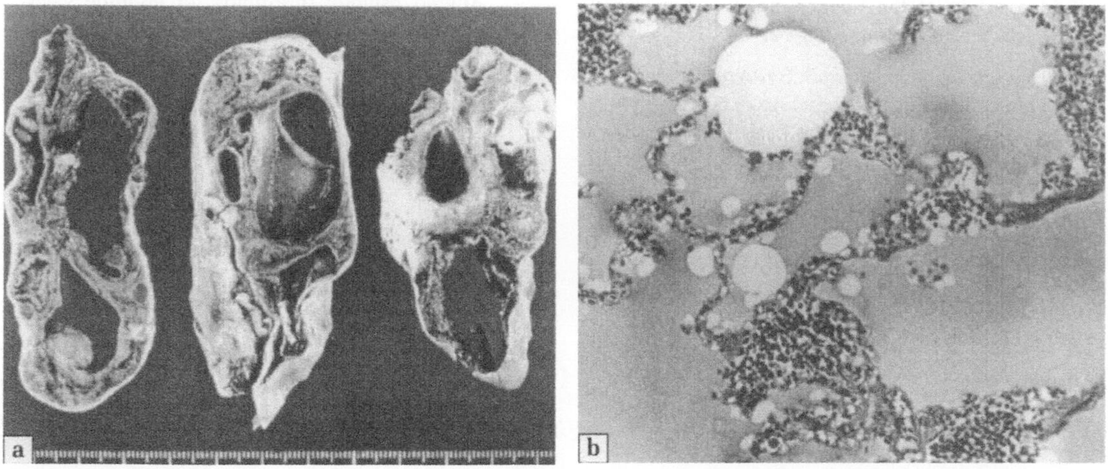

Figure 2 (a) Images of cut surface of ovary of OHSS patient and (b) edema of the alveoli of the lungs of same patient. Reproduced from reference 11, with permission

compartments. In the most severe form of OHSS, this process also leads to systemic manifestations.

In addition to the shift of fluid to extravascular spaces, OHSS is consistently associated with marked arteriolar vasodilatation.

The site and mechanism of arterial vasodilatation and increased permeability are not elucidated. A link between arterial vasodilatation and capillary leakage may exist because arteriolar dilatation induces the formation of interstitial edema by increasing the capillary surface area and capillary hydrostatic pressure.

Various authors have performed renowned and fascinating studies to document these hypotheses; Chapter 10 details these observations.

REFERENCES

1. Polishuk WZ, Schenker JG. Ovarian overstimulation syndrome. Fertil Steril 1969; 20: 443–50.
2. Yarali H, Fleige-Zahradka BG, Yuen BH, et al. The ascites in the ovarian hyperstimulation syndrome does not originate from the ovary. Fertil Steril 1993; 59: 657–61.
3. Goldsman MP, Pedram A, Dominguez CE, et al. Increased capillary permeability induced by human follicular fluid: a hypothesis for an ovarian origin of the hyperstimulation syndrome. Fertil Steril 1995; 63: 268–72.
4. Delvigne A, Rozenberg S. Systematic review of data concerning etiopathology of ovarian hyperstimulation syndrome. Int J Fertil Womens Med 2002; 47: 211.
5. Daniel Y, Geva E, Amit A, et al. Levels of soluble vascular cell adhesion molecule-1 and soluble intercellular adhesion molecule-1 are increased in women with ovarian hyperstimulation syndrome. Fertil Steril 1999; 71: 896–901.
6. Daniel Y, Geva E, Amit A, et al. Soluble endothelial and platelet selectins in serum and ascitic fluid of women with ovarian hyperstimulation syndrome. Am J Reprod Immunol 2001; 45: 54–60.
7. Ogawa S, Minakami H, Araki S, et al. A rise of the serum level of von Willebrand factor occurs before clinical manifestation of the severe form of ovarian hyperstimulation syndrome. J Assist Reprod Genet 2001; 18: 114–19.
8. Todorow S, Schricker ST, Siebzehnruebl ER, et al. von Willebrand factor: an endothelial marker to monitor in-vitro fertilization patients with ovarian hyperstimulation syndrome. Hum Reprod 1993; 8: 2039–46.
9. Balasch J, Arroyo V, Fabregues F, et al. Neurohormonal and hemodynamic changes in severe cases of the ovarian hyperstimulation syndrome. Ann Intern Med 1994; 121: 27–33.
10. Evbuomwan IO, Davison JM, Baylis PM, et al. Altered osmotic thresholds for arginine vasopressin secretion and thirst during superovulation and in the ovarian hyperstimulation syndrome (OHSS): relevance to the pathophysiology of OHSS. Fertil Steril 2001; 75: 933–41.
11. Semba S, Moriya T, Youssef EM, Sasano H. An autopsy case of ovarian hyperstimulation syndrome with massive pulmonary edema and pleural effusion. Pathol Int 2000; 50: 549–52.

CHAPTER 10

Role of vascular endothelial growth factor in the pathophysiology of ovarian hyperstimulation syndrome

Joseph Neulen

CLINICAL SITUATION

The main symptom of ovarian hyperstimulation syndrome (OHSS) is third-space fluid sequestration due to generalized capillary leakage[1]. The loss of serum causes hemoconcentration and kidney failure from hypovolemic shock[2]. Symptoms of OHSS are aggravated by an increase in von Willebrand factor, resulting in thrombosis in atypical parts of the body or in embolism of the lung or brain[3,4]. Human chorionic gonadotropin (hCG) exacerbates all symptoms[5]. This severe condition after controlled ovarian stimulation (COS) results from substances which are obviously produced by the ovaries[6]. Bilateral ovariectomy will immediately resolve this critical situation[7].

CHARACTERISTICS OF VASCULAR ENDOTHELIAL GROWTH FACTOR

In 1979, Dvorak *et al.* described a factor from hepatocarcinoma cell lines which increased vascular permeability[8]. This factor was designated as vascular permeability factor (VPF)[9]. Ferrara and Henzel isolated from follicular stellate cells of the pituitary gland a highly specific endothelial cell mitogen which they named vascular endothelial growth factor (VEGF)[10]. Eventually, it became apparent that VPF and VEGF were different names for the same protein[11]. VEGF is now the mainly accepted label for this growth factor. Recently, specific forms of VEGF from different gene loci have been found. The original VEGF is therefore also dubbed VEGF-A.

VEGF comprises a family of proteins of about 45 000 Da which originate from a single gene located on chromosome 6p21.3[12]. The human VEGF gene is organized into eight exons, separated by seven introns. From this gene a variety of five different proteins are processed by alternative splicing. These proteins are labeled $VEGF_{121}$, $VEGF_{145}$, $VEGF_{165}$, $VEGF_{189}$ and $VEGF_{206}$, according to their respective numbers of amino acids. $VEGF_{121}$ and $VEGF_{165}$ are the most prominent forms. $VEGF_{121}$ is freely secreted. It lacks residues from exons 6 and 7, and is strongly acidic in the way it reacts. $VEGF_{165}$ is partially secreted, reacts basically and possesses a heparin binding site. It lacks the residue from exon 6[13]. $VEGF_{145}$ is predominantly produced in the endometrium. It contains residues from exons 1–6 and 8[14]. The larger

VEGF forms, 189 and 206, react highly basically and remain cell-associated within the extracellular matrix[15].

The expression of VEGF is strongly induced by hypoxia[16,17]. Furthermore, VEGF expression can be up-regulated by a series of cytokines including other growth factors, e.g. epidermal growth factor (EGF) or keratinocyte growth factor (KGF)[18]. Even heterozygous VEGF gene-deficient mice do not survive the 12th day *in utero*, indicating that there is no substitute for the angiogenic effects of VEGF[19].

Two VEGF receptor tyrosine kinases have been identified. Both represent transmembranous phosphokinase receptors with seven antibody-like loops as extracellular domains. Fms-like tyrosine receptor (flt-1) is associated with VEGF receptor-1 (VEGFR-1). Kinase domain-inserted receptor (KDR) corresponds to VEGF receptor-2 (VEGFR-2). Both receptors are confined to endothelial cells[20]. VEGFR-1 exhibits a dissociation constant (K_D) for $VEGF_{165}$ of 20 pmol/l[21], and VEGFR-2 a K_D for $VEGF_{165}$ of 100 pmol/l[22]. Mice embryos knocked out for one of the two receptor types die *in utero* between days 8.5 and 9.5[23,24]. Signal transduction through the VEGFR-2 leads to mitogenic activity in endothelial cells and enhances vascular permeability within minutes[25,26]. In adults, no such immediate effects can be observed after the activation of VEGFR-1[27]. VEGFR-1 regulates endothelial cell morphology and tissue factor production in endothelial cells, as well as monocyte attraction by these cells. Fibroblast growth factor (FGF) expression[28] or asphyxia[29] causes an increased expression of both receptor types[30].

A third specific receptor is confined to lymphatic endothelial cells. It is designated as flt-4 or VEGFR-3[31]. This receptor can also be stimulated with VEGF. However, the specific ligand seems to be VEGF-C[32].

THE VEGF SUPERFAMILY

VEGF belongs to the superfamily of platelet derived growth factor (PDGF) together with further growth factors which all have some common genetic symmetry[33].

Placental growth factor (PlGF) is produced in villous trophoblast cells, and occurs in two forms arising from alternative splicing[34]. The gene is localized on chromosome 14q24[35]. Its biological function is unknown. PlGF knock-out mice develop normally[36]. It exhibits only a specific binding affinity to VEGFR-1 and cannot activate any other VEGF receptors.

In the attempt to determine the gene for MEN-1, VEGF-B was found[37], and localized to chromosome 11q13[38]. Again, it occurs in two isoforms arising from alternative splicing. VEGF-B has a high affinity to VEGFR-1, but lacks any affinity for VEGFR-2 or -3.

As a specific ligand for VEGFR-3, VEGF-C is described. It possesses only about 30% homology with $VEGF_{165}$. The K_D for VEGFR-3 is 135 pmol/l, whereas the affinity to VEGFR-2 occurs at about 410 pmol/l[39]. Its gene is found on chromosome 4q34[38]. It promotes the growth of lymphatic endothelial cells. By activation of VEGFR-2 it can also induce vascular permeability in blood vessels as well as in lymphatic vessels[40].

Closely related to VEGF-C is VEGF-D. Due to its structural similarity it also binds and activates VEGFR-3[41].

THE VEGF/VEGFR COMPLEX

Usually, VEGFs occur as dimers. Dimerization can happen between different forms of VEGF. Therefore, the receptor specificity may vary in *in vivo* experiments. To obtain a maximum biological response, i.e. proliferation of endothelial cells, receptors also develop into dimers, with optimal results from the dimerization of VEGFR-1 and VEGFR-2. However, VEGF tends to leave the receptor fairly rapidly. To obtain optimal activation, the VEGF/VEGFR complex has to be stabilized by neuropilins on the cell surface[42]. Neuropilins themselves do not show any specific intracellular effects after binding the VEGF/VEGFR complex.

IMPORTANCE OF VEGF ACTIVITIES

The physiological task of VEGF is the induction of endothelial cell proliferation. This occurs normally during wound-healing processes[43]. In the adult organism, there are only two organs where angiogenesis can be observed regularly: in the cyclic endometrium and in the ovary during follicular development and corpus luteum formation[44]. VEGF enables fenestration of the endothelial barrier in small venules and capillaries[45]. In some organs, VEGF is obviously needed for specific endothelial maintenance, e.g. lung or kidney[46].

In some pathological conditions, VEGF expression is elevated. This can be observed in retinopathy[47] or rheumatic arthritis[48]. The most dramatic growth induction of endothelial cells can be observed in malignant tumors. Here, VEGF expression is usually extremely high[43]. Therefore, many attempts are made to block angiogenesis in tumors.

VEGF EFFECTS *IN VIVO* ASSOCIATED WITH OHSS

VEGF can induce all the processes which are typical of clinical symptoms of OHSS. A major effect is the fenestration of vessels, increasing vascular permeability[49]. von Willebrand factor production in endothelial cells can be increased by VEGF[50]. Therefore, the idea that VEGF may elicit OHSS is challenging.

The hypothesis could be strengthened if the source of VEGF in the ovaries is determined. Analyzing the clinical course of OHSS, it becomes clear that a risk exists only after ovulation and during corpus luteum formation[51]. Before ovulation, patients may complain of discomfort due to enlarged cystic ovaries, but there is no generalized capillary leakage producing ascites or pleural effusion.

VEGF EFFECTS *IN VITRO*

In 1993, luteinized granulosa cells became the most interesting suspects. It could be demonstrated that VEGF mRNA was expressed in this cell population *in vitro*[52]. Granulosa cells expressed $VEGF_{121}$ and $VEGF_{165}$[53]. Moreover, hCG could be confirmed to induce the mRNA expression rate dose-dependently. The hCG-dependent secretion of VEGF from granulosa cells *in vitro* could also be validated[54]. Recent data indicate that progesterone is able to support hCG-dependent VEGF production[55]. Granulosa cells of patients with polycystic ovarian syndrome exhibit a greater capacity to express and secrete VEGF, explaining the higher risk for these individuals to develop OHSS after COS[56].

VEGF CONCENTRATIONS IN URINE, ASCITES, SERUM AND FOLLICULAR FLUID

In vivo data showed that ascites from OHSS patients contained large amounts of VEGF[57]. The urinary excretion of VEGF was higher in patients suffering from OHSS than in healthy women undergoing COS[58]. Quantification of VEGF in follicular fluid suggested higher concentrations in patients at risk for OHSS[59]. Also, serum contents of VEGF were elevated[60].

Unfortunately, this simple hypothesis did not endure for long. It became feasible that after COS, with comparable results in ovarian performance, granulosa cells from these individual patients exhibited a wide range of VEGF expression. There was no straight correlation between symptoms of OHSS and the intensity of VEGF expression[53]. VEGF quantification in blood serum was compromised by thrombocyte contributions which could not be exactly calculated[61]. Improved systems to measure VEGF produced conflicting results regarding VEGF concentrations in follicular fluid and serum[62,63].

VEGF RECEPTORS

Finally, other substances were identified which interfere with the biological effects of VEGF. The VEGF–VEGFR system exemplifies a paracrine organization in the ovary[64]. VEGF produced by the growing follicle or in the corpus luteum activates endothelial cell growth in the vicinity of the maturing follicle. A dense capillary network provides sufficient nutrient supply for the oocyte. Endocrine signals from the follicle or corpus luteum are transported into the circulation. However, VEGFR-1 poses a very important capacity.

SOLUBLE VEGF RECEPTOR-1

Endothelial cells can produce a soluble, freely secreted form of VEGFR-1 by alternative splicing of the common VEGFR-1 mRNA[65]. This soluble receptor (sVEGFR-1) acts as a natural VEGF antagonist[66–69]. The situation is comparable to that of growth hormone and its receptor.

sVEGFR-1 AS VEGF ANTAGONIST

It was demonstrated that sVEGFR-1 can effectively inhibit corpus luteum formation in primates[70]. Soluble VEGFR-1 was detected in follicular fluid. Results demonstrated that high amounts of sVEGFR-1 in follicular fluid corresponded to a poor responder, whereas low sVEGFR-1 concentrations coincided with high ovarian response and elevated risk for OHSS[53]. Only the concentration of free VEGF was linked to clinical OHSS[71]. In rats, the use of luteinizing hormone (LH) instead of hCG for ovulation induction could prevent vascular permeability by reducing VEGF production[72]. Similar results could be obtained by GnRH-agonist ovulation induction[73], accounting for lower biologically active VEGF concentrations. Coasting during COS also reduced the amount of total and free VEGF in the peripheral blood[74,75].

REGULATION OF sVEGFR-1 SECRETION

Substances which regulate the production of sVEGFR-1 are unknown. From *in vitro* experiments it became clear that follicular fluid or granulosa cell-conditioned media could reduce the production of sVEGFR-1 in human umbilical venous endothelial cells (HUVEC). Messenger RNA expression of VEGFR-1 or sVEGFR-1 remained unchanged, indicating that this effect is related to post-transcriptional processes. This observation suggested that granulosa cells enhance VEGF effects by down-regulating sVEGFR-1 production in endothelial cells. The paracrine signal by which granulosa cells can influence sVEGFR-1 production remains to be identified[76].

CONCLUSIONS

VEGF remains the main suspect in the pathophysiology of OHSS. However, it is obvious that other substances produced by endothelial cells and granulosa cells affect the clinical course of this condition. From this interesting research on OHSS, profound knowledge about the regulation of angiogenesis can be expected.

REFERENCES

1. McElhinney B, McClure N. Ovarian hyperstimulation syndrome. Baillière's Best Pract Res Clin Obstet Gynaecol 2000; 14: 103–22.
2. Demey HE, Daelemans R, Galdermans D, et al. Acute oligo-anuria during ovarian hyperstimulation syndrome. Acta Obstet Gynecol Scand 1987; 66: 741–3.
3. Todorow S, Schricker ST, Siebzehnruebl ER, et al. von Willebrand factor: an endothelial marker to monitor in-vitro fertilization patients with ovarian hyperstimulation syndrome. Hum Reprod 1993; 8: 2039–46.
4. Ogawa S, Minakami H, Araki S, et al. A rise of the serum level of von Willebrand factor occurs before clinical manifestation of the severe form of ovarian hyperstimulation syndrome. J Assist Reprod Genet 2001; 18: 114–19.
5. Rizk B, Smitz J. Ovarian hyperstimulation syndrome after superovulation using GnRH agonists for IVF and related procedures. Hum Reprod 1992; 7: 320–7.
6. Yarali H, Fleige-Zahradka BG, Yuen BH, et al. The ascites in the ovarian hyperstimulation syndrome does not originate from the ovary. Fertil Steril 1999; 59: 657–61.
7. Amarin ZO. Bilateral partial oophorectomy in the management of severe ovarian hyperstimulation syndrome. An aggressive, but perhaps life-saving procedure. Hum Reprod 2003; 18: 659–64.
8. Dvorak HF, Orenstein NS, Carvalho AC, et al. Induction of a fibrin-gel investment: an early event in line 10 hepatocarcinoma growth mediated by tumor secreted products. J Immunol 1979; 122: 166–74.
9. Senger DR, Galli SJ, Dvorak AM, et al. Tumor cells secrete a vascular permeability factor that promotes accumulation of ascites fluid. Science 1983; 219: 983–5.
10. Ferrara N, Henzel WJ. Pituitary follicular cells secrete a novel heparin-binding growth factor specific for vascular endothelial cells. Biochem Biophys Res Commun 1989; 161: 851–8.
11. Ferrara N, Houck K, Jakeman L, et al. Molecular and biological properties of the vascular endothelial growth factor family of proteins. Endocr Rev 1992; 13: 18–32.
12. Vincenti V, Cassano C, Rocchi M, et al. Assigment of the vascular endothelial growth factor gene to human chromosome 6p21.3. Circulation 1996; 93: 1493–5.
13. Houck KA, Ferrara N, Winer J, et al. The vascular endothelial growth factor family: identification of a fourth molecular species and characterization of alternative splicing of RNA. Mol Endocrinol 1991; 5: 1806–14.
14. Poltorak Z, Cohen T, Sivan R, et al. VEGF145: a secreted vascular endothelial growth factor isoform that binds to the extracellular matrix. J Biol Chem 1997; 272: 7151–8.
15. Park JE, Keller HA, Ferrara N. The vascular endothelial growth factor isoforms: differential deposition into the subepithelial extracellular matrix and bioactivity of extracellular matrix-bound VEGF. Mol Biol Cell 1993; 4: 1317–26.
16. Minchenko A, Baur T, Salceda S, et al. Hypoxic stimulation of vascular endothelial growth factor expression in vivo and in vitro. Lab Invest 1994; 71: 374–9.
17. Tuder RM, Flook BE, Voelkel NF. Increased gene expression for VEGF and VEGF receptors KDR/Flk and Flt in lungs exposed to acute or to chronic hypoxia. Modulation of gene expression by nitric oxide. J Clin Invest 1995; 95: 1798–807.
18. Frank S, Hubner G, Breier G, et al. Regulation of VEGF in cultured keratinocytes. Implications for normal and impaired wound healing. J Biol Chem 1995; 270: 12607–13.
19. Carmeliet P, Ferreira V, Breier G, et al. Abnormal blood vessel development and lethality in embryos lacking a single VEGF allele. Nature 1996; 380: 435–9.
20. Tammela T, Enholm B, Alitalo K, et al. The biology of vascular endothelial growth factors. Cardiovasc Res 2005; 65: 550–63.
21. DeVries C, Escobedo JA, Ueno H, et al. The fms-like tyrosine kinase, a receptor for vascular endothelial growth factor. Science 1992; 255: 989–91.

22. Terman BI, Dougher-Vermazen M, Carrion ME, et al. Identification of the KDR tyrosine kinase as a receptor for vascular endothelial growth factor. Biochem Biophys Res Commun 1992; 187: 1579–86.

23. Fong GH, Rossant J, Gerstenstein M, et al. Role of the Flt-1 receptor tyrosine kinase in regulating the assembly of vascular endothelium. Nature 1995; 376: 66–70.

24. Shalaby F, Rossant J, Yamaguchi TP, et al. Failure of blood-island formation and vasculogenesis in Flk-1 deficient mice. Nature 1995; 376: 62–6.

25. Wang D, Donner DB, Warren RS. Homeostatic modulation of cell surface KDR and Flt1 expression and expression of the vascular endothelial cell growth factor (VEGF) receptor mRNAs by VEGF. J Biol Chem 2000; 275: 15905–11.

26. Dvorak HF, Nagy JA, Berse B, et al. Vascular permeability factor, microvascular hyperpermeability, and angiogenesis. Am J Pathol 1992; 146: 1029–39.

27. Peters KG, deVries C, Williams LT. Vascular endothelial growth factor receptor expression during embryogenesis and tissue repair suggests a role in endothelial differentiation and blood vessel growth. Proc Natl Acad Sci USA 1993; 90: 8915–19.

28. Gabler C, Plath-Gabler A, Killian GJ, et al. Expression pattern of fibroblast growth factor (FGF) and vascular endothelial growth factor (VEGF) system members in bovine corpus luteum endothelial cells during treatment with FGF-2, VEGF or oestradiol. Reprod Domest Anim 2004; 39: 321–7.

29. Brogi E, Schatteman G, Wu T, et al. Hypoxia-induced paracrine regulation of vascular endothelial growth factor receptor expression. J Clin Invest 1996; 97: 469–76.

30. Ferrara N, Davis-Smyth T. The biology of vascular endothelial growth factor. Endocrine Rev 1997; 18: 4–25.

31. Pajusola K, Aprelikova O, Korhonen J, et al. FLT4 receptor tyrosine kinase contains seven immunoglobin-like loops and is expressed in multiple human tissue and cell lines. Cancer Res 1992; 52: 5738–43.

32. Joukov V, Sorsa T, Kumar V, et al. Proteolytic processing regulates receptor specificity and activity of VEGF-C. EMBO J 1997; 16: 3898–911.

33. Heldin C, Ostman A, Westermark B. Structure of platelet-derived growth factor: Implication for functional properties. Growth Factor 1993; 8: 245–52.

34. Vuorela P, Hatva E, Lymbousaki A, et al. Expression of vascular endothelial growth factor and placental growth factor in human placenta. Biol Reprod 1997; 56: 489–94.

35. Di Palma T, Tucci M, Russo G, et al. The placental growth factor gene of the mouse. Mammalian Genome 1996; 7: 6–12.

36. Carmeliet P, Collen D. Genetic analysis of blood vessel formation: role of endothelial versus smooth muscle cells. Trends Cardiovasc Med 1997; 8: 271–81.

37. Grimmond K, Lagercrantz J, Drinkwater C, et al. Cloning and characterization of a novel human gene related to vascular endothelial growth factor. Genome Res 1996; 6: 124–31.

38. Paavonen K, Horelli-Kuitunen N, Chilov D, et al. Novel human vascular endothelial growth factor genes VEGF-B and VEGF-C localize to human chromosome 11q13 and 4q34, respectively. Circulation 1996; 93: 1079–82.

39. Joukov V, Pajusola K, Kaipainen A, et al. A novel endothelial growth factor, VEGF-C, is a ligand for Flt-4 (VEGFR-3) and KDR (VEGFR-2) receptor tyrosine kinase. EMBO J 1996; 15: 290–8.

40. Joukov V, Kumar V, Sorsa T, et al. A recombinant mutant vascular endothelial growth factor C that has lost vascular endothelial growth factor receptor-2 binding, activation and vascular permeability activities. J Biol Chem 1998; 273: 6599–602.

41. Achen MG, Jeltsch M, Kukk E, et al. Vascular endothelial growth factor D (VEGF-D) is a ligand for tyrosine kinase VEGF receptor 2 (flk 1) and VEGF receptor 3 (flt 4). Proc Natl Acad Sci USA 1998; 95: 548–53.

42. Soker S, Takashima S, Quan Miao H, et al. Neuropilin-1 is expressed by endothelial tumor cells as an isoform-specific receptor for vascular

endothelial growth factor. Cell 1998; 92: 735–45.

43. Folkman J. Angiogenesis in cancer, vascular, rheumatic and other disease. Nat Med 1995; 1: 27–31.

44. Shweiki D, Itin A, Neufeld G, et al. Patterns of expression of vascular endothelial growth factor (VEGF) and VEGF receptors in mice suggest a role in hormonally-mediated angiogenesis. J Clin Invest 1993; 91: 2235–43.

45. Roberts WG, Palade GE. Neovasculature induced by vascular endothelial growth factor is fenestrated. Cancer Res 1997; 57: 765–72.

46. Monacci WT, Merrill MJ, Oldfield EH. Expression of vascular permeability factor/vascular endothelial growth factor in normal rat tissue. Am J Physiol 1993; 264: C995–1002.

47. Aiello LP, Avery RL, Arrigg PG, et al. Vascular endothelial growth factor in ocular fluid of patients with diabetic retinopathy and other retinal disorders. N Engl J Med 1994; 331: 1480–7.

48. Koch AE, Harlow L, Haines GK, et al. Vascular endothelial growth factor: a cytokine modulating endothelial function in rheumatoid arthritis. J Immunol 1994; 152: 4149–56.

49. Senger DR, Perruzzi CA, Feder J, et al. A highly conserved vascular permeability factor secreted by a variety of human and rodent tumor cell lines. Cancer Res 1986; 46: 5629–32.

50. Zanetta L, Marcus SG, Vasile J, et al. Expression of von Willebrand factor, an endothelial cell marker, is up-regulated by angiogenesis factors: a potential method for objective assessment of tumor angiogenesis. Int J Cancer 2000; 85: 281–8.

51. Davis JS, Rueda BR, Spanel-Borowski K. Microvascular endothelial cells of the corpus luteum. Reprod Biol Endocrinol 2003;1: 89.

52. Yan Z, Weich HA, Bernart W, et al. Vascular endothelial growth factor (VEGF) messenger ribonucleic acid (mRNA) expression in luteinized human granulosa cells in vitro. J Clin Endocrinol Metab 1993; 77: 1723–5.

53. Neulen J, Raczek S, Pogorzelski M, et al. Secretion of vascular endothelial growth factor/vascular permeability factor from human luteinized granulosa cells is human chorionic gonadotrophin dependent. Mol Hum Reprod 1998; 4: 203–6.

54. Neulen J, Wenzel D, Hornig C, et al. Poor responder–high responder: the importance of soluble vascular endothelial growth factor receptor 1 in ovarian stimulation protocols. Hum Reprod 2001; 16: 621–6.

55. Ishikawa K, Ohba T, Tanaka N, et al. Organ-specific production control of vascular endothelial growth factor in ovarian hyperstimulation syndrome-model rats. Endocr J 2003; 50: 515–25.

56. Agrawal R, Jacobs H, Payne N, et al. Concentration of vascular endothelial growth factor released by cultured human luteinized granulosa cells is higher in women with polycystic ovaries than in women with normal ovaries. Fertil Steril 2002; 78: 1164–9.

57. McClure N, Healy DL, Rogers PA, et al. Vascular endothelial growth factor as capillary permeability agent in ovarian hyperstimulation syndrome. Lancet 1994; 344: 235–6.

58. Robertson D, Selleck K, Suikkari AM, et al. Urinary vascular endothelial growth factor concentrations in women undergoing gonadotrophin treatment. Hum Reprod 1995; 10: 2478–82.

59. Lee A, Christenson LK, Patton PE, et al. Vascular endothelial growth factor production by human luteinized granulosa cells in vitro. Hum Reprod 1997; 12: 2756–61.

60. Krasnow JS, Berga SL, Guzick DS, et al. Vascular permeability factor and vascular endothelial growth factor in ovarian hyperstimulation syndrome: a preliminary report. Fertil Steril 1996; 65: 552–5.

61. Gunsilius E, Petzer A, Stockhammer G, et al. Thrombocytes are the major source for soluble vascular endothelial growth factor in peripheral blood. Oncology 2000; 58: 169–74.

62. Geva E, Amit A, Lessing JB, et al. Follicular fluid levels of vascular endothelial growth factor. Are they predictive markers for ovarian hyperstimulation syndrome? J Reprod Med 1999; 44: 91–6.

63. Mathur R, Hayman G, Bansal A, et al. Serum vascular endothelial growth factor levels are

poorly predictive of subsequent ovarian hyperstimulation syndrome in highly responsive women undergoing assisted conception. Fertil Steril 2002; 78: 1154–8.

64. Yan Z, Neulen J, Raczek S, et al. Vascular endothelial growth factor (VEGF)/vascular permeability factor (VPF) production by luteinized human granulosa cells in vitro; a paracrine signal in corpus luteum formation. Gynecol Endocrinol 1998; 12: 149–53.

65. He Y, Smith SK, Day KA, et al. Alternative splicing of vascular endothelial growth factor (VEGF)-R1 (FLT-1) pre-mRNA is important for the regulation of VEGF activity. Mol Endocrinol 1999; 13: 537–45.

66. Kendall RL, Thomas KA. Inhibition of vascular endothelial cell growth factor activity by an endogenously encoded soluble receptor. Proc Natl Acad Sci USA 1993; 90: 10705–9.

67. Kendall RL, Wang G, Thomas KA. Identification of a natural soluble form of the vascular endothelial growth factor receptor, FLT-1, and its heterodimerization with KDR. Biochem Biophys Res Commun 1996; 226: 324–8.

68. Hornig C, Weich HA. Soluble VEGF receptors. Angiogenesis 1999; 3: 33–9.

69. Hornig C, Barleon B, Ahmad S, et al. Release and complex formation of soluble VEGFR-1 from endothelial cells and biological fluids. Lab Invest 2000; 80: 443–54.

70. Xu F, Hazzard TM, Evans A, et al. Intraovarian actions of anti-angiogenic agents disrupt periovulatory events during the menstrual cycle in monkeys. Contraception 2005; 71: 239–48.

71. Ludwig M, Jelkmann W, Bauer O, et al. Prediction of severe ovarian hyperstimulation syndrome by free serum vascular endothelial growth factor concentration on the day of human chorionic gonadotrophin administration. Hum Reprod 1999; 14: 2437–41.

72. Gomez R, Lima I, Simon C, et al. Administration of low-dose LH induces ovulation and prevents vascular hyperpermeability and vascular endothelial growth factor expression in superovulated rats. Reproduction 2004; 127: 483–9.

73. Kitajima Y, Endo T, Manase K, et al. Gonadotropin-releasing hormone agonist administration reduced vascular endothelial growth factor (VEGF), VEGF receptors, and vascular permeability of the ovaries of hyperstimulated rats. Fertil Steril 2004; 81 (Suppl 1): 842–9.

74. Garcia-Velasco JA, Zuniga A, Pacheco A, et al. Coasting acts through downregulation of VEGF gene expression and protein secretion. Hum Reprod 2004; 19: 1530–8.

75. Tozer AJ, Iles RK, Iammarrone E, et al. The effects of 'coasting' on follicular fluid concentrations of vascular endothelial growth factor in women at risk of developing ovarian hyperstimulation syndrome. Hum Reprod 2004; 19: 522–8.

76. Berghaus D, Gummer R, Weich H, et al. Modulation of sVEGFR-1 secretion by follicular fluid. Hum Reprod 2004; 19 (Suppl 1): i156–7.

CHAPTER 11

The renin–angiotensin system in the pathophysiology of ovarian hyperstimulation syndrome

Maria José Teruel and Isabel Hernández García

INTRODUCTION

Ovarian hyperstimulation syndrome (OHSS) normally manifests itself as a serious complication of ovulation induction treatments, although there have also been reports of spontaneous and familial OHSS, associated with pregnancy[1,2]. The pathogenesis of this syndrome has not been fully clarified, although the description of two spontaneous cases with familial association suggests that a certain genetic predisposition may prove necessary to induce the disorder. Human chorionic gonadotropin (hCG) probably stimulates the ovarian secretion of vasoactive factors that in turn increase vascular permeability and contribute to third-compartment fluid accumulation, these being characteristic physiopathological features of OHSS. Many substances have been suggested as possible mediators of the syndrome, including serotonin, histamine, prolactin, estrogens and prostaglandins, although the renin–angiotensin system (RAS) and certain cytokines (interleukin-2 and -8) produced by the ovaries have been proposed as the main factors implicated in OHSS physiopathology. Thus, the renin–angiotensin system (RAS) is one of the mechanisms presumed to participate in ovarian hyperstimulation syndrome.

In the mid-1980s, Haning *et al*. suggested that OHSS results from excessive secretion of the hormone in charge of regulating peritoneal fluid during the normal menstrual cycle. They found the syndrome to be characterized by an increase in serum aldosterone associated with an increase in plasma renin activity. Initially, it was considered that intravascular fluid displacement to the peritoneum stimulated renin and aldosterone production, secondary to the hypotension implied by the loss of plasma volume. As a result, the increases in these hormones would simply constitute a reaction to ascites[3].

Subsequently, Navot *et al*. suggested participation of the RAS based on their studies in women with OHSS, in which a direct relationship was found between plasma renin activity and the severity of ovarian hyperstimulation syndrome[4].

An increase in plasma renin concentration has also been observed in one of the documented cases of recurrent and familial OHSS[5].

RENIN–ANGIOTENSIN SYSTEM: MECHANISM OF ACTION

The main function of the RAS in maintaining arterial pressure seems to be regulation of the balance between ingestion and excretion of salt.

Renin acts upon angiotensinogen (a plasma protein synthesized in the liver), converting it to angiotensin I (a scantly active molecule) which, at small vessel level, is converted to angiotensin II. This conversion is mediated by angiotensin-converting enzyme (ACE) located mainly in the pulmonary capillaries.

The principal effects of angiotensin comprise arteriolar vasoconstriction (resulting in an increase in total peripheral resistance) and venous constriction (thus increasing venous return), a reduction in the renal elimination of sodium and water, and stimulation of aldosterone by the adrenal glands (Figure 1).

The RAS is stimulated by different mechanisms. Thus, an increase in central venous pressure has been shown to reduce both renin and angiotensin levels, while sympathetic stimulation exerts the opposite effect. In turn, the RAS exerts a response independent of the central nervous system, characterized by direct vasoconstrictive action affording compensation for arterial pressure reductions of up to 65%.

Angiotensin II is a potent vasoconstrictor that acts directly upon the tubular resorption of sodium, and indirectly by modifying the hydrostatic and oncotic forces. In experimental animals it has been shown that angiotensin II, at physiological concentrations, increases fluid resorption in the proximal renal tubuli, while at high concentrations it inhibits sodium excretion. Angiotensin therefore seems to reduce renal blood flow through vasoconstriction, or possibly by modifying the glomerular filtration coefficient. In this context, it reduces the glomerular filtration rate by approximately 20%. This effect, and the increase in sodium resorption, modifies the pressure–natriuresis balance. Such action is a consequence of renal cortical vasoconstriction, while medullary flow does not seem to be modified. In this way, angiotensin modifies the pressure–diuresis curve, shifting it to the right. This in turn implies that a higher arterial pressure is needed to excrete the same amount of water and sodium. Aldosterone in turn increases net sodium resorption in the distal tubuli, thereby increasing the extracellular volume and therefore arterial pressure.

The mechanisms described for pressure control are decisive for long-term control, although short-term arterial pressure adjustments are principally mediated by the nervous system, which modifies total peripheral resistance and cardiac output.

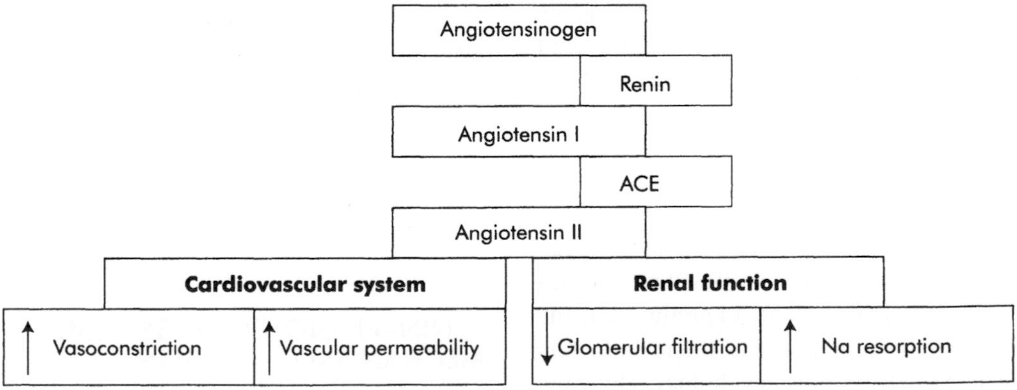

Figure 1 Cardiovascular and renal effects of the renin–angiotensin system. ACE, angiotensin-converting enzyme

On the other hand, recent studies[6,7] have demonstrated that angiotensin II increases vascular permeability that may be mediated by vascular endothelial growth factor (VEGF). In cultured human aortic smooth muscle cells, it was shown that angiotensin II induces expression of the messenger RNA (mRNA) encoding for a glycoprotein known as vascular permeability factor or VEGF (see also Chapters 10 and 14). In this same study it was also found that selective losartan-induced inhibition of angiotensin type I (AT_1) receptors prevents increases in angiotensin II and expression of mRNA encoding VEGF. Likewise, Hernandez *et al.* have recently published a study in rats in which AT_1 receptor block with losartan attenuates the increase in vascular permeability induced by the inhibition of nitric oxide (NO) synthesis via the administration of N^{ω}-nitro-L-arginine methyl ester (L-NAME). All these data suggest that angiotensin II may play an important role in regulating vascular permeability under different pathophysiological conditions[6].

THE OVARIAN RENIN–ANGIOTENSIN SYSTEM

Since the mid-20th century it has been known that plasma renin activity (PRA) varies in the course of the normal ovarian cycle[8]. Later, the existence of an ovarian RAS was demonstrated. This system is activated by gonadotropins and is independent from the renal RAS[9]. In the course of an ovarian cycle, an increase in angiotensin II has been observed in the follicular fluid of the preovulatory follicle[10]. In 1990, Blankenstijn *et al.*, after studying the RAS in nephrectomized women, confirmed that prorenin (the inactive precursor of renin) is secreted by the ovary in response to luteinizing hormone (LH) and hCG[11]. On the other hand, since the studies of *in vitro* fertilization (IVF) cycles, it has been known that prorenin is found in concentrations 12-fold greater in follicular fluid than in plasma, and that hCG administration increases the plasma concentration of prorenin[12]. Later still, Morris and Paulson found that in addition to synthesizing prorenin, the ovaries also contain the entire enzyme system needed to transform prorenin into angiotensin II. The studies of this research group also suggested that angiotensin may modulate steroid synthesis, oocyte maturation, ovulation and formation of the luteal body[13].

Different studies have confirmed the existence of specific angiotensin II receptors in ovarian follicles[10,12–17], thereby defining the functionality of the ovarian RAS. Thus, studies in rabbit ovaries have revealed the presence of AT_1 receptors in the granulosa and theca of preovulatory follicles[18]. On the other hand, AT_2 receptors have been identified in atretic rat follicles, the induction of apoptosis being attributed to stimulation of these receptors[19]. The various studies conducted to date have shown the ovaries to contain a complete and intrinsic RAS, as well as receptors for angiotensin II. These elements and other ovarian modulators contribute to establish ovarian function. This ovarian RAS participates fundamentally in atresia, formation of the dominant follicle, and ovulation – although the underlying intrinsic mechanisms are not known.

RENIN–ANGIOTENSIN SYSTEM AND OHSS

At present it is known that during ovarian hyperstimulation syndrome both the ovarian and plasma RAS are activated (Figure 2). Delbaere *et al.* found that women who develop OHSS have significantly greater concentrations of renin and prorenin in ascitic fluid than in plasma, while the aldosterone levels were higher in plasma than in ascitic fluid. These authors therefore suggested that the greater renin and prorenin levels in ascitic fluid imply activation of the ovarian RAS, while the high

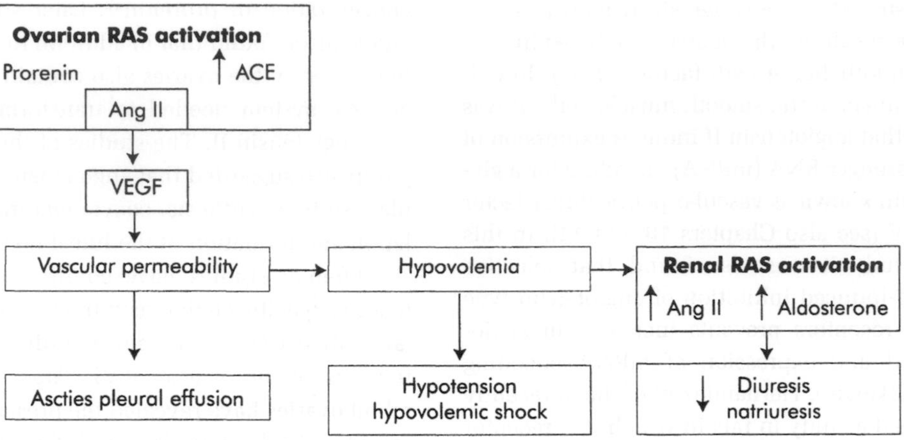

Figure 2 Postulated mechanisms of the renin-angiotensin system (RAS) implication in pathophysiology of ovarian hyperstimulation syndrome. ACE, angiotensin-converting enzyme; Ang, angiotensin; VEGF, vascular endothelial growth factor

serum levels of active renin and aldosterone reflect activation of the renal RAS[20].

Other studies have shown increases in the plasma concentrations of prorenin, renin and aldosterone in women with severe OHSS[21,22], as well as increments in renin and angiotensin activity in both plasma and ascitic fluid obtained from women with OHSS[23–27]. There have also been reports of an increase in angiotensin-converting enzyme (ACE) activity in another woman with this same syndrome[23]. According to these data, OHSS appears to be characterized by stimulation of all RAS components.

The results of studies conducted with ACE inhibitors (ACEIs) in experimental models of OHSS reveal participation of the RAS in the pathophysiology of the syndrome, and more specifically in the production of ascites. Thus, the administration of enalapril (an ACEI) reduced ascites by 40% in female rabbits treated with gonadotropins[28]. Gul *et al.* found that rabbits treated with enalapril showed a significant reduction in aldosterone concentration, with no significant differences in relation to the volume of ascitic fluid[28]. In the same way, Teruel *et al.* found that treatment with captopril (another ACEI) did not modify ovarian size in rabbits, although it did reduce the percentage of animals with ascites (80% vs. 50%) and also the volume of ascitic fluid in those animals that presented ascites[29].

When OHSS manifests itself, the affected patients show both ovarian and renal RAS activation, with elevated prorenin, renin activity, active renin and angiotensin II values. These values in turn are even higher in ascitic and pleural fluid than in plasma – thus reflecting activation of the ovarian RAS[20,23,25]. Plasma renin activity normalizes after the acute phase of the syndrome, in coincidence with patient clinical normalization. In this way, in a documented case of OHSS with internal jugular vein thrombosis, increased plasma renin activity was seen to decrease in parallel with resolution of the thrombus[30].

CLINICAL CHARACTERISTICS

Modifications associated with OHSS

Increased vascular permeability

Different authors attribute the observed increase in vascular permeability to the substances secreted by the corpus luteum after the administration of hCG[31,32].

Studies in experimental animal models have shown that ascites is produced by a generalized increase in vascular permeability, and does not originate in the ovary[33]. The authors reached this conclusion after exteriorizing the ovaries from the peritoneum of rabbits that subsequently underwent ovulation induction with gonadotropins. Both the production of ascites and the plasma hormone levels were found to be no different in these animals compared with the non-operated controls.

Nevertheless, according to Goldsman *et al.*, some substances produced by the ovaries play a fundamental role in the induction of OHSS[34]. The application of follicular and peritoneal fluid obtained from women treated with gonadotropins during an IVF cycle to the endothelium of bovine aorta induced vascular permeability *in vitro*. Likewise, a correlation was found between the increase in vascular permeability and the susceptibility of the donating women to the development of OHSS, determined as the stimulation of over 25 follicles[34]. Other authors have studied the modifications in Starling pressure, which determines transcapillary exchange, during ovarian stimulation with gonadotropins. They observed a progressive reduction of plasma colloidosmotic pressure, together with an increase in interstitial colloidosmotic pressure, thus implying a gradual reduction of the transcapillary colloidosmotic gradient (i.e. the difference between plasma colloidosmotic pressure and interstitial colloidosmotic pressure), and therefore an increase in vascular permeability to proteins during increasing ovarian stimulation[35].

The studies conducted in experimental models have corroborated the hypothesis that angiotensin participates as a mediator in increasing vascular permeability, since ACEI administration reduces the incidence and severity of the syndrome[35,36]. The administration of captopril during ovarian hyperstimulation with gonadotropins reduces both the appearance of ascites and the vascular permeability index, as determined by the extravasation of albumin dyed with Evans blue stain.

Hemodynamic alterations

On the other hand, according to Balasch *et al.*, women who develop OHSS present circulatory alterations characterized by hypotension, tachycardia, an increased cardiac output and a reduction in peripheral resistance[37]. These authors consider that in addition to the increase in vascular permeability, some other factor is responsible for the hemodynamic alterations. This is because the increase in vascular permeability would give rise to hypovolemia, which in turn would lead to a decrease in cardiac output and hypotension. As a response to hypotension, the sympathetic nervous system would attempt to increase cardiac output, elevating heart rate and peripheral resistance in an attempt to restore arterial pressure. However, in the studies of women with severe ovarian hyperstimulation, Balasch *et al.* found a decrease in total peripheral resistance, and an increase in cardiac output with hypotension. These authors therefore consider that the observed circulatory disorders are secondary to peripheral vasodilatation, with the association of increased vascular permeability. This hyperdynamic circulatory situation is comparable to that observed after the formation of edemas and ascites secondary to liver failure[37]. On the other hand, in a study published by Manau *et al.* in women subjected to ovulation induction and who did not develop OHSS, the increase in plasma estradiol concentrations was associated with a decrease in arterial pressure and peripheral vascular resistance, together with a rise in cardiac output. It was also seen that changes in plasma renin activity paralleled plasma estradiol concentration, and aldosterone increased only at the end of the luteal phase. On the basis of these observations, the authors suggested that circulatory dysfunction develops during ovarian stimulation, affecting all patients, and that OHSS represents the extreme expression of such dysfunction[38].

Other authors, however, have reported hypotension with a decrease in cardiac output, systolic stroke volume and cardiac index[39], together with a drop in central venous pressure[40,41], thus supporting the classical idea (defended by Schenker and Elchalal) whereby diminished intravascular volume secondary to massive displacement towards the third compartment, due to a sudden increase in permeability, leads to hypovolemia which in turn gives rise to hypovolemic shock[42] (Figure 2).

Alterations in renal function

Renal dysfunction is another of the clinical features of severe OHSS, and may even culminate in acute renal failure. As shown by Balasch *et al.*, the most frequent renal alterations are oliguria and sodium retention[43–45], along with a minor reduction in glomerular filtration rate. The same authors reported a significant increase in serum creatinine levels in women with OHSS compared with the creatinine levels recorded following patient normalization. They therefore suggested that the glomerular filtration rate decreases in the course of the syndrome[46]. On the other hand, different authors have reported decreases in sodium excretion in urine in women with this syndrome, with some published cases of undetectable urine sodium levels[47]. As a result, these authors suggest that the hyperstimulation syndrome involves sodium retention[47].

Altered kidney function is indicative of marked disease severity in women with OHSS. Accordingly, in previous classifications of the syndrome, serum creatinine > 1.5 mg/ml, or creatinine clearance < 50 ml/min, was used to define critical OHSS[48].

This modification associated with ovarian hyperstimulation syndrome can also be due in part to RAS activation, since both glomerular filtration and sodium resorption are modified by high angiotensin II levels (Figure 1). On the other hand, studies in rabbits have reported a right shift of the pressure–natriuresis curve in animals with OHSS, thus indicating a tendency toward sodium retention. In this case, ACEI therapy (captopril) normalizes the curve, suggesting that angiotensin II may play an important role in the pathophysiology of OHSS.

RENIN–ANGIOTENSIN AND VASCULAR ENDOTHELIAL GROWTH FACTOR

Another mediator in the development of OHSS is vascular endothelial growth factor (VEGF), a protein belonging to the family of heparin ligands, which acts directly upon the endothelial cells, inducing angiogenesis and increased vascular permeability[49–55].

The implication and possible association of RAS and VEGF in the pathophysiology of OHSS appears to have been confirmed by the different studies conducted to date. Not only do the two mediators increase angiogenesis and vascular permeability, but the production of both is moreover interrelated. Angiotensin II affords potent stimulation of VEGF production in smooth muscle cells, myocardium, retinal epithelium and mesenchymal cells[56]. It has also been shown that angiotensin II induces VEGF expression in endometrial cancer cells[57] and in cervical cancer cells[58]. Angiotensin II is related to VEGF production associated with angiogenesis[59], as a result of which some investigators have proposed administering an ACEI as cotreatment in oncological processes[60]. In the kidney, this relationship between the two mediators has also been observed, with angiotensin regulating VEGF expression[61]. However, other authors, on providing treatment with an ACEI (enalapril) in rats subjected to OHSS induction, have reported no reduction in VEGF expression at the ovarian level[62]. Since angiotensin II exerts multiple effects via specific receptor interaction, and moreover shares many functions with VEGF, both substances may possibly mediate the pathophysiology of OHSS either directly or indirectly.

CONTROVERSIES

The ovarian or renal origin of the high plasma concentration of total renin and renin activity during severe OHSS has been a matter of debate for a long time. Haning *et al.*[3] first suggested that the markedly elevated plasma renin activity was secondary to the hypovolemia accompanying the syndrome. However, hyperstimulated ovaries have been considered as the main source of hyperreninism in OHSS since a direct correlation between plasma renin activity and the severity of the syndrome was observed[4]. Further investigations, performed on the ascites from patients with OHSS, showing total renin and prorenin and angiotensin II concentrations much higher in the ascites than in the plasma, reinforced the hypothesis of a marked stimulation of ovarian RAS in the syndrome[23–25]. On the other hand, the severe forms of the syndrome were shown to be consistently associated with a marked arteriolar vasodilatation and fall in blood pressure[46]. This hemodynamic state leads to a neurohormonal compensatory response that involves rapid activation of the RAS and sympathetic nervous system and non-osmotic release of antidiuretic hormone. In view of the above data, the possibility that stimulation of the ovarian RAS is a primary phenomenon, related to a direct effect of gonadotropin, has to be taken seriously, while, on the other hand, the intense stimulation of the renal RAS is secondary to the hemodynamic changes occurring during the syndrome.

TREATMENT

As has already been mentioned in the course of this chapter, the RAS is implicated in the development of OHSS, and different authors using an ACEI have been able to reduce both the incidence of the syndrome and its severity. All such work has been done in experimental rabbit models[28,36,63] and in women.

Morris *et al.* administered captopril (ACEI) to patients who developed ovarian hyperstimulation syndrome and were oocyte donors[27]. These women showed an increase in plasma estradiol levels and a decrease in progesterone concentration. These results suggest that ovarian angiotensin II may exert a stimulating effect on cytochrome P450 and an inhibitory effect on ovarian aromatase – thus raising the possibility that angiotensin II may tonically inhibit estradiol secretion and increase progesterone secretion. In view of this, Morris *et al.* speculated on the possibility of administering an ACEI as preventive treatment, immediately after ovulation[27]. However, considering the teratogenic potential of the ACEIs (e.g. enalapril produces renal defects when administered in the second and third trimesters of pregnancy), such ACEI therapy cannot be advised – unless the cycle involves no gestation. Nevertheless, it is important to know the pathophysiological particulars of the syndrome and identify the intervening mediators, since this opens the way for exerting action at different therapeutic levels.

CONCLUSION

The renin–angiotensin system (RAS) plays a very important role in ovarian physiology, and angiotensin II intervenes in the modulation of steroid synthesis and in follicle production and maturation, ovulation and follicular atresia. Ovarian hyperstimulation syndrome (OHSS) is secondary to an excessive ovarian response, and simply represents a pathological hyperresponse to ovarian stimulation with gonadotropins. In this context, both the ovarian and systemic renin–angiotensin systems contribute to the syndrome, together with other modulators of ovarian origin.

REFERENCES

1. Ayhan A, Tuncer ZS, Aksu AT. Ovarian hyperstimulation syndrome associated with spontaneous pregnancy. Hum Reprod 1996; 11: 1600–1.
2. Di Carlo C, Bruno PA, Cirillo D, et al. Increased concentrations of renin, aldosterone and Ca^{125} in a case of spontaneous, recurrent, familial, severe ovarian hyperstimulation syndrome. Hum Reprod 1997; 12: 2115–17.
3. Haning R Jr, Strawn E, Nolten W. Pathophysiology of the ovarian hyperstimulation syndrome. Obstet Gynecol 1985; 66: 220–4.
4. Navot D, Margalioth EJ, Laufer N. Direct correlation between plasma renin activity and severity of the ovarian hyperstimulation syndrome. Fertil Steril 1987; 48: 57–61.
5. Suzuki Y, Ruiz-Ortega M, Lorenzo O, et al. Inflammation and angiotensin II. Int J Biochem Cell Biol 2003; 35: 881–900.
6. Williams B, Baker AQ, Gallacher B, et al. Angiotensin II increases vascular permeability factor gene expression by human vascular smooth muscle cells. Hypertension 1995; 25: 913–17.
7. Hernández I, Carbonell LF, Quesada T, et al. Role of angiotensin II in modulating the hemodynamic effects of nitric oxide synthesis inhibition. Am J Physiol 1999; 277: R104–11.
8. Brown JJ, Davies DL, Lever AF, et al. Variation in plasma renin during the menstrual cycle. Br Med J 1964; 52: 209–15.
9. Itkovitz J, Sealey JE. Ovarian prorenin reniangiotensin system. Obstet Gynecol Surv 1987; 42: 545–51.
10. Lightman A, Tarlatzis BC, Rzasa PJ, et al. The ovarian renin–angiotensin system: renin-like activity and angiotensin II/III immunoreactivity in gonadotrophin stimulated and unstimulated human follicuar fluid. Am J Obstet Gynecol 1987; 156: 808–16.
11. Blankenstijn PJ, Derk XFHM, Van Geelen JA, et al. Increase in plasma prorenin during the menstrual cycle of a bilaterally nephrectomised woman. Br J Obstet Gynaecol 1990; 97: 1083–142.
12. Glorioso N, Atlas SA, Laragh JH. Prorenin in high concentration in human ovarian follicular fluid. Science 1986; 233: 1422–4.
13. Morris RS, Paulson RJ. Ovarian derived prorenin–angiotensin cascade in human reproduction. Fertil Steril 1994; 62: 1105–14.
14. Husain A, Bumpus FM, De Silva P, Speth RC. Localization of angiotensin II receptor in ovarian follicles and the identification of angiotensin II in rat ovaries. Proc Natl Acad Sci USA 1987; 84: 2489–93.
15. Pucell AG, Bumpus FM, Husain A, et al. Rat ovarian angiotensin II receptor. J Biol Chem 1987; 262: 7076–80.
16. Speth RC, Husain A. Distribution of angiotensin-converting enzyme and angiotensin II-receptor binding sites in the rat ovary. Biol Reprod 1988; 38: 695–702.
17. Palumbo A, Jones C, Lightman A, et al. Immunohistochemical localization of renin and angiotensin II in human ovaries. Am J Obstet Gynecol 1989; 160: 8–14.
18. Feral C, Benhaim A, Leymarie P. Angiotensin II receptor type 1 on granulosa and thecal cells of rabbit preovulatory follicles. Biochim Biophys Acta 1996; 1284: 221–6.
19. Yamada T, Horiuchi M, Dzau VJ. AngII type 2 receptor mediates programmed cell death. Proc Natl Acad Sci USA 1996; 93: 156–60.
20. Delbaere A, Bergmann PJM, Gervy-Decoster C, et al. Prorenin and active renin concentrations in plasma and ascites during severe ovarian hyperstimulation syndrome. Hum Reprod 1997; 12: 236–40.
21. Ong ACM, Eisen V, Rennie DP, et al. The pathogenesis of the ovarian hyperstimulation

syndrome (OHS) a possible role for ovarian renin. Clin Endocrinol 1991; 34: 43–9.

22. Van de Vrie W, Baggen MG, Visser W, et al. High renin and prorenin in plasma and pleural exudate of a patient with the ovarian hyperstimulation syndrome. Neth J Med 1997; 51: 232–6.

23. Delbaere A, Bergmann PJM, Gervy-Decoster C, et al. Increased angiotensin II in ascites during severe ovarian hyperstimulation syndrome: role of early pregnancy and ovarian gonadotropin stimulation. Fertil Steril 1997; 67: 1038–45.

24. Rosemberg ME, McKenzie JK, McKenzie IR, et al. Increased ascitic fluid prorenin in the ovarian hyperstimulation syndrome. Am J Kidney Dis 1994; 23: 427–9.

25. Delbaere A, Bergmann PJM, Gervy-Decoster C, et al. Angiotensin II immunoreactivity is elevated in ascites during severe ovarian hyperstimulation syndrome: implications for pathophysiology and clinical management. Fertil Steril 1994; 62: 731–7.

26. Morris RS, Paulson RJ. Increased angiotensin-converting enzyme activity in a patient with severe ovarian hyperstimulation syndrome. Fertil Steril 1999; 71: 562–3.

27. Morris RS, Wong IL, Kirkman E, et al. Inhibition of ovarian-derived prorenin to angiotensin cascade in the treatment of ovarian hyperstimulation syndrome. Hum Reprod 1995; 10: 1355–8.

28. Gul TC, Posaci C, Caliskan S. The role of enalapril in the prevention of ovarian hyperstimulation syndrome: a rabbit model. Hum Reprod 2001;16:2253–7.

29. Teruel MJG, Carbonell LF, Llanos MC, et al. Hemodynamic state and the role of angiotensin II in ovarian hyperstimulation syndrome in the rabbit. Fertil Steril 2002; 77: 1256–60.

30. Chang FW, Chan CC, Yin CS, et al. Predicted value of renin activity in a woman who had severe hyperstimulation syndrome with internal jugular vein thrombosis. Fertil Steril 2004; 82: 937–9.

31. Polishuk WZ, Schenker JG. Ovarian hyperstimulation syndrome. Fertil Steril 1990; 20: 443–50.

32. Schenker JG, Weinstein D. Ovarian hyperstimulation syndrome: a current survey. Fertil Steril 1978; 30: 255–68.

33. Yarali H, Fleige-Zahradka BG, Ho Juen B, et al. The ascites in the hyperstimulation syndrome does not originate from the ovary. Fertil Steril 1993; 59: 657–61.

34. Goldsman MP, Ciuffardi I, Pedram A, et al. Increased capillary permeability induced by human follicular fluid: a hypothesis for an ovarian origin of the hyperstimulation syndrome. Fertil Steril 1995; 63: 268–72.

35. Tollan A, Holst N, Forsdahl F, et al. Transcapillary fluid dynamics during ovarian stimulation for in vitro fertilization. Am J Obstet Gynecol 1990; 162: 554–8.

36. Teruel MJG, Carbonell LF, Teruel MG, et al. Effect of angiotensin-converting enzyme inhibitor of renal function in ovarian hyperstimulation syndrome in the rabbit. Fertil Steril 2001; 76: 1232–7.

37. Balasch J, Fábregues F, Arroyo V. Peripheral arterial vasodilation hypothesis: a new insight into the pathogenesis of ovarian hyperstimulation syndrome. Hum Reprod 1998; 13: 2718–30.

38. Manau D, Balasch J, Arroyo V, et al. Circulatory dysfunction in asymptomatic in vitro fertilization patients. Relationship with hyperestrogenemia and activity of endogenous vasodilators. J Clin Endocrinol Metab 1999; 83: 1489–93.

39. Ryuko K, Takahanshi K, Okada M, et al. Cardiac output measurement by thoracic electrical bioimpedance in a patient with ovarian hyperstimulation syndrome. Gynecol Obstet Invest 1996; 41: 140–2.

40. Goldchmit R, Elchalal U, Zalel Y. Hypovolaemic shock as a presenting sign of severe hyperstimulation syndrome following in vitro fertilization and embryo transfer (IVF-ET). J Assist Reprod Genet 1993; 10: 480–2.

41. Grochowski D, Sola E, Kulikowski M. Successful outcome of severe ovarian hyperstimulation syndrome (OHSS) with 27 litres of ascitic fluid removed by paracentesis. J Assist Reprod Genet 1995; 12: 394–6.

42. Elchalal U, Schenker JG. The pathophysiology of ovarian hyperstimulation syndrome – views and ideas. Hum Reprod 1997; 12: 1129–37.

43. Balasch J, Carmona F, Llach J, et al. Acute prerenal failure and liver dysfunction in a patient

with severe ovarian hyperstimulation syndrome. Hum Reprod 1990; 5: 348–51.

44. Balasch J, Arroyo V, Carmona F, et al. Severe ovarian hyperstimulation syndrome: role of peripheral vasodilation. Fertil Steril 1991; 56: 1077–83.

45. Balasch J, Arroyo V, Fábregues F, et al. Immunoreactive endothelin plasma levels in severe ovarian hyperstimulation syndrome. Fertil Steril 1995; 64: 65–8.

46. Balasch J, Arroyo V, Fábregues F, et al. Neurohormonal and hemodynamic changes in severe cases of the ovarian hyperstimulation syndrome. Ann Intern Med 1994; 121: 27–33.

47. Cremisi HD, Mitch WE. Profound hypotension and sodium retention with the ovarian hyperstimulation syndrome. Am J Kidney Dis 1994; 24: 854–7.

48. Navot D, Bergh PA, Laufer N. Ovarian hyperstimulation syndrome in novel reproductive technologies: prevention and treatment. Fertil Steril 1992; 58: 249–61.

49. Ferrara N, Henzel WJ. Pituitary follicular cells secrete a novel heparin-binding growth factor specific for vascular endothelial cells. Biochem Biophys Res Commun 1989; 161: 851–8.

50. Lee A, Christenson LK, Patton PE, et al. Vascular endothelial growth factor production by human luteinized granulosa cells in vitro. Hum Reprod 1997; 12: 2756–61.

51. Robertson D, Selleck K, Suikkari AM, et al. Urinary vascular endothelial growth factor concentrations in women undergoing gonadotrophin treatment. Hum Reprod 1995; 10: 2478–82.

52. McClure N, Healy DL, Rogers PAW, et al. Vascular endothelial growth factor as capillary permeability agent in ovarian hyperstimulation syndrome. Lancet 1994; 344: 235–6.

53. Abramov Y, Barak V, Nisman B, et al. Vascular endothelial growth factor plasma levels correlate to the clinical picture in severe ovarian hyperstimulation syndrome. Fertil Steril 1997; 67: 261–5.

54. Kitajima Y, Endo T, Manase K, et al. Gonadotropin-releasing hormone agonist administration reduced vascular endothelial growth factor (VEGF), VEGF receptors, and vascular permeability of the ovaries of hyperstimulated rats. Fertil Steril 2004; 81: 842–9.

55. Gomez R, Lima I, Simon C, et al. Administration of low-dose LH induces ovulation and prevents vascular hyperpermeability and vascular endothelial growth expression in superovulated rats. Reproduction 2004; 127: 483–9.

56. Shihab FS, Bennett WM, Isaac J, et al. Angiotensin II regulation of vascular endothelial growth factor and receptors Flt-1 and KDR/F1k-1 in cyclosporine nephrotoxicity. Kidney Int 2002; 62: 422–33.

57. Watanabe Y, Shibata K, Kikkawa F, et al. Adipocyte-derived leucine aminopeptidase suppresses angiogenesis in human endometrial carcinoma via renin–angiotensin system. Clin Cancer Res 2003; 15: 6497–503.

58. Kikkawa F, Mizuno M, Shibata K, et al. Activation of invasiveness of cervical carcinoma cells by angiotensin II. Am J Obstet Gynecol 2004; 190: 1258–63.

59. Fujita M, Hayashi I, Yamashina S, et al. Angiotensin type 1a receptor signaling-dependent induction of vascular endothelial growth factor in stroma is relevant to tumor-associated angiogenesis and tumor growth. Carcinogenesis 2005; 26: 271–9.

60. Yoshiji H, Kuriyama S, Noguchi R, et al. Angiotensin-I converting enzyme inhibitiors as potential anti-angiogenic agents for cancer therapy. Curr Cancer Drug Targets 2004; 4: 555–67.

61. Feliers D, Duraisamy S, Barnes JL, et al. Translational regulation of vascular endothelial growth factor expression in renal epithelial cells by angiotensin II. Am J Physiol Renal Physiol 2005; 288: F521–9.

62. Ozcakir HT, Gulsen S, Kemal M, et al. Effect of angiotensin-converting enzyme-inhibiting therapy on the expression of vascular endothelial growth factor in hyperstimulated rat ovary. Fertil Steril 2004; 82: 1127–32.

63. Ratnapalan S, Koren G. Taking ACE inhibitors during pregnancy. Is it safe? Can Fam Physician 2002; 48: 1047–9.

CHAPTER 12

Immunological aspects of ovarian hyperstimulation syndrome

Anders Enskog and Mats Brännström

INTRODUCTION

The main pathophysiological mechanism of ovarian hyperstimulation syndrome (OHSS) is increased vascular leakage from the ovaries as well as within the peritoneal lining of the abdominal and thoracic sinuses. This pronounced plasma leakage to the third compartment induces hypovolemia, and because of secondary tissue hypoperfusion, the syndrome may escalate to multiple organ failure. There may also be activation of the coagulation cascade, with the development of thrombosis in large vessels.

The increased permeability is also a hallmark of inflammation, and it has been suggested that there is a major role of inflammatory events during the development and establishment of OHSS. The risk factors for OHSS that also have a strong association with inflammation are polycystic ovarian syndrome (PCOS)[1,2], allergy[3] and suppressed interleukin (IL)-10 production[4]. Their proposed mechanisms of action in OHSS pathophysiology are discussed in detail in this chapter. Moreover, the possible roles of inflammation-associated regulatory T cells (TR) and local glucocorticoid activation in the pathophysiology of OHSS are mentioned.

In our large cohort study, more than 400 patients in one *in vitro* fertilization (IVF) program were prospectively followed, with blood samples taken throughout gonadotropin stimulation[3]. Eighteen patients (about 3%) developed severe OHSS. Matched (for age, number of follicles and pregnancy) controls from the study group were selected and compared with cases with severe OHSS. There was an increased prevalence of hypersensitivity (allergy) in the OHSS group, suggesting a link between an overactive immune response and the increased inflammatory events during the development of OHSS[3]. Moreover, the OHSS group had lower levels of the immunosuppressive cytokine IL-10 at the early stages of gonadotropin stimulation, with a negative correlation between the numbers of follicles and IL-10 levels at the time of oocyte aspiration, seen only in the OHSS patients[4]. The OHSS patients showed increased IL-10 levels at later stages of gonadotropin stimulation, indicating a natural immune response to counteract and thereby control the increasing inflammatory events.

Taking the above results into consideration, it seems as if immunological dysregulation is central in the events occurring in the ovary during OHSS development, and this dysregulation may be present during the follicular phases (folliculogenesis, ovulation/luteinization). This imbalance may cause enhanced inflammatory changes in the ovary, thereby increasing the risk for OHSS.

This review is based on our current hypothesis that women with inherent dysregulation of the immune system are more prone to develop OHSS during gonadotropin stimulation. Dysregulation can take the form of increased proinflammatory activation, decreased anti-inflammatory activity or a combination of both. The increased inflammatory response can be exemplified by hypersensitivity/allergy and the decreased anti-inflammatory response by an altered IL-10 response.

INFLAMMATION AND HYPERSENSITIVITY

Since inflammation is a central event in the pathophysiology of OHSS, and also because inflammation is an integral part of the cycle-dependent ovarian phases, a brief overview of the general mechanisms of inflammation is given below. The clinical hallmarks of inflammation are swelling (tumor), redness (rubor), heat (calor), pain (dolor) and loss of function of the affected area. These are the obvious signs of tissue protection, modulation and remodulation upon stimulation. Today we have considerable knowledge about the cellular and biochemical changes that explain these gross changes, and they can generally be described in terms of the non-specific as well as the specific inflammatory response.

Non-specific inflammatory response

Cells of phagocytic lineage (macrophages/monocytes, Langerhans cells, dendritic cells, neutrophils) are important components of the non-specific immune response, since they have a general capacity to ingest and destroy cells or threatening organisms. Other active cells, such as basophils, eosinophils and mast cells, release opsonins, which enhance phagocytosis, as well as cytotoxic factors that kill cells or bacteria. The natural killer (NK) cell acts on altered membranes of abnormal cells, and destroys the target cell by puncture of the cell membrane.

In inflammation, granulocytes and monocytes play the initiating roles. A general early inflammatory phenomenon is that the endothelial cells of the capillaries around the inflammatory site are induced to express adhesion molecules, enabling transmigration of leukocytes through the vascular wall to the affected site. By this mechanism, polymorphonucleated (PMN) leukocytes accumulate during the first 30–60 min at the site, using their capacity to phagocytose damaged cells or intruders, along with release of lysosomal enzymes. The activation of macrophages starts soon after PMN activation. Activated macrophages release large quantities of tissue-remodeling enzymes, eicosanoids and cytokines. The cytokines typically act in a cytokine network to induce specific responses. The release of IL-1, IL-6 and tumor necrosis factor-α (TNFα) induces further extravasation and activation of neutrophils, monocytes and lymphocytes by up-regulation of adhesion molecules, and also increases permeability directly by the release of vasoactive agents. The result is massive accumulation of activated leukocytes and edema. Macrophages also produce tissue factor, the counterpart of activated coagulation factor VII, to induce coagulation through the extrinsic pathway. Today, this pathway is known to be the most important way to induce the coagulation cascade *in vivo*.

The cytokines that are released from macrophages also induce the production of locally and systemically acting acute-phase proteins. The local response is in part generated by activation of the coagulation, kinin-forming and fibrinolytic pathways. Acute-phase proteins also increase vascular permeability and the expression of adhesion molecules, with the ability to induce contraction of vascular endothelial cells[5].

Specific inflammatory response

This response is induced after the initial non-specific response. Cellular processing to activate humoral (B cells) and cell-mediated (T cells) lymphocytes depends on specific antigen-presenting cells (APCs). APCs are dendritic cells, Langerhans cells, monocytes, macrophages and, in some cases, B cells. The APCs carry human leukocyte antigen (HLA) class II on their surfaces. HLA class I molecules are expressed on all nucleated cells, in contrast to HLA class II. T lymphocytes, that express CD3, are subdivided into T helper (T_H) cells expressing CD4, which recognize HLA class II, and T cytotoxic (T_C) cells expressing CD8, which recognize cells expressing HLA class I together with the antigen expressed on their surface. APCs have the capacity, after ingestion of material, to expose an antigen, together with HLA class II on their cell membranes, to T_H cells. This activation of T_H ($CD4^+$) cells results in the production of specific combinations of cytokines to drive the immune response in certain directions. This entire process takes place in the lymph node, where APCs enter to find a specific T_H cell that responds to the specific antigen.

When activated, T_H cells divide to enhance the production of cytokines that activate other cells such as monocytes/macrophages, T_C ($CD8^+$) cells that are involved in cytotoxic events and B cells that proliferate and differentiate into antibody-producing plasma cells, recognizing the same specific antigen. When B cells differentiate into plasma cells, the organization of the cytokine milieu will determine the type of antibodies that are produced.

T_H1 and T_H2

There exist principally two subgroups of T_H cells arising from naive (T_H0) cells, dependent on their specific cytokine profile produced[6], which can be more cytotoxic (T_H1) or a more immunoglobulin E (IgE)-mediated (T_H2) response. Recent data also indicate other populations of T_H cells with a regulating function (T_R). In development of the polarization of T_H cells, which takes place in the lymph node[7], the pivotal cytokines that stimulate T_H1 production are IL-12 and interferon-γ (IFNγ). The important cytokine concerning T_H2 development is IL-4.

The T_H1 cytokines IFNγ and IL-12 signal through different cellular pathways, activating the transcription factors (tf) STAT 1 and STAT 4, respectively. As a result of activating STAT 1 there will be a production of the master tf T-bet, which together with STAT 4 activation, increases the production of IFNγ. In contrast, activation of the IL-4 receptor in T_H2 development induces tf STAT 6, with production of the master tf GATA-3, and this results in increased production of IL-4 and IL-5[7]. Together, this indicates a delicate balance between T_H1 and T_H2 T-lymphocytes with their different cytokine profiles.

The result of the specific T_H1 cytokine response is activation of T_C cells, NK cells and macrophages involved in cell-mediated effects, but also switching of B cell activity towards some subgroups of IgG production. The T_H2 cells produce cytokines that trigger B cells to switch to IgE production and that also activate eosinophils.

A central cytokine in the activation of T cells is IL-2, which is mostly produced by T_H1 and T_C cells[8]. IL-2 is a proliferation factor for activated T cells, and stimulates the development of a subgroup of regulatory T cells. The IL-2 receptor exists as low-, intermediate- and high-affinity receptor subtypes. The high-affinity receptor (100-fold increased affinity compared with the low-affinity subtype) is expressed shortly after stimulation of the T cell receptor, with the resulting production of IL-2.

Hypersensitivity

Hypersensitivity, or an allergic reaction, differs from the protective immune response in that it is inappropriate to the host. The reaction includes activation of the humoral and/or cell-mediated immune response.

Hypersensitivity reactions are divided into four different types. Classification into types I, II and III depends on the specific type of antibody that reacts with the antigen challenge. The type I reaction is a T_H2-dependent reaction, which includes activation via IgE antibodies of mast cells and basophils and a release of histamine and other mediators. Activation of eosinophils causes airway inflammation and asthmatic hyperresponsiveness[9]. Other forms of type I hypersensitivity reactions are rhinitis and atopic dermatitis. The switch to IgE production and the accumulation of eosinophils are under control of the T_H2 cytokines IL-4 and IL-5, respectively. Other T_H2 cytokines such as IL-9 and IL-13 contribute to airway hypersensitivity in asthma[9].

In hypersensitivity types II and III, the antibodies involved are of non-IgE type, and these activate complement factors or bind to inflammatory cells (monocytes/macrophages and NK cells), which do not release histamine and other related substances.

Type IV hypersensitivity (delayed hypersensitivity reaction) is mediated by T_H1 cells. The antigen is processed by APCs, and following stimulation by cytokines from APCs the T_H1 is activated and produces cytokines that induce accumulation and activation of monocytes/macrophages. This reaction also involves induction and activation of cytotoxic T cells (T_C).

POSSIBLE INFLAMMATION-RELATED PATHOPHYSIOLOGICAL MECHANISMS IN OHSS

There are several endogenous ways to modulate the inflammatory response indirectly and directly or in terms of prolongation/shortening of the inflammation. Those that have been described in the context of OHSS are discussed below.

IL-10

A typical inflammatory response with the production of proinflammatory cytokines such as IL-1, IL-2 and TNFα is followed by IL-10 production with a latency of a few hours. The delayed secretion of IL-10 secures that the inflammatory response in time will be down-regulated. The isolated induction of IL-10 without preceding secretion of proinflammatory cytokines seems to be a rare event[10]. A delay of IL-10 increase during ovarian stimulation was seen in patients who later developed OHSS[4].

The cytokine IL-10 is a non-covalent homodimer with a molecular weight of 17–18 kDa[11]. There are two different IL-10 receptors described that cooperate in IL-10 binding. They are expressed on most hemopoietic cells. IL-10 is produced by $CD4^+$ and $CD8^+$ T cells, macrophages, B cells, dendritic cells[11,12] and keratinocytes[11]. The action of IL-10 includes a broad repertoire with multiple effects on many different cell types to induce an overall anti-inflammatory effect.

Inhibitory effects of IL-10 on APCs[13–16] occur by a decrease of the expression of costimulatory molecules[17,18]. Cytokine production (IL-1α and -β, IL-6, IL-10, IL-12, IL-18, granulocyte colony-stimulating factor (G-CSF), macrophage (M)-CSF, GM-CSF and TNFα) from activated monocytes/macrophages is inhibited by IL-10[11], which also inhibits the production of chemokines, reducing the recruitment of leukocytes[19–22]. The IL-10 effect on T cells is that IL-10 partially inhibits the production of cytokines such as IFNγ, TNFα and IL-4. This results in decreased activation of T_H1 and T_H2 cells. An important effect is the reduction of cyclo-oxygenase (COX)-2 expression and thereby prostaglandin production by a suppressive effect on nuclear factor kappa B (NFκB)[23].

In the human it is proposed that IL-10 is important to control autoimmune disease[24–26]. The net effect of lack of IL-10 function can be seen in mice with deletion of IL-10, typically with increased T_H1 response and increased clearance of infections[27]. Interestingly, the mice develop exaggerated allergic and asthmatic responses and will develop enterocolitis comparable to Crohn's disease.

The increase in coagulation capacity during any inflammation depends on the increased production of acute-phase proteins including coagulation factors such as activated factor VII and tissue factor. IL-10 reduces the amount of tissue factor produced by monocytes, thereby reducing the procoagulatory activity[28].

Vascular endothelial growth factor (VEGF) is the most potent inducer of vascular leakage[29], and has been proposed as a major factor involved in the development of OHSS[30], and in angiogenesis in the corpus luteum[31]. Nitric oxide (NO), also a vascular leakage factor, increases in the systemic blood circulation during gonadotropin stimulation[32], and is also upregulated by the expression of inducible NO synthetase (iNOS) enzyme abundant in monocytes/macrophages. Both VEGF and iNOS are down-regulated by IL-10[33,34], and IL-10 has the capacity to regulate the vascular leakage component induced by these factors.

Regulatory T cells and IL-2

Regulatory T cells (T_R), a subset of T_H cells[35], can be subdivided into T regulatory cells (Treg) and Tr1. Treg cells ($CD4^+CD25^+$) are unique owing to their expression of the α subunit CD25, which is an essential subunit of the high-affinity IL-2 receptor. The tf FOXP3 is a key regulator in Treg function since it induces the expression of high-affinity IL-2 receptor. The expression of this high-affinity IL-2 receptor makes Treg responsive at low IL-2 concentrations, and functional early in an inflammatory event. Treg works through direct cell contact as opposed to common immune cell interactions, which work mostly through intercellular communication by cytokine production.

The Tr1 cells that produce IL-10 are important for the Treg to gain control of autoreactive and hyperreactive reactions[36]. The Tr1 cells can by their production of IL-10 modulate the inflammatory response in T_H1, T_H2 and APCs[36]. The central role of Tr1 and IL-2 (Treg) in inflammation makes them likely candidates as pathophysiological factors in OHSS.

The above indicates a role for T cell regulation, as $CD8^+$ T cells exist in the ovary[37] and need surveillance. A pronounced cytotoxic response can be controlled by the production of IL-10 from macrophages and Tr1 cells. An OHSS patient with low production of IL-10 could react with increased inflammatory response due to a late increase to the concentration of IL-10 necessary to control the inflammatory response.

Glucocorticoids

Glucocorticoids are well-known anti-inflammatory factors with multiple effects on cells. Glucocorticoids affect the ovary by direct action on glucocorticoid receptors[38]. Cortisol and cortisol-binding protein are present in human follicular fluid[39], and an effect on granulosa cells has been suggested[40]. The follicle by itself regulates glucocorticoid activity by the action of 11β-hydroxysteroid dehydrogenase (11βHSD) type 2, which converts the biologically active cortisol into inactive cortisone and 11βHSD type 1, which in turn converts cortisone into cortisol[40].The mid-cycle luteinizing hormone (LH) surge, or human chorionic gonadotropin (hCG) as in IVF cycles, changes the expression to a marked increase in 11βHSD type 1[41], so that more local ovarian anti-inflammatory action is seen due to increased intrafollicular cortisol levels. A key regulator in this seems to be IL-1, which increases the mRNA levels of 11βHSD type 1 more than 30-fold[42] in ovarian surface epithelial cells.

We propose that defects in the ovarian induction of 11βHSD type 1 at ovulation may decrease the local ovarian anti-inflammatory mechanisms and lead to OHSS development. As one effect of glucocorticoids is the induction of IL-10 in macrophages[43], an impaired glucocorticoid response may result in decreased IL-10 regulation, which could be an important factor in the development of OHSS.

Inflammation in PCOS

Polycystic ovarian syndrome (PCOS) affects approximately 6–10% of reproductive-aged women[44], and the syndrome is one of the most established risk factors for OHSS development during gonadotropin stimulation[45–47]. One of the characteristics of PCOS is abdominal obesity, and this group of obese PCOS women has a risk of about 40%[44] to develop the metabolic syndrome, i.e. dyslipidemia, glucose intolerance or diabetes mellitus type 2 and hypertension[48].

Excess adipose tissue located at the abdomen seems to play a role in the pathophysiology of the metabolic syndrome[49]. An increased amount of white fat tissue results in increased production of proinflammatory cytokines such as TNFα, IL-6 and also IL-10, cytokines produced by monocytes/macrophages. In the white fat tissue of lean people, macrophages constitute < 10% of the cells, whereas in obese people they constitute up to 40% of the cells[50]. The increase in these cytokines in obese women is reduced with changes in lifestyle (increased physical activity, reduced body weight), which in turn reduces the prevalence of the metabolic syndrome[51].

Interestingly, macrophages have the capacity to induce iNOS to produce huge amounts of NO, which together with TNFα and other proinflammatory cytokines is instrumental in the development of dyslipidemia and type 2 diabetes[52]. PCOS *per se* may not increase the risk of developing type 2 diabetes, but the obesity often seen in PCOS may be the key factor for this development[53], since a relationship was seen between increased body mass index (BMI), IL-6 and C-reactive protein (CRP).

High IL-10 concentrations seem to protect against development of the metabolic syndrome both in obese and non-obese women, whereas a low IL-10 predisposes both groups to development of the metabolic syndrome[51]. In summary, a low IL-10 seems to be involved the development of the metabolic syndrome, which is more often seen in PCOS patients. Women with PCOS and low IL-10 production with or without obesity may be in a state of increased inflammation and thereby in a high-risk group to develop severe OHSS.

Inflammation in folliculogenesis

During folliculogenesis, an altered immune response due to differences in IL-10 concentration may be a factor in OHSS development[4]. The total numbers of T cells are low in the surrounding stroma and in the theca layer of growing follicles, but the cytotoxic ($CD8^+$) subtype is present[37]. Taking into account reactions that are dependent on T helper cells type 1 (T_H1), T_H2 lymphocytes and the balancing T_R cells, the situation during normal folliculogenesis can be considered as a balance between these cell types. This notion is based on studies that show the presence of T_H1 cytokines (IFNγ, IL-2), T_H2 cytokines (IL-4, IL-5) and the down-regulatory cytokine IL-10 (mostly produced in Tr1 cells and monocytes/macrophages) in follicular fluid[54]. During OHSS, there seems to be an extremely pronounced T_H1-like response, with high levels of IL-1, IL-2 and IL-6.

In our study of IVF patients, we found that the patients who later developed OHSS had lower IL-10 levels at the start of gonadotropin stimulation[4]. Low IL-10 production could permit an inflammatory response to an increase in T_H1 cytokine production, allowing an enhanced inflammatory response during follicular development.

Immune mechanisms in the ovary may also regulate angiogenesis during folliculogenesis and affect the development of OHSS. Relative hypoxia during rapid growth of the follicle or during inflammatory reactions may be instrumental in angiogenesis in the ovary. Hypoxia induces the expression of growth factors, of which VEGF is the most potent in relation to angiogenesis. IL-10 is also involved in angiogenesis as it down-regulates VEGF production[55].

Inflammation in ovulation/luteinization

The ovulatory cascade involves local alterations in and around the preovulatory follicle, which occur from onset of the LH surge until rupture of the follicle. In controlled gonadotropin stimulation for IVF, hCG is used as a substitute for LH. The triggering of the ovulatory cascade by hCG is obligatory for the development of OHSS, since OHSS will not develop without hCG/LH stimulation.

The cooperative actions of inflammatory mediators, such as plasminogen activator (PA) and plasmin, along with matrix metalloproteinases (MMPs), degrade the collagen fibers at the apex of the follicle and this results in decreased tensility. Simultaneously, vascular leakage and blood flow in the vasculature of the follicle are augmented. Inflammatory mediators such as prostaglandins[56] and leukotrienes[57] are involved in these vascular changes.

Inflammatory cells are also important in ovulation, and several reports have demonstrated that the abundance of various subsets of leukocytes increases in the ovulating follicle. Mast cells are located in the central medullary portion of the ovary[58], and in the thecal layer[59]. A preovulatory increase in histamine content has been observed in the human ovary[60].

The density of neutrophils in the ovary increases after the preovulatory LH surge, clearly described in rats[37], sheep[61] and pigs[62]. In the human these cells accumulate specifically in the tunica albuginea and theca layer of the preovulatory follicle[63]. Several lines of evidence suggest that macrophages are the most prominent leukocyte subtype in the follicle, and that activation of these cells is central for ovulation to occur. Macrophage numbers increase considerably in the human follicle wall at ovulation[63] by transmigration, involving leukocyte–endothelial cell recognition by specific adhesion molecules on endothelial cells of the ovary and adhesion receptors on leukocytes[64]. Macrophages carry the nuclear as well as membrane estrogen receptors, suggesting that they may respond directly to this steroid[65].

Instrumental in this follicular leukocyte extravasation are chemokines, a group of factors of great importance in both ovulation and OHSS. Human theca cells of large antral follicles produce the neutrophil-specific chemokine IL-8[66], and elevated IL-8 levels are seen in follicular fluids of IVF patients and of naturally cycling women after the spontaneous LH surge. The macrophage-specific chemokine monocyte chemotactic protein (MCP)-1 is found in high levels in human follicular fluid[67]. Decreased ovulation was observed when neutrophils were depleted from the peripheral blood of rats during ovulation[68] and when macrophages were depleted from mouse ovaries[68]. Changes in phenotype and secretory activity of some leukocytes to a more proinflammatory, promigratory profile[70,71] are other events in ovulation.

Several cytokines are produced at high levels in the ovary by invading leukocytes or by the theca and granulosa cells. A higher concentration of GM-CSF exists in follicular fluids of hyperstimulated women compared with naturally cycling women, and the receptor as well as the ligand is present in human granulosa-lutein cells[72]. Macrophage colony-stimulating factor (M-CSF) and its receptor (cFMS) are found in high concentrations in the human ovary[73].

Ovarian IL-1 induces ovulation and amplifies the LH-induced ovulatory response in *ex vivo* perfused rat ovaries[74], and the IL-1 receptor antagonist decreases LH-supported ovulation *in vivo*[71]. The effects of IL-1 in facilitating ovulation may be related to its stimulatory function of prostaglandins, MMPs, plasminogen activator activity and nitric oxide production, as well as IL-18[75].

Human granulose-lutein cells secrete IL-2[76], and an effect of IL-2 on the lutenization process has been proposed because of its ability to regulate progesterone production in human granulosa. The IL-2 production could also result in activation of Treg cells and thereby reduce inflammation. As macrophages seem to dominate the cellular response in ovulation/luteinization a regulatory effect of locally produced IL-10 should be taken into consideration.

Inflammation in hyperreactivity

We demonstrated an almost doubled prevalence of hypersensitivity (allergy) in patients with OHSS (36%) in comparison with controls (21%)[3]. Allergy was defined as the presence of documented type I- or type IV-mediated hypersensitivity (see below). The result suggested for the first time that systemic immunological mechanisms could be involved in OHSS development. In the same study we were unable to identify the increased presence of infection or intercurrent autoimmune disease in the OHSS group. We also showed lower levels of IL-10 at the start of gonadotropin stimulation in the OHSS group[4].

The amount of IL-10 produced is controlled to 50–75% by genes[52,77,78], and there also exists an intraindividual variation of about 20%[79]. Eleven promotor and two microsatellite variations have been described[77,78] in the IL-10 genome, together forming 13 common IL-10 haplotypes. Four of these haplotypes dominate, and are found in 75% of the population[80].

The expression of IL-10 increases during the early stages of a healthy pregnancy, whereas reduced amounts are described in the endometrium and placental tissues of women with recurrent spontaneous abortions and preeclampsia[27], and, in infertility, low IL-10 production has been described[81].

Reactivity against potential allergy-inducing antigens can be a normal step in the body, but in patients without overt hypersensitivity this reaction is rapidly down-regulated by Treg cells[82], whereas in the allergic patient this reaction dominates the process.

In hypersensitivity patients, the induction of tolerance by increasing concentrations of the antigen has recently been shown to induce IL-10-producing regulatory T cells[9,83–85].

Earlier studies demonstrated a shift from T_H2 to T_H1 immune response towards the allergen[86,87], with an increase in IgG antibodies and a decrease in the IgE-mediated response[88]. As IL-10 can induce a shift toward the production of IgG_4, this may have an effect on reducing hypersensitivity, which could persist for at least 3–4 years[89].

Other ways to induce hyposensibility include the use of topical or systemic corticosteroids, resulting in the inhibition of T cell activation and T_H2 cytokine expression as well as an increased production of IL-10 by macrophages[43]. *In vitro* studies of the immune response toward allergens shows that vitamin D_3 together with corticosteroids can induce T_R phenotypes, producing IL-10, in turn suppressing the T_H2 response[9,90]. Although clinically effective, corticosteroid therapy does not seems to alter the initial sensitization, as the reaction returns after cancellation of the medication.

In summary, IL-10 is central in regulation of the immune response, and a genetically controlled low production of IL-10 may have a central role in the control of hypersensibility, and control of the inflammatory response as seen in situations such as pregnancy and infectious disease.

CONCLUSION

Based on the restricted knowledge concerning the pathophysiology of OHSS we have today, we propose a simplified working hypothesis of the dysregulated immune functions that contribute to the development of OHSS.

In the normal situation of controlled gonadotropin stimulation, where IL-10 levels are within normal ranges, IL-10 controls and restricts the ovary-related inflammatory response (Figure 1). In contrast, with an inherently low IL-10 production, the ovary-related inflammatory response will escalate and contribute to the development of OHSS (Figure 2).

In this review, several immunological factors in the development of OHSS have been discussed. We acknowledge that the proposed hypothesis is still only a basic description of the complex immune mechanisms in the ovaries of OHSS patients. Rapid expansion of the immunology field, together with growing knowledge about intraovarian regulation of follicular development/ovulation, provides a new and complex research field concerning

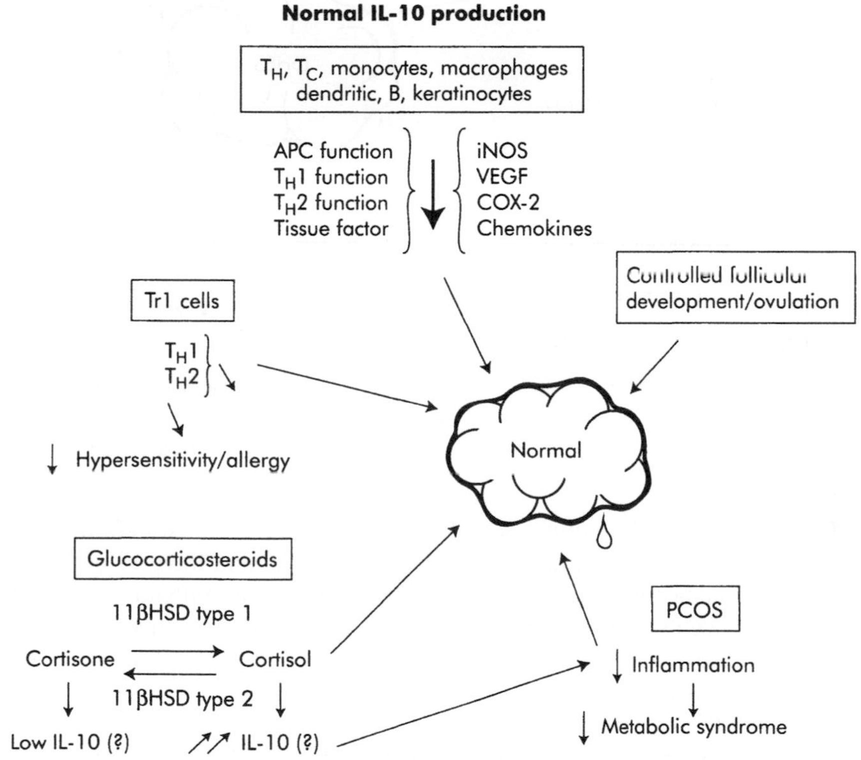

Figure 1 Controlled follicular development/ovulation and avoidance of OHSS due to normal interleukin-10 (IL-10) levels. IL-10 reduces the activation of antigen-presenting cells (APCs) and T helper (T_H) cells and induces a general reduction of vascular endothelial growth factor (VEGF), cyclooxygenase-2 (COX-2), inducible NO synthetase (iNOS), chemokines and tissue factor. T regulatory cells type 1 (Tr1) control T_H1 and T_H2 and thereby diminish hypersensitivity through the production of IL-10. A normal function of 11β-hydroxysteroid dehydrogenase (11βHSD) type 1 increases the potent anti-inflammatory cortisol, which induces IL-10 in macrophages. Normal IL-10 levels reduce polycystic ovarian syndrome (PCOS)-related inflammation. T_C, T cytotoxic cells

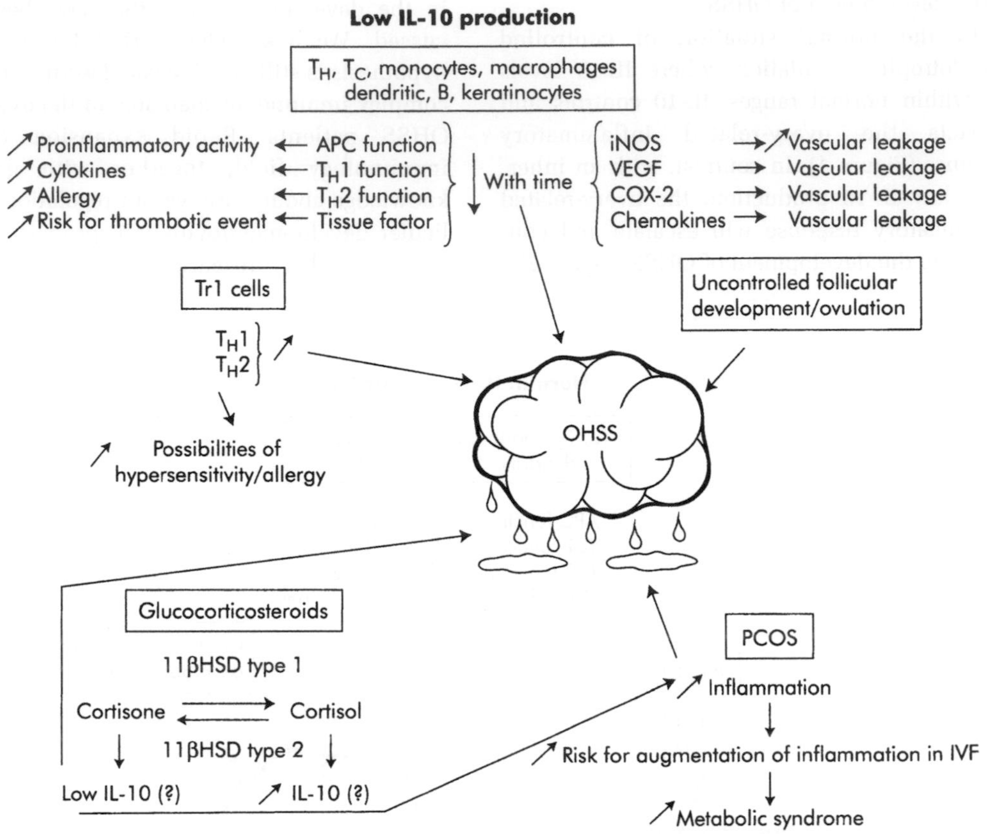

Figure 2 Development of OHSS due to low IL-10 levels (see Figure 1 for definitions). Low IL-10 levels increase the activity of APCs and T_H cells and induce a general increase of VEGF, COX-2, iNOS, chemokines and tissue factor. These changes result in increased proinflammatory activity, cytokines, allergy, thrombotic events and vascular leakage. Tr1 cells cannot control T_H1 and T_H2 cells and increase the possibility of hypersensibility. Increased function of 11βHSD type 2 decreases the potent anti-inflammatory cortisol and increases the amount of fairly inactive cortisone. The net effect is low IL-10 and increased PCOS-related inflammation. During uncontrolled follicular development/ovulation, the intraovarian inflammatory reaction is greatly enhanced. IVF, *in vitro* fertilization

immunology and OHSS. To be able to solve many of the problems concerning the identification of patients at risk for OHSS and its treatment, it is of importance not only to utilize modern molecular biology techniques (for example, gene expression profiling), but also to use material from OHSS patients identified in prospective studies with well-defined OHSS criteria. The significance of all results obtained should be challenged in prospective randomized studies testing different factors that are proposed to interfere in OHSS pathophysiology.

REFERENCES

1. Asch RH, Li HP, Balmaceda JP, et al. Severe ovarian hyperstimulation syndrome in assisted reproductive technology: definition of high risk groups. Hum Reprod 1991; 6: 1395–9.

2. Kelly CC, Lyall H, Petrie JR, et al. Low grade chronic inflammation in women with polycystic ovarian syndrome. J Clin Endocrinol Metab 2001; 86: 2453–5.

3. Enskog A, Henriksson M, Unander M, et al. Prospective study of the clinical and laboratory parameters of patients in whom ovarian hyperstimulation syndrome developed during controlled ovarian hyperstimulation for in vitro fertilization. Fertil Steril 1999; 71: 808–14.

4. Enskog A, Nilsson L, Brannstrom M. Low peripheral blood levels of the immunosuppressive cytokine interleukin 10 (IL-10) at the start of gonadotrophin stimulation indicates increased risk for development of ovarian hyperstimulation syndrome (OHSS). J Reprod Immunol 2001; 49: 71–85.

5. Millan J, Ridley AJ. Rho GTPases and leucocyte-induced endothelial remodelling. Biochem J 2005; 385: 329–37.

6. Mosmann TR, Coffman RL. TH1 and TH2 cells: different patterns of lymphokine secretion lead to different functional properties. Annu Rev Immunol 1989; 7: 145–73.

7. Neurath MF, Finotto S, Glimcher LH. The role of Th1/Th2 polarization in mucosal immunity. Nat Med 2002; 8: 567–73.

8. Gaffen SL, Liu KD. Overview of interleukin-2 function, production and clinical applications. Cytokine 2004; 28: 109–23.

9. Robinson DS, Larche M, Durham SR. Tregs and allergic disease. J Clin Invest 2004; 114: 1389–97.

10. Stenvinkel P, Ketteler M, Johnson RJ, et al. IL-10, IL-6, and TNF-alpha: central factors in the altered cytokine network of uremia – the good, the bad, and the ugly. Kidney Int 2005; 67: 1216–33.

11. Moore KW, de Waal Malefyt R, Coffman RL, et al. Interleukin-10 and the interleukin-10 receptor. Annu Rev Immunol 2001; 19: 683–765.

12. Trinchieri G. Regulatory role of T cells producing both interferon gamma and interleukin 10 in persistent infection. J Exp Med 2001; 194: F53–7.

13. Ding L, Shevach EM. IL-10 inhibits mitogen-induced T cell proliferation by selectively inhibiting macrophage costimulatory function. J Immunol 1992; 148: 3133–9.

14. Fiorentino DF, Zlotnik A, Vieira P, et al. IL-10 acts on the antigen-presenting cell to inhibit cytokine production by Th1 cells. J Immunol 1991; 146: 3444–51.

15. Macatonia SE, Doherty TM, Knight SC, et al. Differential effect of IL-10 on dendritic cell-induced T cell proliferation and IFN-gamma production. J Immunol 1993; 150: 3755–65.

16. Enk AH, Angeloni VL, Udey MC, et al. Inhibition of Langerhans cell antigen-presenting function by IL-10. A role for IL-10 in induction of tolerance. J Immunol 1993; 151: 2390–8.

17. Ding L, Linsley PS, Huang LY, et al. IL-10 inhibits macrophage costimulatory activity by selectively inhibiting the up-regulation of B7 expression. J Immunol 1993; 151: 1224–34.

18. Willems F, Marchant A, Delville JP, et al. Interleukin-10 inhibits B7 and intercellular adhesion molecule-1 expression on human monocytes. Eur J Immunol 1994; 24: 1007–9.

19. Berkman N, John M, Roesems G, et al. Inhibition of macrophage inflammatory protein-1 alpha expression by IL-10. Differential sensitivities in human blood monocytes and alveolar macrophages. J Immunol 1995; 155: 4412–18.

20. Rossi DL, Vicari AP, Franz-Bacon K, et al. Identification through bioinformatics of two new macrophage proinflammatory human chemokines: MIP-3alpha and MIP-3beta. J Immunol 1997; 158: 1033–6.

21. Marfaing-Koka A, Maravic M, Humbert M, et al. Contrasting effects of IL-4, IL-10 and corticosteroids on RANTES production by human monocytes. Int Immunol 1996; 8: 1587–94.

22. Kopydlowski KM, Salkowski CA, Cody MJ, et al. Regulation of macrophage chemokine expression by lipopolysaccharide in vitro and in vivo. J Immunol 1999; 163: 1537–44.

23. Berg DJ, Zhang J, Lauricella DM, et al. Il-10 is a central regulator of cyclooxygenase-2 expression and prostaglandin production. J Immunol 2001; 166: 2674–80.

24. Fillatreau S, Sweenie CH, McGeachy MJ, et al. B cells regulate autoimmunity by provision of IL-10. Nat Immunol 2002; 3: 944–50.

25. Saito I. Structure of IL-10 and its role in autoimmune exocrinopathy. Crit Rev Immunol 2000; 20: 153–65.

26. Yang Z, Chen M, Wu R, et al. Suppression of autoimmune diabetes by viral IL-10 gene transfer. J Immunol 2002; 168: 6479–85.

27. Pestka S, Krause CD, Sarkar D, et al. Interleukin-10 and related cytokines and receptors. Annu Rev Immunol 2004; 22: 929–79.

28. Pajkrt D, van der Poll T, Levi M, et al. Interleukin-10 inhibits activation of coagulation and fibrinolysis during human endotoxemia. Blood 1997; 89: 2701–5.

29. Dvorak HF, Brown LF, Detmar M, et al. Vascular permeability factor/vascular endothelial growth factor, microvascular hyperpermeability, and angiogenesis. Am J Pathol 1995; 146: 1029–39.

30. McClure N, Healy DL, Rogers PA, et al. Vascular endothelial growth factor as capillary permeability agent in ovarian hyperstimulation syndrome. Lancet 1994; 344: 235–6.

31. Ferrara N, Chen H, Davis-Smyth T, et al. Vascular endothelial growth factor is essential for corpus luteum angiogenesis. Nat Med 1998; 4: 336–40.

32. Ekerhovd E, Enskog A, Caidahl K, et al. Plasma concentrations of nitrate during the menstrual cycle, ovarian stimulation and ovarian hyperstimulation syndrome. Hum Reprod 2001; 16: 1334–9.

33. Kohno T, Mizukami H, Suzuki M, et al. Interleukin-10-mediated inhibition of angiogenesis and tumor growth in mice bearing VEGF-producing ovarian cancer. Cancer Res 2003; 63: 5091–4.

34. Huang CJ, Stevens BR, Nielsen RB, et al. Interleukin-10 inhibition of nitric oxide biosynthesis involves suppression of CAT-2 transcription. Nitric Oxide 2002; 6: 79–84.

35. Foussat A, Cottrez F, Brun V, et al. A comparative study between T regulatory type 1 and CD4+CD25+ T cells in the control of inflammation. J Immunol 2003; 171: 5018–26.

36. O'Garra A, Vieira P. Regulatory T cells and mechanisms of immune system control. Nat Med 2004; 10: 801–5.

37. Brannstrom M, Mayrhofer G, Robertson SA. Localization of leukocyte subsets in the rat ovary during the periovulatory period. Biol Reprod 1993; 48: 277–86.

38. Schreiber JR, Nakamura K, Erickson GF. Rat ovary glucocorticoid receptor: identification and characterization. Steroids 1982; 39: 569–84.

39. Andersen CY, Hornnes P. Intrafollicular concentrations of free cortisol close to follicular rupture. Hum Reprod 1994; 9: 1944–9.

40. Michael AE, Gregory L, Walker SM, et al. Ovarian 11 beta-hydroxysteroid dehydrogenase: potential predictor of conception by in-vitro fertilisation and embryo transfer. Lancet 1993; 342: 711–12.

41. Yong PY, Thong KJ, Andrew R, et al. Development-related increase in cortisol biosynthesis by human granulosa cells. J Clin Endocrinol Metab 2000; 85: 4728–33.

42. Gubbay O, Guo W, Rae MT, et al. Anti-inflammatory and proliferative responses in human and ovine ovarian surface epithelial cells. Reproduction 2004; 128: 607–14.

43. Hodge S, Hodge G, Flower R, et al. Methyl-prednisolone up-regulates monocyte interleukin-10 production in stimulated whole blood. Scand J Immunol 1999; 49: 548–53.

44. Apridonidze T, Essah PA, Iuorno MJ, et al. Prevalence and characteristics of the metabolic syndrome in women with polycystic ovary syndrome. J Clin Endocrinol Metab 2005; 90: 1929–35.

45. Lunenfeld B, Insler V. Gonadotrophin. Berlin: Thieme Verlag, 1978.

46. Kemmann E, Tavakoli F, Shelden RM, et al. Induction of ovulation with menotropins in women with polycystic ovary syndrome. Am J Obstet Gynecol 1981; 141: 58–64.

47. Delvigne A, Demoulin A, Smitz J, et al. The ovarian hyperstimulation syndrome in in-vitro

fertilization: a Belgian multicentric study. I. Clinical and biological features. Hum Reprod 1993; 8: 1353–60.

48. Hansen BC. The metabolic syndrome X. Ann NY Acad Sci 1999; 892: 1–24.

49. Lebovitz HE. Insulin resistance: definition and consequences. Exp Clin Endocrinol Diabetes 2001; 109 (Suppl 2): S135–48.

50. Weisberg SP, McCann D, Desai M, et al. Obesity is associated with macrophage accumulation in adipose tissue. J Clin Invest 2003; 112: 1796–808.

51. Esposito K, Pontillo A, Giugliano F, et al. Association of low interleukin-10 levels with the metabolic syndrome in obese women. J Clin Endocrinol Metab 2003; 88: 1055–8.

52. van Exel E, Gussekloo J, de Craen AJ, et al. Low production capacity of interleukin-10 associates with the metabolic syndrome and type 2 diabetes: the Leiden 85-Plus Study. Diabetes 2002; 51: 1088–92.

53. Mohlig M, Spranger J, Osterhoff M, et al. The polycystic ovary syndrome per se is not associated with increased chronic inflammation. Eur J Endocrinol 2004; 150: 525–32.

54. Brannstrom M, Enskog A. Leukocyte networks and ovulation. J Reprod Immunol 2002; 57: 47–60.

55. Huang S, Xie K, Bucana CD, et al. Interleukin 10 suppresses tumor growth and metastasis of human melanoma cells: potential inhibition of angiogenesis. Clin Cancer Res 1996; 2: 1969–79.

56. Larson L, Olofsson J, Hellberg P, et al. Regulation of prostaglandin biosynthesis by luteinizing hormone and bradykinin in rat preovulatory follicles in vitro. Prostaglandins 1991; 41: 111–21.

57. Matousek M, Mitsube K, Mikuni M, et al. Inhibition of ovulation in the rat by a leukotriene B(4) receptor antagonist. Mol Hum Reprod 2001; 7: 35–42.

58. Jones RE, Duvall D, Guillette LJ Jr. Rat ovarian mast cells: distribution and cyclic changes. Anat Rec 1980; 197: 489–93.

59. Nakamura Y, Smith M, Krishna A, et al. Increased number of mast cells in the dominant follicle of the cow: relationships among luteal, stromal, and hilar regions. Biol Reprod 1987; 37: 546–9.

60. Morikawa H, Okamura H, Takenaka A, et al. Histamine concentration and its effect on ovarian contractility in humans. Int J Fertil 1981; 26: 283–6.

61. Cavender JL, Murdoch WJ. Morphological studies of the microcirculatory system of periovulatory ovine follicles. Biol Reprod 1988; 39: 989–97.

62. Standaert FE, Zamora CS, Chew BP. Quantitative and qualitative changes in blood leukocytes in the porcine ovary. Am J Reprod Immunol 1991; 25: 163–8.

63. Brannstrom M, Pascoe V, Norman RJ, et al. Localization of leukocyte subsets in the follicle wall and in the corpus luteum throughout the human menstrual cycle. Fertil Steril 1994; 61: 488–95.

64. Bonello N, Norman RJ. Soluble adhesion molecules in serum throughout the menstrual cycle. Hum Reprod 2002; 17: 2272–8.

65. Willis C, Morris JM, Danis V, et al. Cytokine production by peripheral blood monocytes during the normal human ovulatory menstrual cycle. Hum Reprod 2003; 18: 1173–8.

66. Runesson E, Bostrom EK, Janson PO, et al. The human preovulatory follicle is a source of the chemotactic cytokine interleukin-8. Mol Hum Reprod 1996; 2: 245–50.

67. Arici A, Oral E, Bukulmez O, et al. Monocyte chemotactic protein-1 expression in human preovulatory follicles and ovarian cells. J Reprod Immunol 1997; 32: 201–19.

68. Brannstrom M, Bonello N, Norman RJ, et al. Reduction of ovulation rate in the rat by administration of a neutrophil-depleting monoclonal antibody. J Reprod Immunol 1995; 29: 265–70.

69. Van der Hoek KH, Maddocks S, Woodhouse CM, et al. Intrabursal injection of clodronate liposomes causes macrophage depletion and inhibits ovulation in the mouse ovary. Biol Reprod 2000; 62: 1059–66.

70. Leslie CA, Dubey DP. Increased PGE2 from human monocytes isolated in the luteal phase of the menstrual cycle. Implications for immunity? Prostaglandins 1994; 47: 41–54.

71. Simon C, Tsafriri A, Chun SY, et al. Interleukin-1 receptor antagonist suppresses human chorionic gonadotropin-induced ovulation in the rat. Biol Reprod 1994; 51: 662–7.

72. Jasper MJ, Brannstrom M, Olofsson JI, et al. Granulocyte-macrophage colony-stimulating factor: presence in human follicular fluid, protein secretion and mRNA expression by ovarian cells. Mol Hum Reprod 1996; 2: 555–62.

73. Shinetugs B, Runesson E, Bonello NP, et al. Colony stimulating factor-1 concentrations in blood and follicular fluid during the human menstrual cycle and ovarian stimulation: possible role in the ovulatory process. Hum Reprod 1999; 14: 1302–6.

74. Brannstrom M, Wang L, Norman RJ. Ovulatory effect of interleukin-1 beta on the perfused rat ovary. Endocrinology 1993; 132: 399–404.

75. Tsuji Y, Tamaoki TH, Hasegawa A, et al. Expression of interleukin-18 and its receptor in mouse ovary. Am J Reprod Immunol 2001; 46: 349–57.

76. Wang LJ, Robertson S, Seamark RF, et al. Lymphokines, including interleukin-2, alter gonadotropin-stimulated progesterone production and proliferation of human granulosa-luteal cells in vitro. J Clin Endocrinol Metab 1991; 72: 824–31.

77. Westendorp RG, Langermans JA, Huizinga TW, et al. Genetic influence on cytokine production and fatal meningococcal disease. Lancet 1997; 349: 170–3.

78. Reuss E, Fimmers R, Kruger A, et al. Differential regulation of interleukin-10 production by genetic and environmental factors – a twin study. Genes Immun 2002; 3: 407–13.

79. van der Linden MW, Huizinga TW, Stoeken DJ, et al. Determination of tumour necrosis factor-alpha and interleukin-10 production in a whole blood stimulation system: assessment of laboratory error and individual variation. J Immunol Meth 1998; 218: 63–71.

80. Kurreeman FA, Schonkeren JJ, Heijmans BT, et al. Transcription of the IL10 gene reveals allele-specific regulation at the mRNA level. Hum Mol Genet 2004; 13: 1755–62.

81. Westendorp RG, van Dunne FM, Kirkwood TB, et al. Optimizing human fertility and survival. Nat Med 2001; 7: 873.

82. Cavani A, Nasorri F, Ottaviani C, et al. Human CD25+ regulatory T cells maintain immune tolerance to nickel in healthy, nonallergic individuals. J Immunol 2003; 171: 5760–8.

83. Sundstedt A, O'Neill EJ, Nicolson KS, et al. Role for IL-10 in suppression mediated by peptide-induced regulatory T cells in vivo. J Immunol 2003; 170: 1240–8.

84. Francis JN, Till SJ, Durham SR. Induction of IL-10+CD4+CD25+ T cells by grass pollen immunotherapy. J Allergy Clin Immunol 2003; 111: 1255–61.

85. Chen Y, Kuchroo VK, Inobe J, et al. Regulatory T cell clones induced by oral tolerance: suppression of autoimmune encephalomyelitis. Science 1994; 265: 1237–40.

86. Ebner C, Siemann U, Bohle B, et al. Immunological changes during specific immunotherapy of grass pollen allergy: reduced lymphoproliferative responses to allergen and shift from TH2 to TH1 in T-cell clones specific for Phl p 1, a major grass pollen allergen. Clin Exp Allergy 1997; 27: 1007–15.

87. Jutel M, Pichler WJ, Skrbic D, et al. Bee venom immunotherapy results in decrease of IL-4 and IL-5 and increase of IFN-gamma secretion in specific allergen-stimulated T cell cultures. J Immunol 1995; 154: 4187–94.

88. Platts-Mills T, Vaughan J, Squillace S, et al. Sensitisation, asthma, and a modified Th2 response in children exposed to cat allergen: a population-based cross-sectional study. Lancet 2001; 357: 752–6.

89. Durham SR, Walker SM, Varga EM, et al. Long-term clinical efficacy of grass-pollen immunotherapy. N Engl J Med 1999; 341: 468–75.

90. Barrat FJ, Cua DJ, Boonstra A, et al. In vitro generation of interleukin 10-producing regulatory CD4(+) T cells is induced by immunosuppressive drugs and inhibited by T helper type 1 (Th1)- and Th2-inducing cytokines. J Exp Med 2002; 195: 603–16.

CHAPTER 13

Genetic aspects of ovarian hyperstimulation syndrome

Anne Delbaere, Lucia Montanelli, Guillaume Smits, Sabine Costagliola and Gilbert Vassart

While nearly all cases of ovarian hyperstimulation (OHSS) arise as a complication of ovulation induction therapies, spontaneous forms of the syndrome have been reported in rare instances during pregnancy[1–8]. Several cases were reported during multiple pregnancies[7] or hydatidiform moles, known to be associated with supraphysiological production of human chorionic gonadotropin (hCG)[5]. Other cases were associated with hypothyroidism, and it was proposed that the high levels of thyroid-stimulating hormone (TSH) could stimulate the ovaries[6]. Some cases were recurrent, with development of the syndrome observed in 2–6 consecutive pregnancies[1–4].

MUTATIONS IN THE FOLLICLE STIMULATING HORMONE RECEPTOR GENE IN SPONTANEOUS OHSS

It is in the last category of patients, with recurrent OHSS, that four different mutations were recently identified in exon 10 of the follicle stimulating hormone (FSH) receptor gene (Figure 1)[9–12].

Smits *et al.*[9] identified a heterozygous mutation in the FSH receptor of a patient presenting with spontaneous OHSS during each of her four pregnancies[2]. The mutation consisted of the substitution of an adenine for a guanine at the first base of codon 567 of the FSH receptor gene, resulting in the replacement of an aspartic acid with an asparagine at the cytoplasmic end of transmembrane helix VI in the serpentine domain (mutation D567N) (Figure 1). Vasseur *et al.*[10] identified another heterozygous mutation in a patient who developed OHSS during all of her four pregnancies that went on beyond 6 weeks of gestation. The mutation was also found in the DNA of two of the patient's sisters, who similarly presented with spontaneous OHSS during their pregnancies, but not in that of a third, unaffected sister. It consisted of the substitution of a thymidine for a cytosine at the second base of codon 449, resulting in the substitution of isoleucine for threonine at the upper part of the third transmembrane domain of the receptor (mutation T449I) (Figure 1). More recently, Montanelli *et al.*[11] described a distinct heterozygous mutation in a patient who presented with spontaneous OHSS during each of her two pregnancies. The mutation was also found in the DNA of her sister who developed OHSS during her unique pregnancy[4]. As for the mutation described by Vasseur *et al.*, it also involved codon 449, but at its first base, with substitution of a guanine for an adenine, causing a different amino acid replacement of a

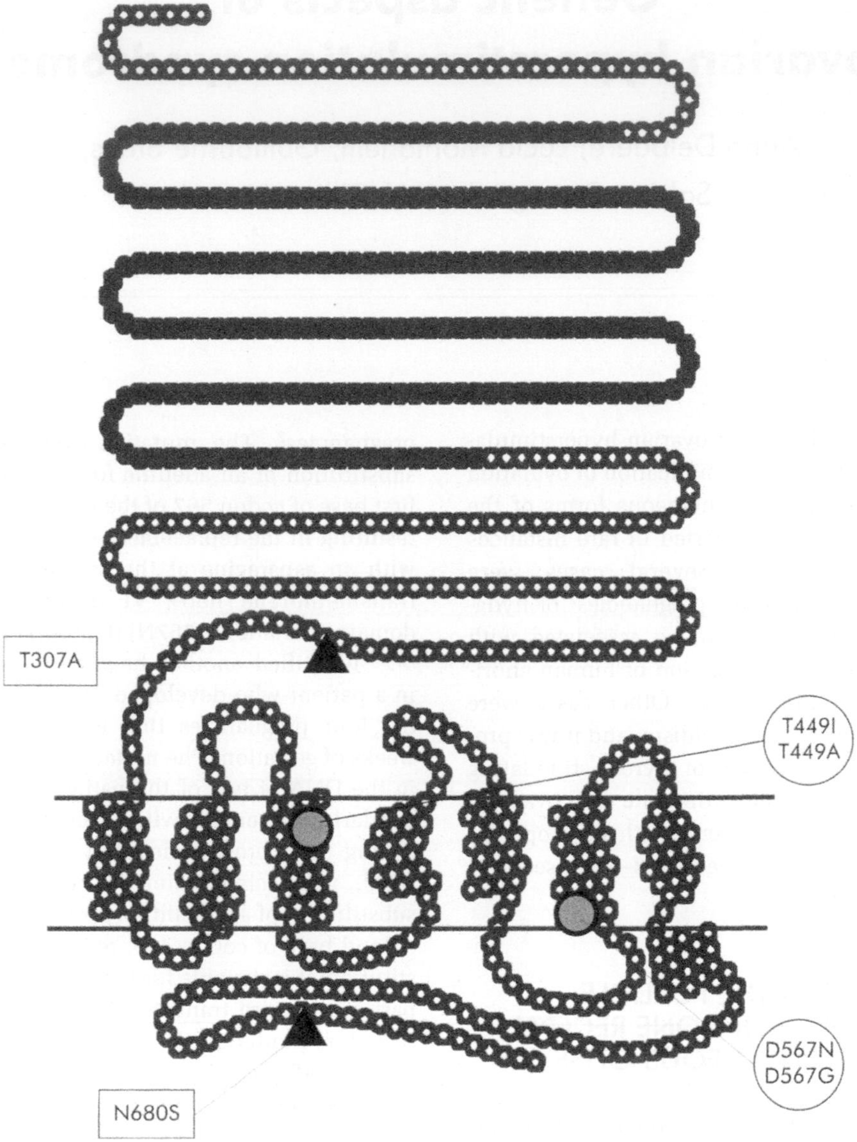

Figure 1 Schematic representation of the follicle stimulating hormone (FSH) receptor with locations of the D567N/G and T449I/A mutations (gray circles) identified in patients presenting spontaneous OHSS. The locations of polymorphisms T307A and N680S of the FSH receptor are represented by black triangles

threonine with an alanine (mutation T449A)[11] (Figure 1). A fourth mutation was identified in a patient diagnosed as having a hyperreactio luteinalis[8]. This clinical condition appears to be similar to spontaneous OHSS when it develops in the first trimester of pregnancy, which was the case in this patient. Similarly to the mutation described by Smits *et al.*,[9] the mutation implicated codon 567 of the FSH receptor gene but at its second base, consisting of the substitution of a guanine for an adenine, which induced the replacement of an aspartic acid with a glycine at the cytoplasmic end of transmembrane helix VI in the serpentine domain (mutation D567G)[12] (Figure 1). This last mutation had been previously reported in a hypophysectomized man, who, despite undetectable serum gonadotropin levels had normal testis volume and semen parameters[13]. It was the first-described activating mutation of the FSH receptor which autonomously sustained spermatogenesis in the absence of gonadotropins[13]. The functional characterization of the mutant FSH receptors in transfection experiments revealed that their sensitivity to FSH was minimally affected, but they all displayed an abnormally high sensitivity to hCG (Figure 2)[9–11,14]. In addition, all mutant receptors also displayed constitutive activity together with an increased sensitivity to TSH[9–11,14]. In the initial report, the T449I mutant receptor appeared to produce similar basal levels of cyclic adenosine monophosphate (cAMP) as the wild-type receptor, and could not be activated by TSH[10]. However, in contrast to the original description, further site-directed mutagenesis and functional experiments demonstrated that the T449I mutant FSH receptor also showed constitutive activity and an abnormal responsiveness to TSH[14]. Unexpectedly, the four mutations reported so far affected the serpentine portion of the FSH receptor rather than the hormone-binding ectodomain of the protein, which is known to be responsible for recognition specificity in glycoprotein hormone receptors[15,16]. This observation led to the hypothesis that the emergence of chorionic gonadotropin (CG) during the evolution of primates has been accompanied by the development of an intramolecular barrier to activation, within the serpentine domain of the FSH receptor, preventing its promiscuous activation by CG[17]. Indeed, study of the phenotype of spontaneous FSH receptor mutants and additional site-directed mutagenesis experiments established a clear relationship between constitutive activity and lowering of specificity in FSH receptor mutants[14]. The increase in sensitivity to hCG is accompanied by a very modest increase in binding affinity. This is consistent with the suggestion that the gain of sensitivity of the mutants to hCG would be due to lowering of an intramolecular barrier to activation rather than to an increase in binding affinity[17], with the consequence that a physiological concentration of hCG would become an effective FSH receptor stimulus during early pregnancy. Interestingly, it seems that protection of the TSH receptor against stimulation by hCG has evolved differently, relying on the hormone-binding ectodomain to avoid pregnancy hyperthyroidism[15,18].

RELATIONSHIP BETWEEN MUTANT FSH RECEPTORS AND SPONTANEOUS OHSS

The abnormal functionality of the mutant FSH receptors *in vitro* provides a rational explanation for their implication in the development of spontaneous OHSS *in vivo*. During pregnancy, the expression of FSH receptors decreases drastically in the corpus luteum, but remains constant in granulosa cells of developing follicles[19]. These receptors are usually not or very weakly stimulated during pregnancy, as pituitary gonadotropins fall to very low or undetectable levels in the serum. In the presence of a mutation rendering them abnormally sensitive to hCG, these receptors are stimulated under the action of pregnancy-derived hCG, resulting in the recruitment and growth of a follicular

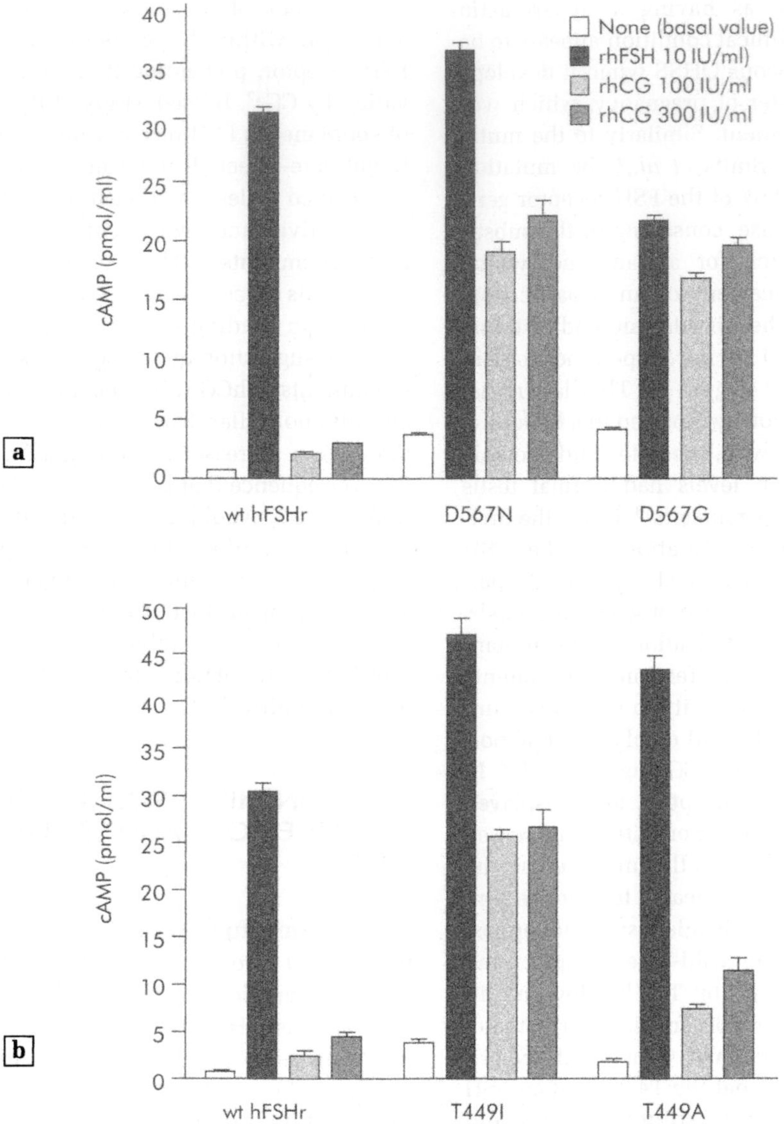

Figure 2 Functional characteristics of the four follicle stimulating hormone (FSH) mutant receptors identified in patients presenting spontaneous OHSS. Levels of cyclic adenosine monophosphate (cAMP) observed using COS-7 cells transfected with wild-type human FSH receptor (wt hFSHr), D567N, D567G mutants (a) and T449I, T449A mutants (b) after stimulation with recombinant human (rh) FSH (10 IU/ml) and increasing concentrations of recombinant human chorionic gonadotropin (rhCG) (100–300 IU/ml). Each graph represents the mean ± SEM of at least two separate experiments

cohort. Accordingly, the follicles enlarge and acquire LH receptors on granulosa cells which are further stimulated by hCG, inducing follicular luteinization together with the secretion of vasoactive molecules responsible for development of the syndrome.

The stimulation of the mutated FSH receptors most likely occurs at a threshold level of hCG which could vary according to the type of mutation, as suggested by *in vitro* site-directed mutagenesis experiments[14]. hCG usually peaks between 8 and 10 weeks of pregnancy and declines thereafter. In the same way, the symptomatology of most spontaneous cases of OHSS develops as of 8 weeks' amenorrhea, culminating at the end of the first trimester of pregnancy. From these findings, it appears that the development of spontaneous OHSS is the result of a non-physiological interaction between pregnancy-derived hCG and the ovarian FSH receptor, either in the presence of normal levels of hCG with a mutated FSH receptor, or in the presence of abnormally high levels of hCG as found in molar or multiple pregnancies, with a presumably normal FSH receptor[20]. Indeed, it has been shown recently that hCG was able to stimulate the FSH receptor in conditions that mimic a high ligand concentration[15,21]. This interaction between hCG and the FSH receptor is likely to be a prerequisite in the development of spontaneous OHSS, and could explain why symptoms in spontaneous cases of OHSS appear later than in iatrogenic OHSS, in which follicular recruitment and enlargement occur during ovarian stimulation with exogenous FSH[20] (Figure 3). Hence, spontaneous forms of OHSS generally occur between 8 and 14 weeks' amenorrhea, differing from iatrogenic OHSS starting usually between 3 and 5 weeks' amenorrhea.

FROM SPONTANEOUS TO IATROGENIC OHSS

Although differing by the timing of their occurrence, spontaneous and iatrogenic OHSS share similar pathophysiological sequences: massive recruitment and growth of ovarian follicles, extensive luteinization provoked by hCG and oversecretion of vasogenic molecules by luteinized corpora lutea (Figure 3). FSH receptor mutations being directly implicated in the development of spontaneous OHSS, it was tempting to consider the possibility that such mutations or polymorphisms in the FSH receptor gene could constitute risk factors in the development of the much more frequent iatrogenic OHSS.

In contrast to naturally occurring mutations which appear to be rather rare, the FSH receptor and its promoter display some very common single-nucleotide polymorphisms. Two non-synonymous polymorphisms have been described in exon 10 of the FSH receptor[22]. The first is located at nucleotide position 919, occupied either by adenine or by guanine, leading to either threonine or alanine at position 307 of the receptor (T307A), just before the beginning of the first transmembrane helix (Figure 1)[22]. The second is located at nucleotide position 2039 occupied either by adenine or guanine, leading to either asparagine or serine at position 680 of the receptor (N680S), located intracellularly at the end of its C-terminal tail (Figure 1). In the Caucasian population, the two FSH polymorphisms in exon 10 almost invariably occur in two haplotypes, leading to two allelic variants: threonine307–asparagine680 (allele TN) and alanine307–serine680 (allele AS)[23]. Recent reports suggest that the FSH receptor genotype could play a role *in vivo* in the ovarian response to FSH stimulation. Analysis of the FSH receptor polymorphism at position 680 showed that patients homozygous for serine in position 680 (SS) displayed a slightly higher basal FSH level[24–26]. In addition, higher requirements of exogenous FSH were necessary to achieve successful ovarian stimulation for *in vitro* fertilization (IVF) in patients with the SS680 genotype compared with patients with the NS680 or NN680 genotype[24]. In another retrospective

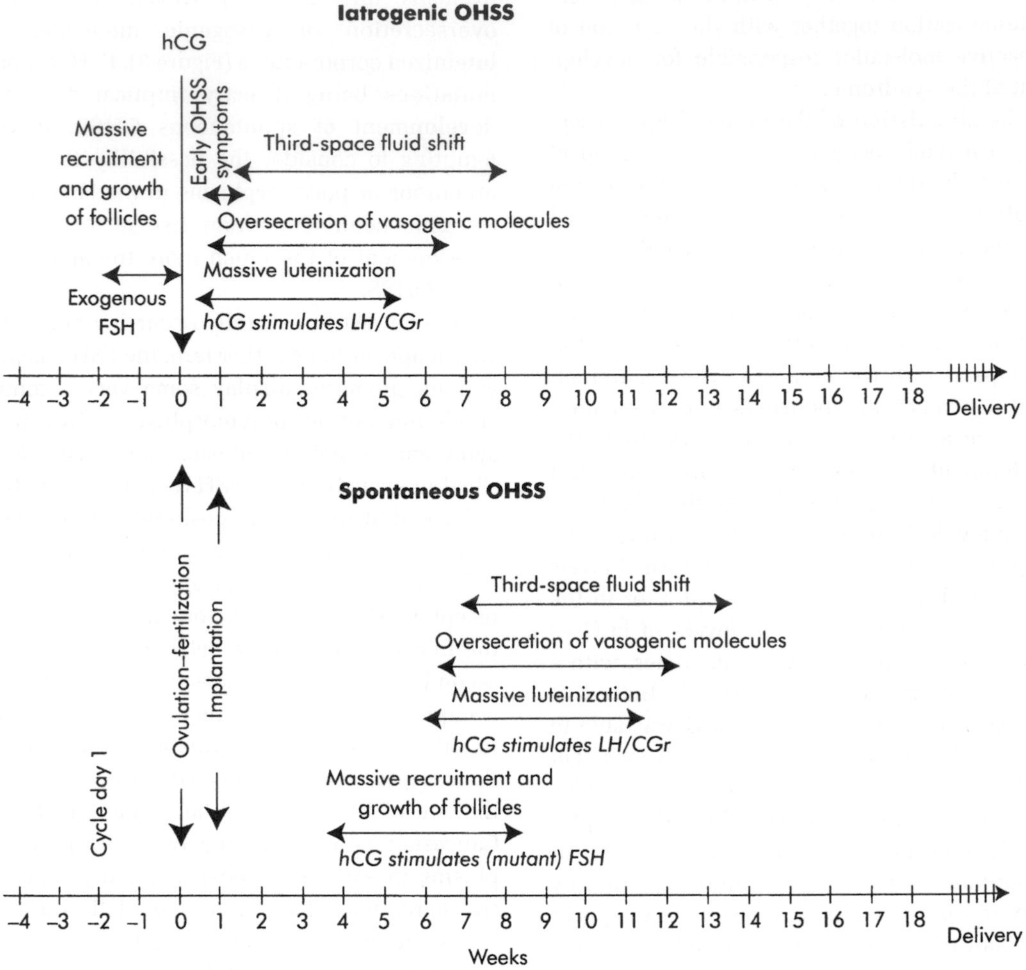

Figure 3 Pathophysiological sequences of iatrogenic and spontaneous OHSS. In the iatrogenic form, follicular recruitment and enlargement occur during ovarian stimulation with exogenous follicle stimulating hormone (FSH). In the spontaneous form, follicular recruitment and enlargement occur later through promiscuous stimulation, by pregnancy-derived human chorionic gonadotropin (hCG), of a mutated FSH receptor (abnormally sensitive to hCG) or a wild-type receptor (in the presence of abnormally high levels of hCG). In both forms, massive luteinization of enlarged stimulated ovaries ensues, inducing the release of vasoactive mediators, leading to development of the symptoms. CG, chorionic gonadotropin; LH, luteinizing hormone; r, receptor. From reference 20 ©European Society of Human Reproduction and Embryology. Reproduced by permission of Oxford University Press/Human Reproduction

study, the presence of serine in position 680 was associated with poor responses to gonadotropin stimulation in IVF, suggesting that individuals with the SS680 genotype could be associated with decreased FSH sensitivity[27]. However, a study conducted among normogonadotropic anovulatory patients resistant to clomiphene citrate could not establish associations between FSH receptor genotype and ovarian sensitivity during ovulation induction with exogenous FSH[26]. It is possible that these discrepancies are related to differences in the ovarian stimulation protocols: in anovulatory patients, the treatment aims at monofollicular development, while for IVF, it aims at multifollicular development. The supraphysiological doses of FSH used during IVF stimulation protocols could therefore reveal differences in ovarian response according to FSH receptor genotype, which could not be manifest in more physiological conditions.

Analysis of the FSH receptor polymorphism was recently performed among patients who developed iatrogenic OHSS[28]. This pilot study involved 37 Caucasian patients who developed OHSS after an IVF cycle compared with a control IVF population (130 patients who did not develop OHSS after an IVF cycle) and with a Caucasian control population (99 patients)[28]. The OHSS population, as well as the control IVF population, displayed higher allelic frequencies of S680 in the FSH receptor gene than those observed in the Caucasian control population. Although not fully explained, this difference could be related to the inclusion of patients presenting ovulatory disorders in the IVF control population and in the OHSS group[25,26]. No significant difference could be established for the S680N polymorphism of the FSH receptor between the OHSS group and the IVF control population[28]. However, a significant enrichment in the N680 allele was observed as the severity of the syndrome increased[28]. This difference persisted when the analysis was performed between mild, moderate and severe OHSS patients who were pregnant. Bearing in mind the limitations of the small number of patients studied, which could introduce potential sample biases, these data suggested that the FSH receptor genotype could not predict iatrogenic OHSS, but that the N680 allele of the FSH receptor could be a predictor of severity of symptoms among OHSS patients[28].

More clinical data are required to determine further the exact relationship between FSH receptor genotypes and the severity of OHSS symptoms after ovarian stimulation. In addition, further experimental data are necessary to understand the *in vivo* association of FSH receptor alleles and the response to ovarian stimulation. So far, the *in vitro* functional characterization of the two FSH receptor variants (alleles TN and AS) in transfection experiments could not show significant differences in binding affinity, either in the production of cAMP or inositol phosphate after stimulation with FSH[23,25]. Several hypotheses have been proposed, such as different expression of the variants at the cell surface, differences in their turnover or in their down-regulation rate, or different affinity for various FSH isoforms[24]. On the other hand, the S680N polymorphism of the FSH receptor could play no direct functional role in the development of OHSS, but instead be in linkage disequilibrium with other polymorphisms in the same or neighboring gene(s).

CONCLUSIONS AND PERSPECTIVES

The identification of mutations in the FSH receptor of patients presenting spontaneous OHSS provides for the first time a molecular basis for the physiopathology of spontaneous forms of the syndrome, and opens new perspectives to understand the development of iatrogenic OHSS. Being able to predict the individual ovarian response to exogenous FSH remains a challenge for IVF teams. While a mutation in the FSH receptor gene should be sought in the presence of recurrent or familial spontaneous OHSS, future work should aim to identify susceptibility genes in the development of iatrogenic OHSS. The individual response to controlled ovarian hyperstimulation is most likely a polygenic trait, as recently suggested by de Castro *et al.*, who provided evidence of genetic interactions between the FSH receptor and estrogen receptors α and β genes in relation to controlled ovarian hyperstimulation outcome[29]. The genetic background of the patient probably also plays a role in susceptibility to the increase of vascular permeability. Two clinical entities have been described in iatrogenic OHSS: early forms occurring 3–7 days after triggering of ovulation by hCG, and late forms developing 12–17 days after ovulation in close association with an initiated pregnancy[30,31]. The early pattern is related to an excessive response to gonadotropin stimulation, while the late pattern is more likely to be severe and is induced by endogenous hCG in conception cycles. Although the clinical sequences of the syndrome are very similar in both forms, it is possible that susceptibility to one or the other form differs between both patterns: in the early form, the genetic background of the patient could influence the ovarian hyperresponse to exogenous FSH, while in the late form, it would be more implicated in stimulation of the corpora lutea by hCG. OHSS can indeed be viewed as a tremendous exaggeration of the local inflammatory-like reactions which accompany angiogenesis during corpus luteum formation in a normal menstrual cycle, with a massive release of vasoactive molecules such as vascular endothelial growth factor[32,33], angiotensin II[34,35] and various interleukins[36]. As the release of these molecules reaches a threshold, physiological control mechanisms can be overstretched, leading to development of the symptoms of the syndrome. The respective genes of these vasoactive molecules could also constitute candidate susceptibility genes in the development of iatrogenic OHSS. These association studies will require large series of patients, which will most probably only be obtained through multicentric studies. The identification of patients susceptible to elicit a hyperresponse to standard stimulation treatments would allow adaptation of their treatment and avoidance, if not completely at least to a large extent, of OHSS, which remains a frequent and potentially life-threatening complication of IVF.

ACKNOWLEDGMENTS

We thank members of the Laboratory of Research on Human Reproduction and of the Institut de Recherche Interdisciplinaire en Biologie Humaine et Moléculaire (IRIBHM) for helpful support and discussion.

REFERENCES

1. Zalel Y, Orvieto R, Ben Rafael Z, et al. Recurrent spontaneous ovarian hyperstimulation syndrome associated with polycystic ovary syndrome. Gynecol Endocrinol 1995; 9: 313–15.
2. Olatunbosun OA, Gilliland B, Brydon LA, et al. Spontaneous ovarian hyperstimulation syndrome in four consecutive pregnancies. Clin Exp Obstet Gynecol 1996; 23: 127–32.
3. Edi-Osagie EC, Hopkins RE. Recurrent idiopathic ovarian hyperstimulation syndrome in pregnancy. Br J Obstet Gynaecol 1997; 104: 952–4.
4. Di Carlo C, Bruno P, Cirillo D, et al. Increased concentrations of renin, aldosterone and Ca125 in a case of spontaneous, recurrent, familial, severe ovarian hyperstimulation syndrome. Hum Reprod 1997; 12: 2115–17.
5. Ludwig M, Gembruch U, Bauer O, et al. Ovarian hyperstimulation syndrome (OHSS) in a spontaneous pregnancy with fetal and placental triploidy: information about the general pathophysiology of OHSS. Hum Reprod 1998; 13: 2082–17.
6. Nappi RG, Di Naro E, D'Aries AP, et al. Natural pregnancy in hypothyroid woman complicated

by spontaneous ovarian hyperstimulation syndrome. Am J Obstet Gynecol 1998; 178: 610–11.

7. Check JH, Choe JK, Nazari A. Hyperreactio luteinalis despite the absence of a corpus luteum and suppressed serum follicle stimulating concentrations in a triplet pregnancy. Hum Reprod 2000; 15: 1043–5.

8. Suzuki S. Comparison between spontaneous ovarian hyperstimulation syndrome and hyperreactio luteinalis. Arch Gynecol Obstet 2004; 269: 227–9.

9. Smits G, Olatunbosun O, Delbaere A, et al. Ovarian hyperstimulation syndrome due to a mutation in the follicle-stimulating hormone receptor. N Engl J Med 2003; 349: 760–6.

10. Vasseur C, Rodien P, Beau I, et al. A chorionic gonadotropin-sensitive mutation in the follicle-stimulating hormone receptor as a cause of familial gestational spontaneous ovarian hyperstimulation syndrome. N Engl J Med 2003; 349: 753–9.

11. Montanelli L, Delbaere A, Di Carlo C, et al. A mutation in the follicle-stimulating hormone receptor as a cause of familial spontaneous ovarian hyperstimulation syndrome. J Clin Endocrinol Metab 2004; 89: 1255–8.

12. Delbaere A, Smits G, De Leener A, et al. Understanding ovarian hyperstimulation syndrome. Endocrine 2005; 26: 285–90.

13. Gromoll J, Simoni M, Nieschlag E. An activating mutation of the follicle-stimulating hormone receptor autonomously sustains spermatogenesis in a hypophysectomized man. J Clin Endocrinol Metab 1996; 81: 1367–70.

14. Montanelli L, Van Durme JJ, Smits G, et al. Modulation of ligand selectivity associated with activation of the transmembrane region of the human follitropin receptor. Mol Endocrinol 2004; 18: 2061–73.

15. Smits G, Campillo M, Govaerts C, et al. Glycoprotein hormone receptors: determinants in leucine-rich repeats responsible for ligand specificity. EMBO J 2003; 22: 2692–703.

16. Fan QR, Hendrickson WA. Structure of human follicle-stimulating hormone in complex with its receptor. Nature 2005; 433: 269–77.

17. Vassart G, Pardo L, Costagliola S. A molecular dissection of the glycoprotein hormone receptors. Trends Biochem Sci 2004; 29: 119–26.

18. Rodien P, Bremont C, Sanson ML, et al. Familial gestational hyperthyroidism caused by a mutant thyrotropin receptor hypersensitive to human chorionic gonadotropin. N Engl J Med 1998; 339: 1823–6.

19. Simoni M, Gromoll J, Nieschlag E. The follicle-stimulating hormone receptor: biochemistry, molecular biology, physiology, and pathophysiology. Endocr Rev 1997; 18: 739–73.

20. Delbaere A, Smits G, Olatunbosun O, et al. New insights into the pathophysiology of ovarian hyperstimulation syndrome. What makes the difference between spontaneous and iatrogenic syndrome? Hum Reprod 2004; 19: 486–9.

21. Vischer HF, Granneman JC, Noordam MJ, et al. Ligand selectivity of gonadotropin receptors. Role of the beta-strands of extracellular leucine-rich repeats 3 and 6 of the human luteinizing hormone receptor. J Biol Chem 2003; 278: 15505–13.

22. Simoni M, Nieschlag E, Gromoll J. Isoforms and single nucleotide polymorphisms of the FSH receptor gene: implications for human reproduction. Hum Reprod Update 2002; 8: 413–21.

23. Simoni M, Gromoll J, Hoppner W, et al. Mutational analysis of the follicle-stimulating hormone (FSH) receptor in normal and infertile men: identification and characterization of two discrete FSH receptor isoforms. J Clin Endocrinol Metab 1999; 84: 751–5.

24. Perez MM, Gromoll J, Behre HM, et al. Ovarian response to follicle-stimulating hormone (FSH) stimulation depends on the FSH receptor genotype. J Clin Endocrinol Metab 2000; 85: 3365–9.

25. Sudo S, Kudo M, Wada S, et al. Genetic and functional analyses of polymorphisms in the human FSH receptor gene. Mol Hum Reprod 2002; 8: 893–9.

26. Laven JS, Mulders AG, Suryandari DA, et al. Follicle-stimulating hormone receptor polymorphisms in women with normogonadotropic anovulatory infertility. Fertil Steril 2003; 80: 986–92.

27. De Castro F, Ruiz R, Montoro L, et al. Role of follicle-stimulating hormone receptor Ser680Asn polymorphism in the efficacy of follicle-stimulating hormone. Fertil Steril 2003; 80: 571–6.
28. Daelemans C, Smits G, de Maertelaer V, et al. Prediction of severity of symptoms in iatrogenic ovarian hyperstimulation syndrome by follicle-stimulating hormone receptor Ser680Asn polymorphism. J Clin Endocrinol Metab 2004; 89: 6310–15.
29. De Castro F, Moron FJ, Montoro L, et al. Human controlled ovarian hyperstimulation outcome is a polygenic trait. Pharmacogenetics 2004; 14: 285–93.
30. Lyons CA, Wheeler CA, Frishman GN, et al. Early and late presentation of the ovarian hyperstimulation syndrome: two distinct entities with different risk factors. Hum Reprod 1994; 9: 792–9.
31. Papanikolaou EG, Tournaye H, Verpoest W, et al. Early and late ovarian hyperstimulation syndrome: early pregnancy outcome and profile. Hum Reprod 2005; 20: 636–41.
32. McClure N, Healy DL, Rogers PA, et al. Vascular endothelial growth factor as capillary permeability agent in ovarian hyperstimulation syndrome. Lancet 1994; 344: 235–6.
33. Levin ER, Rosen GF, Cassidenti DL, et al. Role of vascular endothelial cell growth factor in ovarian hyperstimulation syndrome. J Clin Invest 1998; 102: 1978–85.
34. Delbaere A, Bergmann PJ, Gervy-Decoster C, et al. Angiotensin II immunoreactivity is elevated in ascites during severe ovarian hyperstimulation syndrome: implications for pathophysiology and clinical management. Fertil Steril 1994; 62: 731–7.
35. Delbaere A, Bergmann PJ, Gervy-Decoster C, et al. Prorenin and active renin concentrations in plasma and ascites during severe ovarian hyperstimulation syndrome. Hum Reprod 1997; 12: 236–40.
36. Abramov Y, Schenker JG, Lewin A, et al. Plasma inflammatory cytokines correlate to the ovarian hyperstimulation syndrome. Hum Reprod 1996; 11: 1381–6.

CHAPTER 14

Potential new treatment implications derived from recent molecular developments in ovarian hyperstimulation syndrome

Raul Gómez, Ralf Zimmermann, Juan A García-Velasco,
José Remohi, Carlos Simon and Antonio Pellicer

INTRODUCTION: THE VASCULAR ENDOTHELIAL GROWTH FACTOR SYSTEM IN OVARIAN HYPERSTIMULATION SYNDROME

It is known that common symptoms of ovarian hyperstimulation syndrome (OHSS) such as ascites and anasarca are a consequence of the extravasation of fluid from leaky vessels into body cavities, where it accumulates. Due to this extravasation a deficit in circulating volume develops, which can lead to hemoconcentration and/or prerenal failure. It is clear that increased vascular permeability (iVP) after gonadotropin administration is the main factor causing OHSS, but as human chorionic gonadotropin (hCG) itself has no vasoactive properties, its actions must be mediated by other specific vasoactive factors. It is likely that hCG induces the release of one or several ovarian substances that have potent and direct systemic effects on the vascular system, and is therefore responsible for the pathophysiology and its clinical presentations[1].

It is likely that these mediators are of ovarian origin, produced in excess during induction of ovulation, because the syndrome resolves quickly in OHSS patients after oophorectomy or does not develop at all when the formation of an active corpus luteum is prevented (or does not occur). This is very interesting, as it implies that hCG + ovary is an absolute requirement for the development of OHSS. Both oophorectomy and withholding hCG to prevent ovulation are effective, but not specific, approaches to prevent the formation of OHSS. Most efforts regarding OHSS research have been focused on trying to identify the ovarian vasoactive substance(s) induced by the effect of hCG.

Over the years, many substances involved in the regulation of vascular permeability have been implicated in causing OHSS. Some of them are still under investigation, the list of potential mediators including: estradiol[2], histamines[3], prostaglandins[4], the ovarian renin–angiotensin system[5], interleukin (IL)-6, IL-2 and IL-8[6], angiogenin[7], insulin[8] and the ovarian kinin–kallikrein system[9] among others.

However, vascular endothelial growth factor (VEGF) has emerged as the main angiogenic factor responsible for increased vascular permeability (iVP), leading to the extravasation of protein-rich fluid and, subsequently, the full appearance of OHSS. Both its vasoactive properties and its increased ovarian expression during the development of OHSS suggest that VEGF plays a major role in the development of this syndrome.

VEGF was originally described as a tumor-secreted protein which caused substantial vascular leakage[10]. It is a homodimer of relative molecular mass (M_r) ~ 46 000 which is produced by many cell types[11], including a variety of tumors, folliculostellate cells, macrophages, possibly podocytes, capsular epithelial cells in the renal glomeruli and granulosa cells[12], among others. VEGF (vascular permeability factor (VPF) is a potent enhancer of endothelial permeability, being 50 000 times more potent than histamine[13]. VEGF increases capillary and venular leakage, as a result of opening intercellular junctions between neighboring endothelial cells, as well as other morphological modifications that can rapidly occur 10 min after topical application, such as the induction of fenestrae in venular and capillary endothelia which normally are not fenestrated[14].

There are several findings which support the role of VEGF in the development of OHSS. Serum VEGF levels increase after hCG administration in superovulated women at risk of developing OHSS[15]. In fact, a rise in serum VEGF levels has been used as a marker for subsequent development of OHSS[16]. Moreover, VEGF plasma levels correlate with the clinical picture of OHSS[17], and changes of VEGF levels in ascites have been correlated with the clinical course of OHSS[18].

In women who develop OHSS, VEGF is over-expressed and produced by granulosa-lutein cells[19–23] and released into the follicular fluid in response to hCG[24], inducing increased capillary permeability[24–26]. Similarly, we have shown that hCG stimulates the release of VEGF in human endothelial cells which, in turn, acts in an autocrine manner, increasing vascular permeability[27]. Thus, both the granulosa and endothelial cells may be involved in the production and release of VEGF in women treated with gonadotropins who develop OHSS. If the endothelium is certainly involved in the production of VEGF, we still do not know whether only the vessels of the ovary, or the entire vascular tree, participates in the production of VEGF, leading to OHSS.

The human VEGF gene has been mapped to chromosome 6p12[28] and is made up of eight exons. Exons 1–5 and 8 are always present in VEGF mRNA, while the expression of exons 6 and 7 is regulated by alternative splicing. This process allows the formation of various VEGF isoforms differing in length, all VEGF products having a common region. In humans, five different VEGF mRNAs have been detected encoding the isoforms $VEGF_{121}$, $VEGF_{145}$, $VEGF_{165}$, $VEGF_{189}$ and $VEGF_{206}$[29]. Isoforms $VEGF_{121}$ and $VEGF_{165}$ appear to be mainly involved in the process of angiogenesis[30], and are in fact the only ones that the ovary is able to secrete[25].

The VEGF gene shows the same exonic structure in rodents and humans[26]. Murine-expressed VEGF isoforms $VEGF_{120}$, $VEGF_{144}$, $VEGF_{164}$, $VEGF_{188}$ and $VEGF_{205}$ are only one amino acid less in length when compared with human VEGF isoforms, and there is 95% protein homology between these two[31]. Similar to the human[19–24,27], hybridization studies in the rat ovary have demonstrated significant VEGF mRNA expression seen mostly after the luteinizing hormone (LH) surge[32].

Receptors for VEGF are present on the endothelial cell surface and belong to the tyrosine kinase receptor family[33]. They are also present in the inner theca of human follicles[12,23]. Two specific endothelial cell membrane receptors for VEGF have been identified: VEGFR-1 (Flt-1) and VEGFR-2 (Flk-1/KDR)[33,34]. The receptor Flk-1/KDR appears to be mainly involved in regulating vascular permeability, angiogenesis and vasculogenesis[35,36]. Targeting the Flk-1/KDR receptor has been a goal for researchers working in gynecological oncology. Different specific VEGFR-2 blockers have been used in animal models which reduce tumor growth and ascites[37,38]. Although the mechanism of ascites formation may be different in neoplasms and OHSS[39], nobody had tried so far to reverse ascites formation in OHSS, targeting the VEGF system. This has been our main goal during the past few years.

Based on the above information, we basically describe in this chapter:

(1) The development of an OHSS animal model in order to demonstrate functionally the *increased signaling through the VEGF/VEGFR-2 pathway as a key factor in the development of OHSS* and how inactivation of this pathway by a variety of means can specifically and effectively block the iVP which underlies development of the syndrome;

(2) How new *clinical strategies* may effectively *treat OHSS by targeting the VEGF system;*

(3) Recent findings identifying women at increased risk and finally *developing OHSS based on the up-regulation and bioavailability of VEGF.*

UP-REGULATION OF VEGF PATHWAY AS KEY TO DEVELOPMENT OF INCREASED VASCULAR PERMEABILITY IN OHSS

Development of OHSS in an animal model

Our goal was to understand the pathophysiology of OHSS in order to expand treatment options beyond expectant management by directly influencing the VEGF/VEGFR-2 pathway.

We developed an *in vivo* rodent model which allows induction of OHSS, consistently including the two main characteristics: ovarian enlargement and increased vascular permeability leading to ascites. In immature rats, the hypothalamic–pituitary axis is inactive; therefore, follicle development is nearly inactive as these animals lack endogenous LH production, but it can be induced by the exogenous administration of gonadotropins. Follicle development was induced with pregnant mare's serum gonadotropin (PMSG), 10 IU, during 4 consecutive days. On the 5th day these animals were injected with hCG, 30 IU, in order to trigger ovulation. In agreement with previous results from Ujioka *et al.*[40], OHSS manifestations developed, including ascites and iVP, in these animals. The quantification of vascular permeability in such an animal model can be carried out objectively with the measurement of extravasation of a previously injected dye. Time-course experiments were performed to analyze vascular permeability by injecting Evans blue dye into the femoral vein, and quantifying the amount of dye recovered after irrigating the abdominal cavity with a fixed volume of saline 30 min later[41]. The results of these experiments (Figure 1) validated the animal model employed, because iVP values during the time course were observed in animals superovulated with PMSG if hCG was administered to trigger ovulation. No OHSS was observed in animals which received PMSG without hCG. This first experiment also provided useful information for later functional experiments showing maximal iVP at 48 h after hCG in all the PMSG + hCG-treated animals.

Increased permeability correlates with overexpression of VEGF and VEGFR-2

In addition to the vascular permeability experiments, the expression of whole VEGF mRNA in the mesentery and ovaries employing the reverse transcriptase polymerase chain reaction (RT-PCR) was also measured to determine the tissue source(s) of VEGF. The reason for selecting the ovary or mesentery to measure VEGF expression was related to the possible ovarian or systemic origin of the syndrome, based on the presence of hCG receptors in both the ovary and endothelial cells. Hence, the ovary and the mesentery, as highly vascularized tissue, were selected as representative of an ovarian or systemic origin of the syndrome, respectively. The

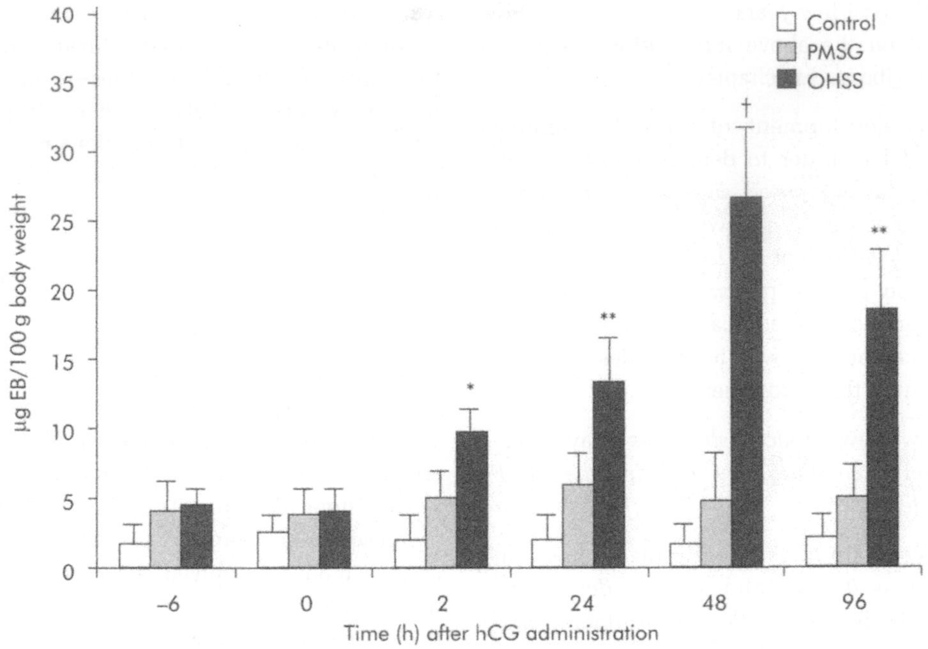

Figure 1 Vascular permeability in three groups of animals injected with saline during 5 consecutive days (control group), 10 IU pregnant mare's serum gonadotropin (PMSG group) or PMSG and 10 IU human chorionic gonadotropin (hCG) (OHSS group). EB, Evans blue

results of these experiments showed that in narrow correlation to vascular permeability (Figure 1), ovarian mRNA VEGF expression increased during the time course, reaching peak values after 48 h, whereas no significant change in expression was observed in the mesentery (Figure 2). To demonstrate further the ovarian origin of VEGF, we showed that vascular permeability was not altered when ovariectomized rats were treated with PMSG + hCG[41].

In addition, we also analyzed which of the VEGF isoforms were expressed by the ovaries of hyperstimulated animals with specific primers for conventional RT-PCR. The ovary expressed $VEGF_{120}$ and $VEGF_{164}$ isoforms. We showed that there was also an increase of VEGFR-2 expression in the ovaries, coincidental in time with maximal vascular permeability[42], demonstrating the involvement of the VEGF/VEGFR-2 system in OHSS. Immunohistochemistry showed VEGF in granulosa and in the zona pellucida of preovulatory and atretric follicles, and in granulosa-lutein and endothelial cells of whole corpus luteum[41,42].

In summary, these experiments showed that the VEGF system (ligand and receptor 2) is upregulated in the ovaries of hyperstimulated animals, coincidental in time with maximal vascular permeability, clearly suggesting a crucial role for locally (ovary)-produced VEGF in OHSS. Although VEGF measurements in the serum/plasma of these animals would have provided us with more evidence to confirm the role of VEGF in OHSS, unfortunately VEGF

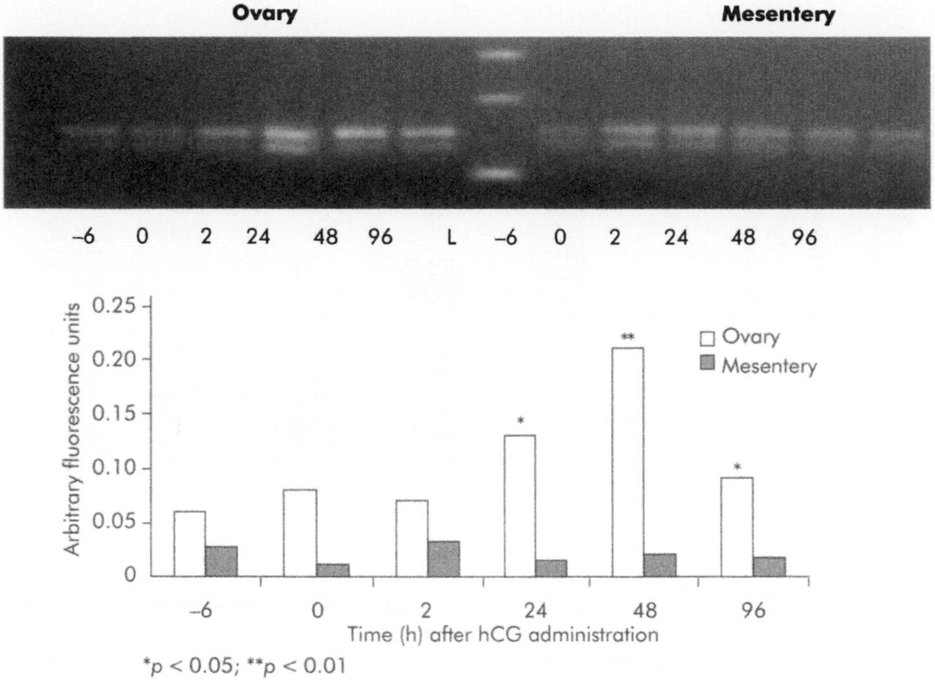

Figure 2 Vascular endothelial growth factor (VEGF) mRNA expression in ovary and mesentery of OHSS animals. Adapted from reference 41. hCG, human chorionic gonadotropin

measurements in the serum of these animals were (are) in all cases below the limit of detection of the most sensitive enzyme-linked immunosorbent assay (ELISA) kits used.

Prevention of development of OHSS by interference with VEGF pathway

After the role of VEGF in establishing vascular permeability was demonstrated, a series of blocking experiments was designed through the administration of SU5416, a VEGFR-2 inhibitor, as a new strategy to prevent and treat OHSS by inhibiting an increase of vascular permeability. Since this was a totally new concept, primarily designed to be employed as an antiangiogenic approach in cancer patients, we attempted several protocols of SU5416 administration in order to block iVP in our OHSS animal models. We found that SU5416 should be administered after hCG, with a single injection of hCG being as effective as multiple injections[41] (Figure 3). The reasons for this behavior can be found in the observation that the syndrome develops only during corpus luteum formation after the ovulation process.

In any case, the ability to reverse hCG action on vascular permeability by targeting the VEGFR-2 employing SU5416 not only confirmed the key role of VEGF in OHSS, but also provided new insights into the development of strategies to prevent and treat the syndrome based on its pathophysiological mechanism, rather than using empirical approaches as we do today. In fact, tumor growth, neoangiogenesis

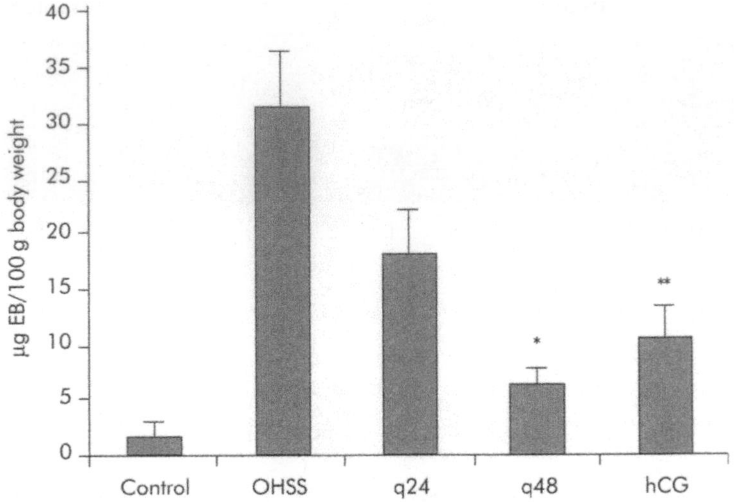

*p < 0.005; **p < 0.05

Figure 3 Reversal of increased vascular permeability employing SU5416 (48 h after human chorionic gonadotropin (hCG) administration). Adapted from reference 41. EB, Evans blue; q24, injection of SU5416 every 24 h; q48, injection of SU5416 every 48 h; hCG, injection of SU5416 just after hCG administration

and ascites formation have been prevented in animals with different ovarian neoplasms by targeting the VEGF system[43,44], and specifically the Flk-1 receptor with SU5416[45]. Herein, we present evidence that the same approach can be used in the OHSS model.

Gene expression in hyperstimulated ovaries

In the previous experiments, we showed that inhibition of VEGF action was accompanied by reduced vascular permeability. However, the use of such strategies employing antiangiogenic drugs (in cancer patients) has been abandoned in women due to side-effects of these compounds[46–48]. Aiming to find a specific non-toxic treatment for OHSS, we reverted to our hypothesis utilizing microarray technology in order to investigate all the genes potentially involved in the development of OHSS. We looked at the expression of gene products regulated under OHSS conditions. This approach resulted in the development of new approaches to block the onset of the syndrome by employing dopamine agonists.

Microarray technology has become one of the most powerful techniques to check, in a single experiment, all the possible genes which are up- or down-regulated under the effects of administration of one or several compounds. We compared ovarian gene expression in animals subjected to different regimens of gonadotropins, including control animals and stimulated rats developing OHSS[49]. Forty-eight hours after hCG, vascular permeability was measured, and mRNA from ovaries extracted to perform gene expression profiles in microarray filters containing 14 000 genes. In the microarray technology, RNA was reverse transcribed and transferred to nylon membrane filters under radioactive conditions. Clusters of 5 × 5 spot signals were analyzed using specific software, and the expression paired with other groups after background signal substraction. Only genes with a three-fold up- or down-regulation were considered to be significantly regulated. The hybridization results were confirmed by quantitative fluorescence (QF)-PCR employing the same RNA in an ABI PRISM® 7700 thermocycler to amplify three up-regulated and three down-regulated genes. Also, immunostaining and cluster analysis were done. Gene expression showed 80 up-regulated and seven down-regulated genes in OHSS as compared with mild stimulation and controls. Up-regulated genes were grouped into five families: cholesterol synthesis, VEGF signal transduction, prostaglandin synthesis, oxidative stress process and cell cycle regulation. The down-regulation of tyrosine hydroxylase (TH, enzyme responsible for dopamine synthesis) was considered a characteristic of OHSS as well.

Dopamine agonists to block OHSS

Taking together the results described above, it was realized that targeting the up-regulated genes could compromise basic cellular or physiological processes, such as estradiol and progesterone production, and ovulation. Hence, we focused on the down-regulated genes, hypothesizing that they could act as natural inhibitors of the angiogenic processes which then needed to be enhanced or up-regulated.

Tyrosine hydroxylase, the key enzyme responsible for dopamine synthesis, was down-regulated, suggesting that perhaps dopamine could act as an antiangiogenic factor in the ovary; a deficit in its production after PMSG + hCG administration in the OHSS animal model could be involved in iVP which characterizes the syndrome. In fact, several reports showed that dopamine administration could decrease vascular permeability in *in vitro*[50] and *in vivo*[51] cancer models by decreasing VEGFR-2 phosphorylation, which is the first step in VEGF downstream signaling leading to iVP after VEGF binding to this receptor[52]. Although the mechanism by which dopamine is able to decrease VEGFR-2 phosphorylation still remains unknown, we wondered whether the administration of dopamine to experimental OHSS rats could be as effective for inhibiting iVP.

Thus, we performed a second series of experiments in which the dopamine agonist bromocriptine (Br2) was employed in OHSS animals in order to study its effects on vascular permeability. Different doses of Br2 (0.1, 0.5, 1, 5, 10 and 25 mg/kg) were administered on the day of hCG injection in the form of pellets that continuously released the product. Vascular permeability was measured 48 h after hCG. In OHSS animals it was significantly reduced when 10 and 25 mg Br2 were employed (Figure 4), demonstrating the efficacy of this approach.

Thus, we concluded that OHSS is associated with the up- and down-regulation of several families of genes in the ovaries. In addition to VEGF, the finding of up- and down-regulation of genes encoding for prolactin and dopamine expression encouraged the successful use of Br2 to prevent increased vascular permeability[49]. Bearing in mind the few toxic and absent teratogenic effects associated with dopamine agonist administration, these experiments provide the rationale to test Br2 as a safe and possible effective medication in the prevention/treatment of OHSS.

Several main questions remain unanswered after these experiments. One is whether dopamine really affects VEGFR-2 phosphorylation, because commercial antiangiogenic drugs with this kind of property have been shown to have very serious side-effects[46–48], not observed after dopamine agonist[49] administration. One possible explanation would be that VEGFR-2 inhibition is not toxic *per se*, and side-effects observed with commercial drugs are due to the

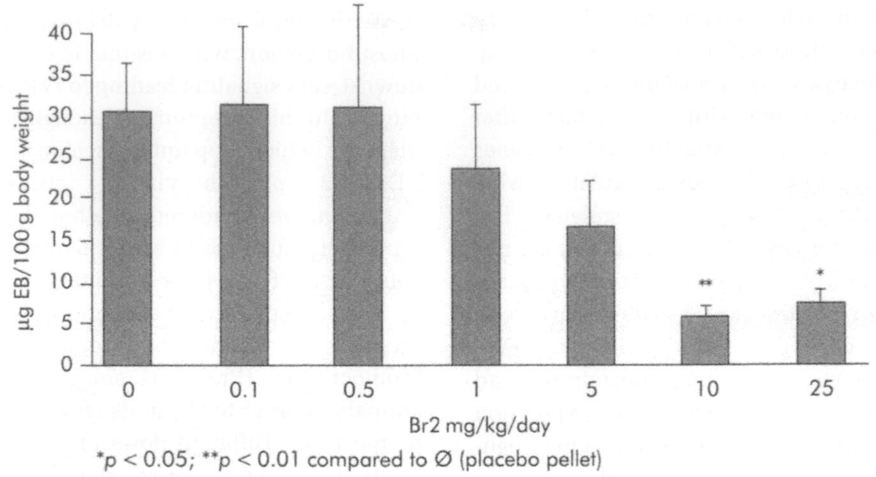

Figure 4 Reversal of increased vascular permeability with bromocriptine (Br2) in rat OHSS model. EB, Evans blue

chemical nature of these drugs and not to the molecular mechanism. Levels of VEGFR-2 phosphorylation in the ovaries of OHSS animals before and after the administration of dopamine agonists are currently being studied. If dopamine agonists are really able to block VEGFR-2 phosphorylation, the next question would be: what is their molecular mechanism of action? We do not know whether dopamine agonists block iVP by competing with VEGF for VEGFR-2 binding, if they directly affect VEGFR-2 conformation or whether these effects are mediated through binding to their own dopamine receptors. As this is a new area of research, more studies are needed in order to elucidate this question.

THE ROLE OF VEGF IN OTHER STRATEGIES USED TO REDUCE OHSS INCIDENCE

Although based on an empirical approach, some clinical strategies developed to reduce the incidence of OHSS, e.g. using different hormones to trigger ovulation, or coasting, have been successful in achieving this purpose. Here, we focus on recent data providing evidence that the effectiveness of both of these approaches is at least partially related to targeting the VEGF system. The rationale for using LH as a trigger for ovulation by reducing VEGF levels and, hence, OHSS is provided by studies performed on OHSS in animal models. Findings regarding the role of VEGF in coasting were made in OHSS patients.

Using hormones other than hCG to trigger ovulation: studies in an animal model

In many mammalian species, including humans, the mid-cycle surge of luteinizing hormone (LH) initiates a series of events included under the term ovulation, comprising oocyte maturation, follicular rupture and luteinization of granulosa and theca cells. The LH surge is accompanied by a follicle stimulating hormone

(FSH) surge which could be relevant to these processes as well. Because of the inconsistency of spontaneous LH surges and the wide use of gonadotropin-releasing hormone (GnRH) analogs, hCG has been clinically employed preferentially. As already mentioned, the clinical use of hCG is associated with some undesirable effects such as OHSS. Whether LH and FSH induce the same phenomenon is not known. Thus, we aimed to study the biological activity of hCG, recombinant LH (rLH) and rFSH in an attempt to find out the minimum effective dose to induce ovulation and prevent OHSS in the rat model.

Immature female rats were treated with 10 IU PMSG for 4 days, and ovulation was triggered with saline, 10 IU hCG, 10 IU FSH, 10 IU LH or 60 IU LH[53]. The number of ovulated oocytes entering the tubes 17–20 h after hCG, as well as vascular permeability and mRNA VEGF expression 48 h after hCG, were evaluated and compared. All the hormones employed to trigger ovulation were equally effective as compared with control rats, in which none was employed. The use of 10 IU LH was associated with a significant reduction in vascular permeability and VEGF expression when compared with the groups treated with 10 IU hCG, 10 IU FSH or 60 IU LH (Figure 5). It was concluded that FSH and hCG, as well as a six-fold dosage of LH, have similar biological activities, including increased vascular permeability due to excessive VEGF expression. The use of lower LH doses resulted in similar rates of ovulation while preventing the undesired changes in permeability and VEGF expression (Figure 5).

Initial multicentric studies in humans have shown that a single dose of 15 000 IU rLH, comparable to 5000 IU hCG, is necessary to achieve optimal oocyte maturation in *in vitro* fertilization (IVF) and is more efficient than 5000 IU rLH[54]. These studies showed a reduced incidence of OHSS when 15 000–30 000 IU rLH was employed, as compared with hCG. A more recent publication, however, obtained the same number of mature oocytes and similar implantation rates in embryos derived from women treated with 5000 IU hCG or rLH[55], suggesting that the dose of rLH necessary to trigger oocyte maturation and avoid OHSS might be lower than initially expected. Moreover, the same authors showed that the hemodynamic changes associated with controlled ovarian stimulation in IVF are less pronounced when rLH is employed, and that the overall incidence of OHSS is reduced[55].

These animal experiments and the still conflicting observations in humans should encourage clinicians to find the optimal dose of LH to be employed in women to trigger ovulation and simultaneously avoid the risk of OHSS, since the medication employed in the experiments is commercially available.

The role of VEGF in coasting

A novel approach to avoid OHSS is to withhold gonadotropin adminstration during ovarian stimulation while continuing pituitary desensitization with GnRH analogs (coasting) until the serum estradiol level drops.[56] The clinical benefit of this approach to reduce the incidence of OHSS without hampering oocyte and/or embryo quality has been shown by our group and others[57–64]. Of all the different options to reduce the incidence of OHSS, coasting is the first choice among physicians, as shown in a recent survey[65]. However, there are no experimental data offering a plausible biological explanation why coasting could be effective. Probably, mature follicles will survive for a few days without exogenous FSH/human menopausal gonadotropin (hMG) while smaller follicles will enter apoptosis/necrosis, reducing the potential granulosa cell population that will release vascular mediators after hCG administration.

The aims of the study we review were:

(1) To evaluate the outcome of IVF in coasted cycles as well as the clinical usefulness of the coasting procedure in preventing

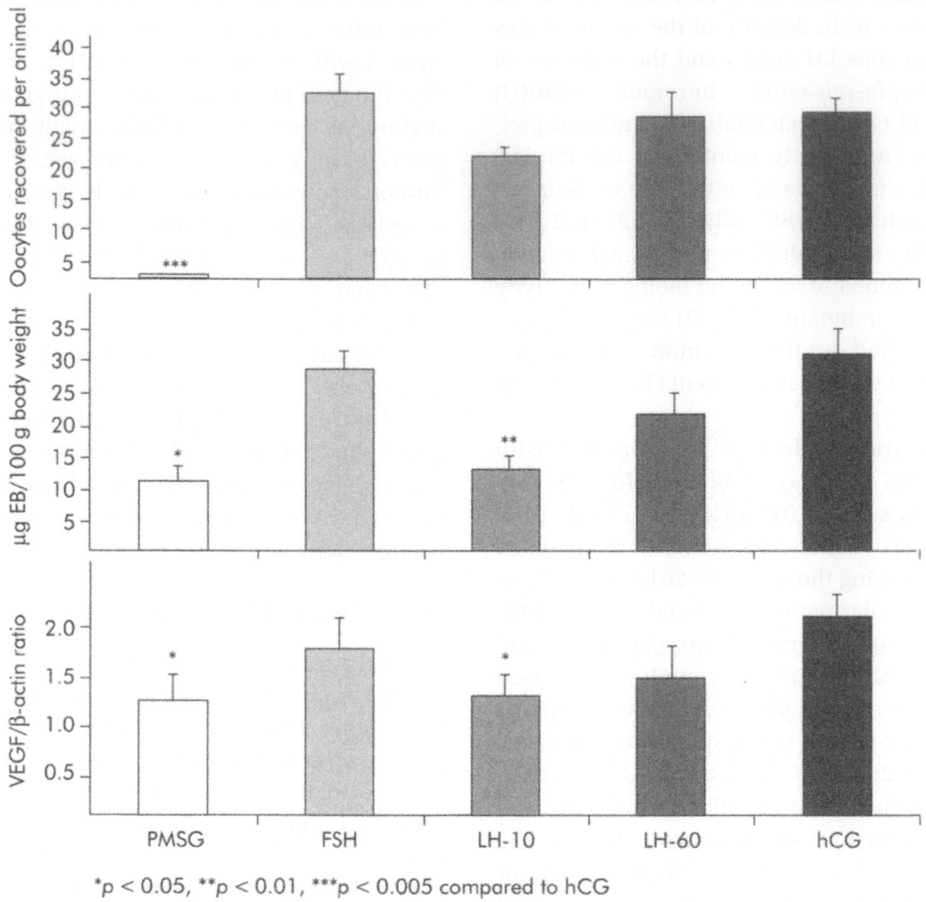

Figure 5 Number of oocytes recovered, vascular permeability and VEGF expression after using different hormones to trigger ovulation. EB, Evans blue; hCG, human chorionic gonadotropin; PMSG, pregnant mare's serum gonadotropin; FSH, follicle stimulating hormone; LH-10, 10 IU luteinizing hormone; LH-60, 60 IU LH

OHSS in women undergoing controlled ovarian stimulation (COS);

(2) To investigate the mechanism by which coasting may act, hypothesizing the possibility that coasting acts through VEGF regulation;

(3) To determine which follicle population is more likely to be affected by coasting.

A total of 160 women (patients and oocyte donors) undergoing coasting and 116 controls were included in the study. Serum, follicular fluid and granulosa cells were collected on the day of oocyte retrieval. VEGF concentrations were determined using ELISA. Real-time PCR was performed to evaluate VEGF gene expression in granulosa cells. Cell death was studied by flow cytometry[66].

Follicular cells aspirated from coasted patients showed a ratio in favor of apoptosis, especially in smaller follicles (48 vs. 26%, $p < 0.05$). Follicular fluid determinations confirmed that coasting reduces VEGF protein secretion (1413 vs. 3538 pg/ml, $p < 0.001$) and gene expression (two-fold decrease) in granulosa cells (Figure 6). Follicular fluid VEGF

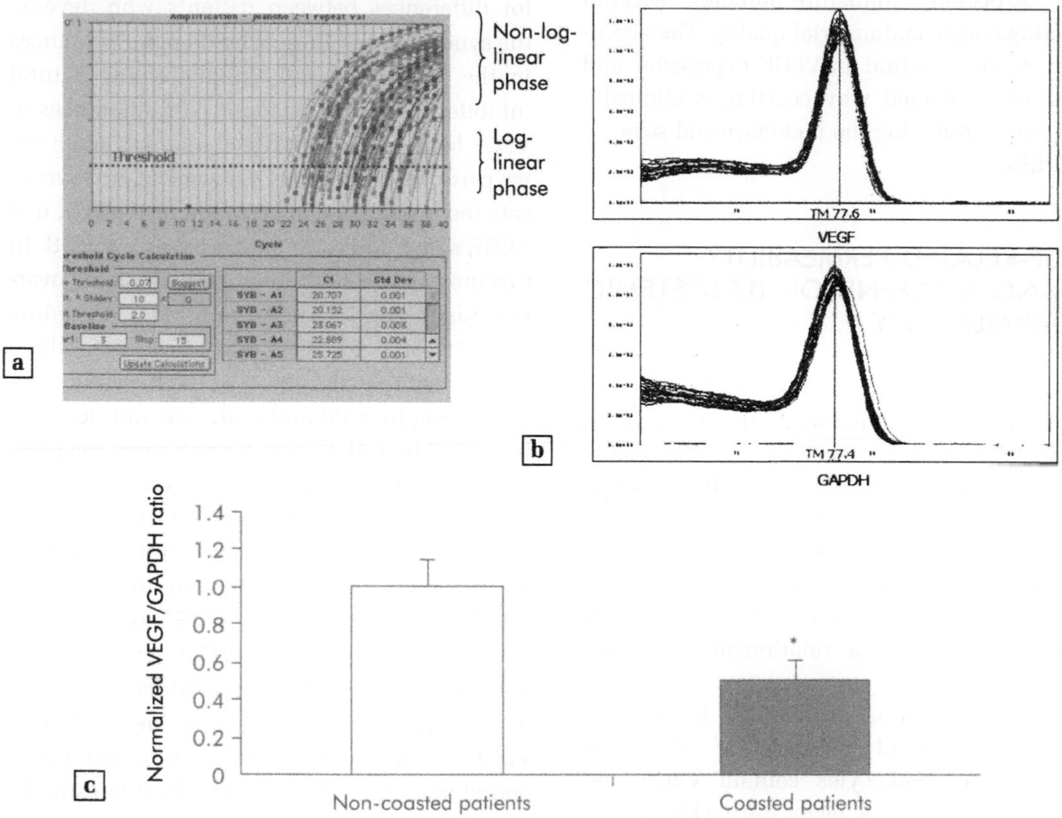

Figure 6 The vascular endothelial growth factor/glyceraldehyde-3-phosphate dehydrogenase (VEGF/GAPDH) ratio was used to compare VEGF expression between coasted and non-coasted patients. (a) Typical logarithmic curve observed during PCR amplification. At the beginning of the reaction increases in cDNA expression are linear (log-linear phase), so quantification is performed during this phase. When the reaction becomes saturated, quantification cannot be performed accurately (non-log-linear phase) as products are overexpressed. (b) Temperature of melting (TM) for the GAPDH and VEGF cDNA PCR products in the fusion curve. As the temperature increases, double DNA strings separate and the dye intercalated between them can be measured. The maximum dye expression coincides with TM which is characteristic for each PCR product. As observed a single peak means that only the one expected product was amplified. (c) VEGF levels are expressed as the VEGF/GAPDH ratio, where GAPDH expression is used to normalize results, so VEGF expression could be compared at the same level. $^{*}p < 0.05$

protein levels correlated positively with follicular size ($r = 0.594$, $p = 0.001$) and estradiol production ($r = 0.558$, $p = 0.038$). Women who underwent coasting showed a comparable IVF cycle outcome[66]. The conclusion seems to be that coasting affected all follicles through apoptosis, especially immature follicles, without affecting oocyte/endometrial quality. The significant decrease found in VEGF expression and secretion explained why coasting is clinically effective in reducing the incidence and severity of OHSS.

VEGF-RELATED PERMEABILITY CHANGES DEPEND ON ITS SYSTEMIC BIOAVAILABILITY

The correlation between VEGF and OHSS has been clearly demonstrated in the animal model[41,42,53], and, similarly, such a relationship seems to hold in humans as well. Although studies trying to find differences in circulating VEGF blood levels between women developing OHSS and those who do not have usually failed to do so, there are several reasons that may explain why such a relationship was not detected.

In many studies, serum VEGF levels were measured to detect the onset of OHSS. As platelets and leukocytes contain VEGF and release this angiogenic factor during blood clotting[67], serum VEGF measurements do not reflect biologically available VEGF in the blood. This also explains why serum concentrations of VEGF are 8–10-fold higher than plasma levels, secondary to the release of VEGF from activated cellular components[68].

The second reason is based on the observation that 90% of the secreted VEGF isoforms remain inactive in the circulation because of binding to the soluble VEGFR-1 (also called sFlt-1). The extracellular domain of VEGFR-1, released by endothelial cells to the circulation, binds VEGF and then inactivates it as well as α_2-macroglobulin (A2M). In fact, higher or lower levels of either A2M[69] or sFlt-1[70] in women at risk for OHSS have been proposed as a reason to explain why some develop OHSS while others do not. Variations in the 'free' and not the 'total' VEGF levels would hence account for differences between patients who develop the syndrome and those who do not. Differences in the expression and activity of the natural inhibitors could be the reason for differences in VEGF biodisponibility. Based on this hypothesis we performed a series of experiments to investigate the implication of systemic total VEGF, free VEGF, sFlt-1 and A2M on the onset of OHSS. In this prospective study, women undergoing ovarian stimulation for IVF were divided according to their risk of developing OHSS into three groups: without risk ($n = 11$), with risk but not developing ($n = 18$) and with risk and developing OHSS ($n = 8$). Factors for risk were: the presence of > 25 follicles at the time of oocyte retrieval, a previous history of OHSS or polycystic ovaries. Blood was drawn from the day of oocyte retrieval each 72 h during the complete luteal phase until day 14. ELISA was used to measure total VEGF, free VEGF and sFlt-1 in plasma, while A2M was measured in serum using nepholometry[71]. We observed that total VEGF levels were similar during the study period in all groups analyzed and, interestingly, free VEGF levels were statistically higher at day 6 after oocyte retrieval in the group who developed OHSS. Free VEGF/A2M and free VEGF/total VEGF ratios were significantly increased in the OHSS risk group at day 6, when compared with the non-risk group and with the group not developing OHSS (Figure 7). It could be concluded that it is likely that free VEGF and not total VEGF in blood is involved in causing vascular permeability, and that the amount of VEGF-binding protein present in blood might influence whether a person will develop OHSS or not.

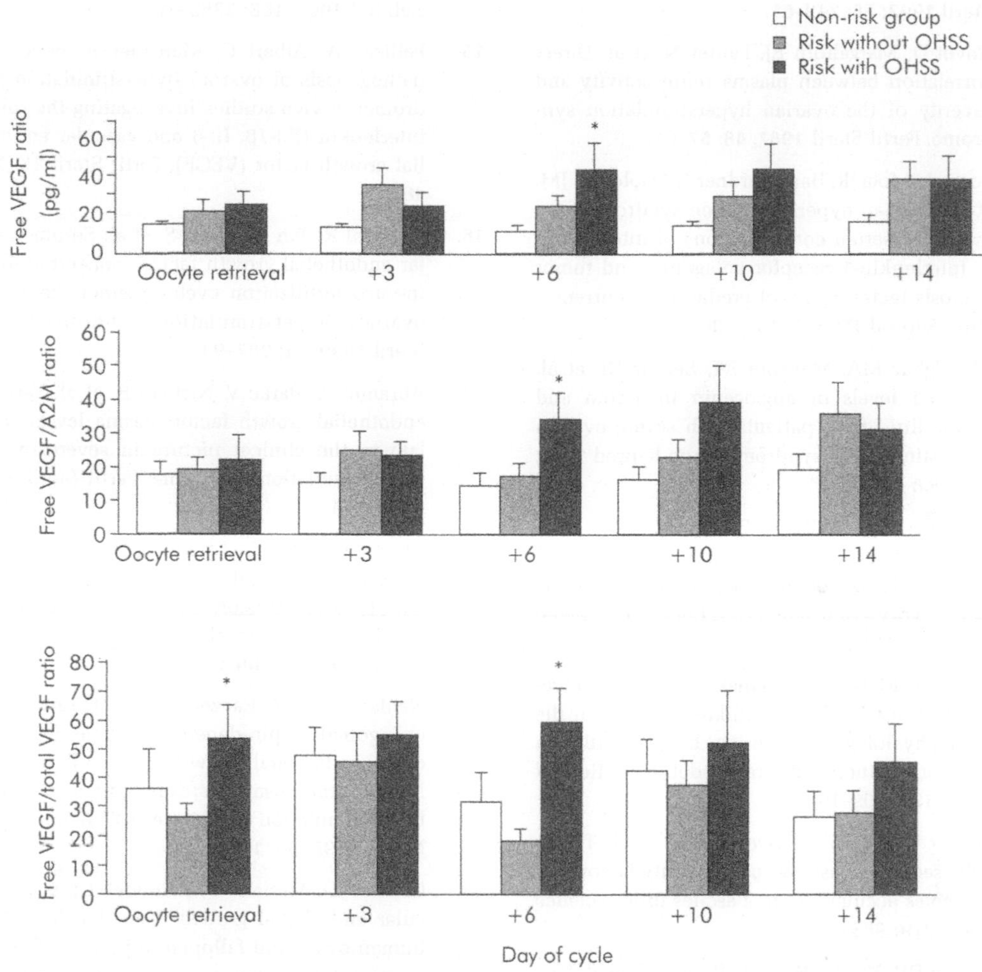

Figure 7 Measurements of free vascular endothelial growth factor (VEGF) and ratios of free VEGF/α_2-macroglobulin (A2M) and free VEGF/total VEGF in non-risk, risk without and risk with OHSS during the time course, 0, 3, 6, 10 and 14 (pregnancy test) days after oocyte retrieval. *$p < 0.05$

REFERENCES

1. Pellicer A, Albert C, Mercader A, et al. The pathogenesis of ovarian hyperstimulation syndrome: in vivo studies investigating the role of interleukin-1, interleukin-6, and vascular endothelial growth factor. Fertil Steril 1999; 71: 482–9.
2. Schenker JG, Weinstein D. Ovarian hyperstimulation syndrome: a current survey. Fertil Steril 1978; 30: 255–68.
3. Knox GE. Antihistamine blockade of the ovarian hyperstimulation syndrome. Am J Obstet Gynecol 1974; 118: 992–4.
4. Navot D, Bergh PA, Laufer N. Ovarian hyperstimulation syndrome in novel reproductive

technologies: prevention and treatment. Fertil Steril 1992; 58: 249–61.

5. Navot D, Margalioth EJ, Laufer N, et al. Direct correlation between plasma renin activity and severity of the ovarian hyperstimulation syndrome. Fertil Steril 1987; 48: 57–61.

6. Loret de Mola JR, Baumgardner GP, Goldfarb JM, et al. Ovarian hyperstimulation syndrome: preovulatory serum concentrations of interleukin-6, interleukin-1 receptor antagonist and tumor necrosis factor-α cannot predict its occurrence. Hum Reprod 1996; 7: 1377–80.

7. Aboulghar MA, Mansour RT, Serour GI, et al. Elevated levels of angiogenin in serum and ascitic fluid from patients with severe ovarian hyperstimulation syndrome. Hum Reprod 1998; 13: 2068–71.

8. Fulghesu AM, Villa P, Pavone V, et al. The impact of insulin secretion on the ovarian response to exogenous gonadotropins in polycystic ovary syndrome. J Clin Endocrinol Metab 1997; 82: 644–8.

9. Ujioka T, Matsuura K, Tanaka N, et al. Involvement of ovarian kinin–kallikrein system in the pathophysiology of ovarian hyperstimulation syndrome: studies in a rat model. Hum Reprod 1998; 13: 3009–15.

10. Senger DR, Galli SJ, Dvorak AM, et al. Tumor cells secrete a vascular permeability factor that promotes accumulation of ascites fluid. Science 1983; 219: 983–5.

11. Senger DR, Van De Water L, Brown LF, et al. Vascular permeability factor (VPF, VEGF) in tumor biology. Cancer Metast Rev 1993; 12: 303–24.

12. Yan Z, Weich HA, Bernart W, et al. Vascular endothelial growth factor (VEGF) messenger ribonucleic acid (mRNA) expression in luteinized human granulosa cells in vitro. J Clin Endocrinol Metab 1993; 77: 1723–5.

13. Senger DR, Connolly DT, Van De Water L, et al. Purification and NH2-terminal amino acid sequence of guinea pig tumor secreted vascular permeability factor. Cancer Res 1990; 50: 1774–8.

14. Roberts WG, Palade GE. Increased microvascular permeability and endothelial fenestration induced by vascular endothelial growth factor J Cell Sci 1995; 108: 2369–79.

15. Pellicer A, Albert C, Mercader A, et al. The pathogenesis of ovarian hyperstimulation syndrome: in vivo studies investigating the role of interleukin (IL)-1β, IL-6 and vascular endothelial growth factor (VEGF). Fertil Steril 1999; 7: 482–9.

16. Agrawal R, Tan SL, Wild S, et al. Serum vascular endothelial growth factor concentrations in in-vitro fertilization cycles predict the risk of ovarian hyperstimulation syndrome. Fertil Steril 1999; 71: 287–93.

17. Abramov Y, Barac V, Nisman B, et al. Vascular endothelial growth factor plasma levels correlate to the clinical picture in severe ovarian hyperstimulation syndrome. Fertil Steril 1997; 67: 261–5.

18. Chen CD, Wu MY, Chen HF, et al. Prognostic importance of serial cytokine changes in ascites and pleural effusion in women with severe ovarian hyperstimulation syndrome. Fertil Steril 1999; 72: 286–92.

19. Neulen J, Yan Z, Raczek S, et al. Human chorionic gonadotropin-dependent expression of vascular endothelial growth factor/VP factor in human granulosa cells: importance in ovarian hyperstimulation syndrome. J Clin Endocrinol Metab 1995; 80: 1967–71.

20. Gordon JD, Mesiano S, Zaloudek CJ, et al. Vascular endothelial growth factor localization in human ovary and fallopian tubes: possible role in reproductive function and ovarian cyst formation. J Clin Endocrinol Metab 1996; 81: 353–9.

21. Otani N, Minami S, Yamoto M, et al. The vascular endothelial growth factor/fms-like tyrosine kinase system in human ovary during the menstrual cycle and early pregnancy. J Clin Endocrinol Metab 1999; 84: 3845–51.

22. Yamamoto S, Konishi I, Tsuruta A, et al. Expression of vascular endothelial growth factor (VEGF) during folliculogenesis and corpus luteum formation in the human ovary. Gynecol Endocrinol 1997; 11: 371–81.

23. Goldsman MP, Pedram A, Domínguez CE, et al. Increased capillary permeability induced by

human follicular fluid: a hypothesis for an ovarian origin of the hyperstimulation syndrome. Fertil Steril 1995; 63: 268–72.

24. Watkins RH, D'Angio CT, Ryan RM, et al. Differential expression of VEGF mRNA splice variants in newborn and adult hyperoxic lung injury. Am J Physiol 1999; 276: 858–67.

25. Olson TA, Mohanraj D, Carson LF, et al. VP factor gene expression in normal and neoplastic human ovaries. Cancer Res 1994; 54: 276–80.

26. McClure N, Healy DL, Rogers PA, et al. Vascular endothelial cell growth factor as permeability agent in ovarian hyperstimulation syndrome. Lancet 1994; 344: 235–6.

27. Albert C, Garrido N, Rao CV, et al. The role of the endothelium in the pathogenesis of ovarian hyperstimulation syndrome. Mol Hum Reprod 2002; 8: 409–18.

28. Wei MH, Popescu NC, Lerman MI, et al. Localization of the human vascular endothelial growth factor gene, VEGF, at chromosome 6p12. Hum Genet 1996; 97: 794–7.

29. Neufeld G, Cohen T, Gengrinovitch S, et al. Vascular endothelial growth factor (VEGF) and its receptors. FASEB J 1999; 13: 9–22.

30. Shima DT, Kuroki M, Deutsch U, et al. The mouse gene for vascular endothelial growth factor. Genomic structure, definition of the transcriptional unit, and characterization of transcriptional and post-transcriptional regulatory sequences. J Biol Chem 1996; 271: 3877–83.

31. Burchardt M, Burchardt T, Chen MW, et al. Expression of messenger ribonucleic acid splice variants for the vascular endothelial growth factor in the penis of adult rats and humans. Biol Reprod 1999; 60: 398–404.

32. Phillips HS, Hains J, Leung DW, et al. Vascular endothelial growth factor is expressed in rat corpus luteum. Endocrinol 1990; 127: 965–7.

33. De Vries C, Escobedo JA, Ueno H, et al. The fms-like tyrosine kinase, a receptor for vascular endothelial growth factor. Science 1992; 255: 989–91.

34. Waltenberger J, Claesson-Welsh L, Siegbahn A, et al. Different signal transduction properties of KDR and Flt1, two receptors for vascular endothelial growth factor. J Biol Chem 1994; 269: 288–95.

35. Shalaby F, Rossant J, Yamaguchi TP, et al. Failure of blood island formation and vasculogenesis in Flk-1-deficient mice. Nature (London) 1995; 376: 62–6.

36. Verheul HM, Hoekman K, Jorna AS, et al. Targeting vascular endothelial growth factor blockade: ascites and pleural effusion formation. Oncologist 2000; 5: 45–50.

37. Xu L, Yoneda J, Herrera C, et al. Inhibition of malignant ascites and growth of human ovarian carcinoma by oral administration of a potent inhibitor of the vascular endothelial growth factor receptor tyrosine kinases. Int J Oncol 2000; 16: 445–54.

38. Yukita A, Asano M, Okamoto T, et al. Suppression of ascites formation and re-accumulation associated with human ovarian cancer by an anti-VPF monoclonal antibody in vivo. Anticancer Res 2000; 20: 155–60.

39. Kobayashi H, Okada Y, Asahina T, et al. The kallikrein–kinin system, but not vascular endothelial growth factor, plays a role in the increased VP associated with ovarian hyperstimulation syndrome. J Mol Endocrinol 1998; 20: 363–74.

40. Ujioka T, Matsuura K, Kawano T, et al. Role of progesterone in capillary permeability in hyperstimulated rats. Hum Reprod 1997; 12: 1629–34.

41. Gómez R, Simón C, Remohi J, et al. Vascular endothelial growth factor receptor-2 activation induces vascular permeability in hyperstimulated rats, and this effect is prevented by receptor blockade. Endocrinology 2002; 143: 4339–48.

42. Gómez R, Simón C, Remohi J, et al. Administration of moderate and high doses of gonadotropins to female rats increases ovarian vascular endothelial growth factor (VEGF) and VEGF receptor-2 expression that is associated to vascular hyperpermeability. Biol Reprod 2003; 68: 2164–71.

43. Brekken RA, Overholser JP, Stastny VA, et al. Selective inhibition of vascular endothelial growth factor (VEGF) receptor 2 (KDR/Flk-1)

activity by a monoclonal anti-VEGF antibody blocks tumor growth in mice. Cancer Res 2000; 60: 5117–24.

44. Wedge SR, Ogilvie DJ, Dukes M, et al. ZD4190: an orally active inhibitor of vascular endothelial growth factor signaling with broad-spectrum antitumor efficacy. Cancer Res 2000; 60: 970–5.

45. Vajkoczy P, Menger MD, Vollmar B, et al. Inhibition of tumor growth, angiogenesis, and microcirculation by the novel Flk-1 inhibitor SU5416 as assessed by intravital multi-fluorescence videomicroscopy. Neoplasia 1999; 1: 31–41.

46. Marx GM, Steer CB, Harper P, et al. Unexpected serious toxicity with chemotherapy and antiangiogenic combinations: time to take stock! J Clin Oncol 2002; 20: 1446–8.

47. Glade-Bender J, Kandel JJ, Yamashiro DJ. VEGF blocking therapy in the treatment of cancer. Expert Opin Biol Ther 2003; 3: 263–76.

48. Kuenen BC, Tabernero J, Baselga J. Efficacy and toxicity of the angiogenesis inhibitor SU5416 as a single agent in patients with advanced renal cell carcinoma, melanoma, and soft tissue sarcoma. Clin Cancer Res 2003; 9: 1648–55.

49. Gómez R, González M, Simón C, et al. Tyroxine hydroxylase (TH) downregulation in hyperstimulated ovaries reveals the dopamine agonist bromocriptine (Br2) as an effective and specific method to block increased vascular permeability (VP) in OHSS. Fertil Steril 2003; 80: 43–4.

50. Basu S, Nagy JA, Pal S, et al. The neurotransmitter dopamine inhibits angiogenesis induced by vascular permeability factor/vascular endothelial growth factor. Nat Med 2001; 7: 569–74.

51. Sarkar C, Chakroborty D, Mitra RB. Dopamine in vivo inhibits VEGF-induced phosphorylation of VEGFR-2, MAPK, and focal adhesion kinase in endothelial cells. Am J Physiol Heart Circ Physiol 2004; 287: H1554–60.

52. Quinn TP, Peters KG, De Vries C, et al. Fetal liver kinase 1 is a receptor for vascular endothelial growth factor and is selectively expressed in vascular endothelium. Proc Natl Acad Sci USA 1993; 90: 7533–7.

53. Gómez R, Lima I, Simón C, et al. Low dose LH administration induces ovulation and prevents vascular hyperpermeability and VEGF expression in superovulated rats. Reproduction 2004; 127: 483–9.

54. The European Recombinant LH Study Group. Recombinant human luteinizing hormone is as effective as, but safer than, urinary human chorionic gonadotropin in inducing final follicular maturation and ovulation in in vitro fertilization procedures: results of a multicenter double-blind study. J Clin Endocrinol Metab 2001; 86: 2607–18.

55. Manau D, Fabregues F, Arroyo V, et al. Hemodynamic changes induced by urinary human chorionic gonadotropin and recombinant luteinizing hormone used for inducing final follicular maturation and luteinization. Fertil Steril 2002; 78: 1261–7.

56. Delvigne A, Rozenberg S. Epidemiology and prevention of ovarian hyperstimulation syndrome (OHSS): a review. Hum Reprod Update 2002; 8: 559–77.

57. Sher G, Salem R, Feinman M, et al. Eliminating the risk of life-endangering complications following overstimulation with menotropin fertility agents: a report on women undergoing in vitro fertilization and embryo transfer. Obstet Gynecol 1993; 81: 1009–11.

58. Benadiva C, Davis O, Kligman I, et al. Withholding gonadotropin administration is an effective alternative for the prevention of ovarian hyperstimulation syndrome. Fertil Steril 1997; 67: 724–7.

59. Tortoriello D, McGovern P, Colon J, et al. Coasting does not affect cycle outcome in a subset of highly responsive in vitro fertilization patients. Fertil Steril 1998; 69: 454–60.

60. Lee C, Tummon I, Martin J, et al. Does withholding gonadotropin administration prevent severe ovarian hyperstimulation syndrome? Hum Reprod 1998; 13: 1157–8.

61. Fluker MR, Hooper WM, Yuzpe AA. Withholding gonadotrophin ('coasting') to minimize the risk of ovarian hyperstimulation during superovulation and in vitro fertilization-embryo transfer cycles. Fertil Steril 1999; 71: 294–301.

62. Waldestrom U, Kahn J, Marsk L, et al. High pregnancy rates and successful prevention of

severe ovarian hyperstimulation syndrome by prolonged coasting of very hyperstimulated patients: a multicentre study. Hum Reprod 1999; 14: 294–7.

63. Al-Shawaf T, Zosmer A, Hussain S, et al. Prevention of severe ovarian hyperstimulation syndrome in IVF with or without ICSI and embryo transfer: a modified coasting strategy based on ultrasound for identification of high-risk patients. Hum Reprod 2001; 16: 24–30.

64. Isaza V, Garcia-Velasco JA, Aragones M, et al. Oocyte and embryo quality after coasting: the experience from oocyte donation. Hum Reprod 2002; 17: 1777–82.

65. Delvigne A, Rozenberg S. Preventive attitude of physicians to avoid OHSS in IVF patients. Hum Reprod 2001; 16: 2491–5.

66. Garcia-Velasco JA, Zuniga A, Pacheco A, et al. Coasting acts through downregulation of VEGF gene expression and protein secretion. Hum Reprod 2004; 19: 1530–8.

67. Jelkmann W. Pitfalls in the measurement of circulating vascular endothelial growth factor. Clin Chem 2001; 47: 617–23.

68. Verheul HM, Hoekman K, Luykx-de-Bakker S, et al. Platelet: transporter of vascular endothelial growth factor. Clin Cancer Res 1997; 3: 2187–90.

69. McElhinney B, Ardill J, Caldwell C, et al. Ovarian hyperstimulation syndrome and assisted reproductive technologies: why some and not others? Hum Reprod 2002; 17: 1548–53.

70. Neulen J, Wenzel D, Hornig C, et al. Poor responder–high responder: the importance of soluble vascular endothelial growth factor receptor 1 in ovarian stimulation protocols. Hum Reprod 2001; 16: 621–6.

71. Alonso I, Gomez R, Pau E, et al. Free VEGF but not total VEGF is responsable for ovarian hyperstimulation syndrome (OHSS) onset. J Soc Gynecol Invest 2005; 12: abstr 6.

CHAPTER 15

Clinical management, ascites management and obstetrical outcome in patients with ovarian hyperstimulation syndrome

Raphael Ron-El, Shevach Friedler, Morey Schachter and Arieh Raziel

INTRODUCTION

Severe ovarian hyperstimulation syndrome (OHSS) is defined as a serious and potentially life-threatening physiological complication classically encountered in patients who undergo controlled ovarian hyperstimulation (COH). It is typically associated with regimens of exogenous gonadotropins and rarely during the administration of clomiphene citrate.

Severe OHSS in *in vitro* fertilization with (IVF) may appear with different timing, early or late[1]. In early-onset OHSS, it occurs within 8 days of initial human chorionic gonadotropin (hCG) exposure relating to 'excessive' preovulatory response to stimulation. In late OHSS it appears after 14–16 days of hCG administration, and depends on the occurrence of pregnancy, where endogenous hCG plays the role. Late OHSS is more likely to be severe, and is only poorly related to preovulatory events.

Much effort has been invested to prevent severe OHSS, as is well reflected by the gradual decline in the incidence of hospitalization for OHSS in our patients, reported over time, from 6.4% in 1994 to 1.5% in the years 1997–99 and less than 1% in 2003–04. Previous studies have reported an incidence of severe OHSS after IVF of approximately 1%, which might be even higher, because of the tendency to under-report[2]. The last European IVF Monitoring Report recorded 1586 OHSS cases in 146 000 assisted reproductive technologies (ART) cycles (1.1%)[3]. Severe OHSS occurred in 0.22% of the ART-treated patients. This gradual reduction reflects a change in our concepts regarding the use of less aggressive protocols for COH, and the change to use of progestogens instead of hCG for luteal support.

PRINCIPLES OF MANAGEMENT

A mild form of OHSS occurs in almost every cycle of COH. In its severe presentation it is characterized by increased vascular permeability, and thus the shift of fluids from the blood vessels to extravascular space. Ninety-five per cent of severe OHSS patients have a hematocrit level of > 45%, 99% are with ascites, 92% are dyspneic, 30% oliguric, 19% with massive pleural effusion, 28% with peripheral edema, 2% with thromboembolic phenomena and 1% of patients have acute renal failure[4]. As such, it often requires hospitalization, and in its critical form may require admission to an intensive-care unit[5].

Admission to hospital should not be in doubt once the patient is dyspneic or complains of vomiting or diarrhea. Normally, such clinical manifestations will be already accompanied by hemoconcentration, with a hematocrit of > 45%. In OHSS patients of whom the degree of clinical severity is unclear, a hematocrit of ≥ 42% is an indication for active monitoring and treatment of the patient, which can only be done under continuous observation. A possible scheme for the management of hospitalized patients with severe OHSS is presented in Figure 1.

The following steps should be performed on admission: recording of vital signs: pulse, blood pressure, number of breaths per minute and fluid balance; measurement of body weight and abdominal circumference; physical examination with emphasis on palpation of the abdomen and lung auscultation; and sonographic examination can be done using abdominal or vaginal ultrasound. Abdominal sonography is preferable for the patient's convenience. It includes measurement of the size of the ovaries and estimation of the quantity of ascitic fluid.

Laboratory tests on admission are: red and white blood count, electrolytes, renal and liver function tests (mainly albumin and total protein) and coagulation tests.

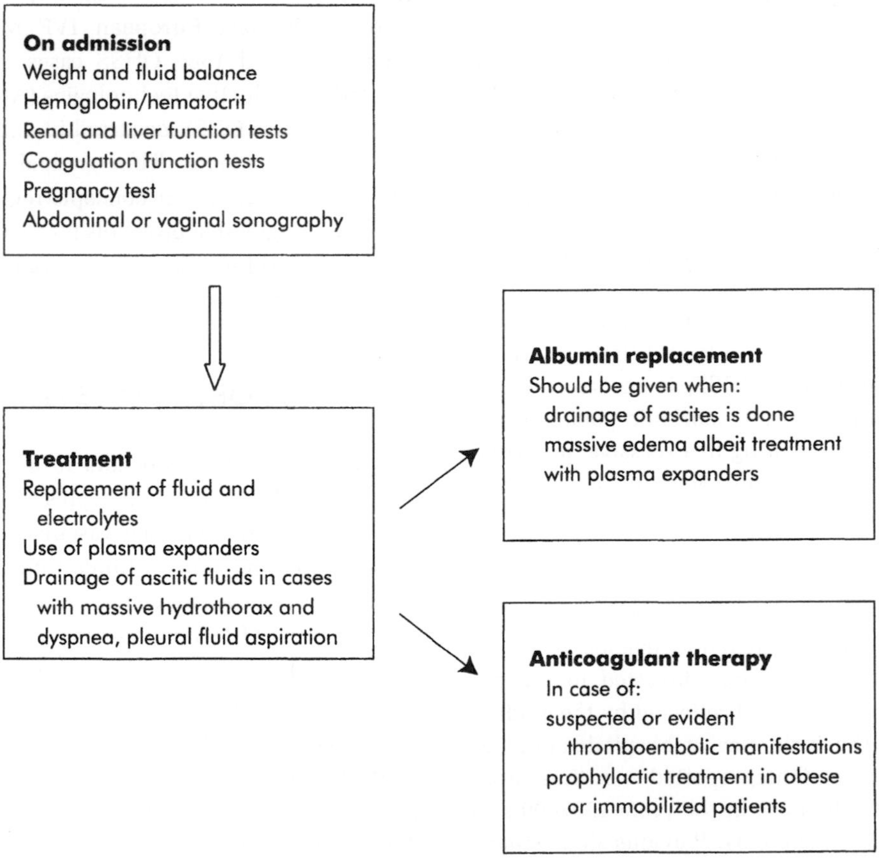

Figure 1 The management of hospitalized patients with severe OHSS

Fluid administration

Principles of treatment are to continue intravascular hydration in order to maintain diuresis, intravascular colloid pressure and electrolyte balance. Intravenous administration includes 2500–3000 ml sodium chloride 0.9% (saline), as the starting dose. Over the next few days the amount of fluid administered should be determined according to the urinary output of the previous day. A combination of saline and dextrose 5% solution by intravenous administration should be given. Fluids should be restricted either when the patient is overloaded with fluids, namely hemoglobin and hematocrit levels are low, or when the patient is in her polyuric phase.

Plasma expanders

The plasma expanders available are dextran and hydroxyethyl starch 6% solution (HES) in isotonic sodium chloride solution (Fresenlus Kabi Deutschland). The maximum daily dose of HES is 33 ml/kg or 250–500 ml per day. It should be used in dropwise and a slow rhythm, to avoid lung congestion.

Albumin administration

Albumin administration should be reserved for a later stage, once hypoalbuminemia is proven, because of: high cost, excessive albumin overload, renal function impairment and risk of viral contamination in general, and viral hepatitis in particular. The administration of albumin is mainly important during drainage of ascites that contains large amounts of proteins. The daily dose is between 25 and 75 g (100–300 ml) per day, according to the severity of hypoalbuminemia and the amount of drained ascitic fluid. The total albumin quantity in the body is measured by multiplying the serum albumin concentration of 30 g/1000 ml by 5000 ml or 5 l of serum, i.e. 150 g. By determining the shortfall between the present albumin value and the anticipated value, the amount needed for intravenous use can be obtained. For example, if the current value of serum albumin is 24 g/1000 ml and the anticipated value is 30 g/1000 ml, then the shortfall of 6 g/1000 ml multiplied by 5000 ml or 5 l defines the need for 30 g albumin. A bottle of 50 ml albumin 25% contains 12.5 g. To achieve 30 g albumin, 120 ml of the above should be administered to the patient (practically two and a half bottles).

Albumin administration is done in equally divided doses during 24 h to increase its effect on urine production in a slow fashion, in order to prevent lung congestion.

A recent comparative study evaluated the effectiveness of 10% dextran 40 infusion (500 ml/day) versus 25% human albumin (100 ml/day). Both infusions were continued for 1–3 days after recovery of hemoconcentration. The recovery from hemoconcentration was much faster in the dextran group compared with the albumin group. Since the occurrence of thromboembolic phenomena of OHSS has been related to the rapid body-fluid shift, leading to hemoconcentration and increased blood viscosity, faster recovery is probably an advantage of dextran use over that of albumin[6].

Anticoagulant administration

We use anticoagulants (such as heparin or low-molecular-weight heparin: Clexan®) when clinical evidence exists of thromboembolic phenomena, in the presence of congenital/acquired thrombophilia and in view of a history of hypercoagulability or thromboembolic events. Anticoagulant use is also considered when the patient is extremely obese or non-mobile. Some clinicians administer anticoagulants on a routine basis. Because of the danger of active bleeding this should be considered with special care while ascitic fluid is drained. Low-dose aspirin (such as pediatric aspirin) use is also an option for the prevention of thromboembolic complications in patients who are scarcely mobile because of obesity or a long immobilization time.

Antiprostaglandin administration

Antiprostaglandin synthetase use (for example, indomethacin) has been suggested in the past to decrease vascular permeability. Although effective in rabbits, its employment in humans has never been effective, and therefore it is of no use today.

Dual renin–angiotensin blockage therapy

Ando *et al.* recently reported the first successful combined use of the angiotensin-converting enzyme (ACE) alacepril 12.5 mg and angiotensin II receptor blocker (ARB) cilexitil 8 mg, with routine cryopreservation, for the prevention of OHSS in four high-risk women for the syndrome[7]. We adopt their final conclusion that dual renin–angiotensin blockage therapy 'would be worth exploring further in a study with more patients and prospective randomized design'.

ASCITES AND PARACENTESIS

Since ascites is very common and is the major reason for discomfort and dyspnea in severe OHSS, its drainage is an integral part of treatment. The decision to drain is sometimes urgent according to the patient's current condition. Drainage of ascitic fluid is mandatory in three conditions: when the patient is dyspneic, when extreme abdominal distension causes great discomfort to the patient and when oliguria is present despite a massive load of fluids and plasma expanders.

Levin *et al.* depicted the advantage of drainage of ascites in OHSS patients[8]. It may cause immediate patient relief by increased venous return to the right heart and increased cardiac output, which leads to renal function improvement caused by increased urinary output, increased creatinine clearance rate and decreased blood urea nitrogen levels.

Padilla *et al.* showed better ventilation of the lower lobes of the lungs and a decrease in pulsatility index (PI)[9] of the uterine artery after drainage of ascites. A shortening of hospitalization duration has been shown by several clinicians[10–12].

Drainage of the ascitic fluid has been described in several publications[10–12]. Ultrasonographic-guided transabdominal drainage is frequently performed[9]. In rare cases, such as in extremely obese patients, the transvaginal route is preferable with the usual ovum pick-up needle[13], or with the insertion of a pigtail catheter as suggested by Raziel *et al.*[14].

Since the factor responsible for increased vascular permeability remains, the ascitic fluid is quickly replaced with new quantities from the vascular bed after paracentesis. Rizk and Aboulghar considered the reaccumulation time to be between 3 and 5 days. Therefore, they drained between 900 and 1400 ml of fluid in one session and, if necessary, repeated the drainage procedure[10]. In our experience, the reaccumulation time of ascitic fluid can be very short, so that the patient becomes dyspneic again within 12–24 h after fluid aspiration. The refilling interval depends on the severity of the case and phase of the disease.

We believe that continuous drainage of ascitic fluid is preferable to intermittent catheterizations. The catheter is introduced through the abdominal wall under ultrasound guidance and remains until drainage stops, or 48–72 h after its insertion. Several types of indwelling catheters have been described. One is a central venous pressure (CVP) catheter (Intracath, short type), as used by our group. A suprapubic bladder drainage catheter (Cystofix; Braun Melsungen, Germany) is easy for use, but seems traumatic when inserted. A closed-system Dawson–Mueller catheter (Cook, USA) has been used by Al-Ramahi[15]. A pigtail catheter

(Boston Scientific, USA) anchored to the skin with a 2–0 silk suture has also been used[14].

The ascitic fluid should be removed in a gradual manner. With too rapid drainage of the fluid the patient may feel extreme weakness and exhaustion. Normally, we drain not more than 4 l within 12 h. When 4 l are already drained, we close the catheter while leaving it *in situ*.

The risk associated with abdominal drainage of ascitic fluid is minimal. The risk of puncturing the ovaries is negligible when it is done under ultrasonographic guidance[12,15]. Loss of proteins is of great concern. With the drainage of large amounts of ascitic fluid there is a huge loss of plasma proteins. A peritoneovenous shunt for the continuous autotransfusion system of ascites (CATSA) was developed in order to overcome the need for massive protein supplementation. CATSA includes a transabdominal 16 g Teflon catheter connected via a peristaltic pump and microfilter to an 18 g Teflon catheter inserted in the antecubital vein. The treatment is performed once a day for 5 h[16].

Another side-effect of drainage is the development of vulvar edema due to either massive drainage of ascitic fluid with inadequate albumin replacement or the creation of fistulous tracts between the peritoneal cavity and the subcutaneous tissues in a lower-abdominal paracentesis. Cellulitis at the area of insertion of the catheter may rarely be encountered.

In rare cases, on the grounds of a deteriorating clinical picture, after failure of the above 'conservative treatments', transvaginal ultrasonographic-guided aspiration of multiple corpora lutea has been reported[17]. Bilateral partial oophorectomy has been offered as an effective approach, due not only to emptying of the contents of the corpora lutea, but also to total excision of the walls of ovarian cysts which incorporate the granulosa cells that are probably the origin of most vasoactive mediators[18].

Although the pathophysiology of OHSS is not clear, appearance of the symptoms is closely related to hCG production. Therefore, in extremely rare cases of critical OHSS, reduction of endogenous hCG by pregnancy termination is the last choice[18].

The clinical courses of two patients hospitalized for severe OHSS are illustrated in Figures 2 and 3.

OBSTETRICAL OUTCOME IN OHSS PATIENTS

Since severe OHSS is a potentially life-threatening, iatrogenic complication in a basically healthy young woman desiring fertility, much effort is made to prevent it[2,4,19,20]. Naturally, in such an acute situation, the endangering syndrome is focused upon and the anticipated pregnancy is of secondary importance.

Since women with severe OHSS are in a lower age group (28.4 ± 4.5 years) than the average age of IVF patients (35.2 ± 4.5 years) and with a higher number of aspirated oocytes per cycle, it is logical that the pregnancy rate in this specific group will be much higher than in the general IVF program. Indeed, the clinical pregnancy rate among 104 severe OHSS patients in our study reached 58%, compared with 23% in our general IVF program[19], or 73% vs. 14% among 142 severe OHSS patients of a multicenter study[21]. These results were in concordance with a Swedish study published by Enskog *et al.*, which included 428 IVF patients who received controlled ovarian hyperstimulation during a 6-month follow-up period[22].

The multiple pregnancy rates among the patients with OHSS were higher than found in the general ART population. The multiple pregnancy rate in the above-mentioned multicenter study was 58%, 39% twins and 17% triplets[21]. However, the study was conducted during the years 1987–96. Nowadays, such a high multiple pregnancy rate would not be acceptable.

The miscarriage rate was significantly higher among severe OHSS cases than that found in non-OHSS IVF patients (38% vs. 15%,

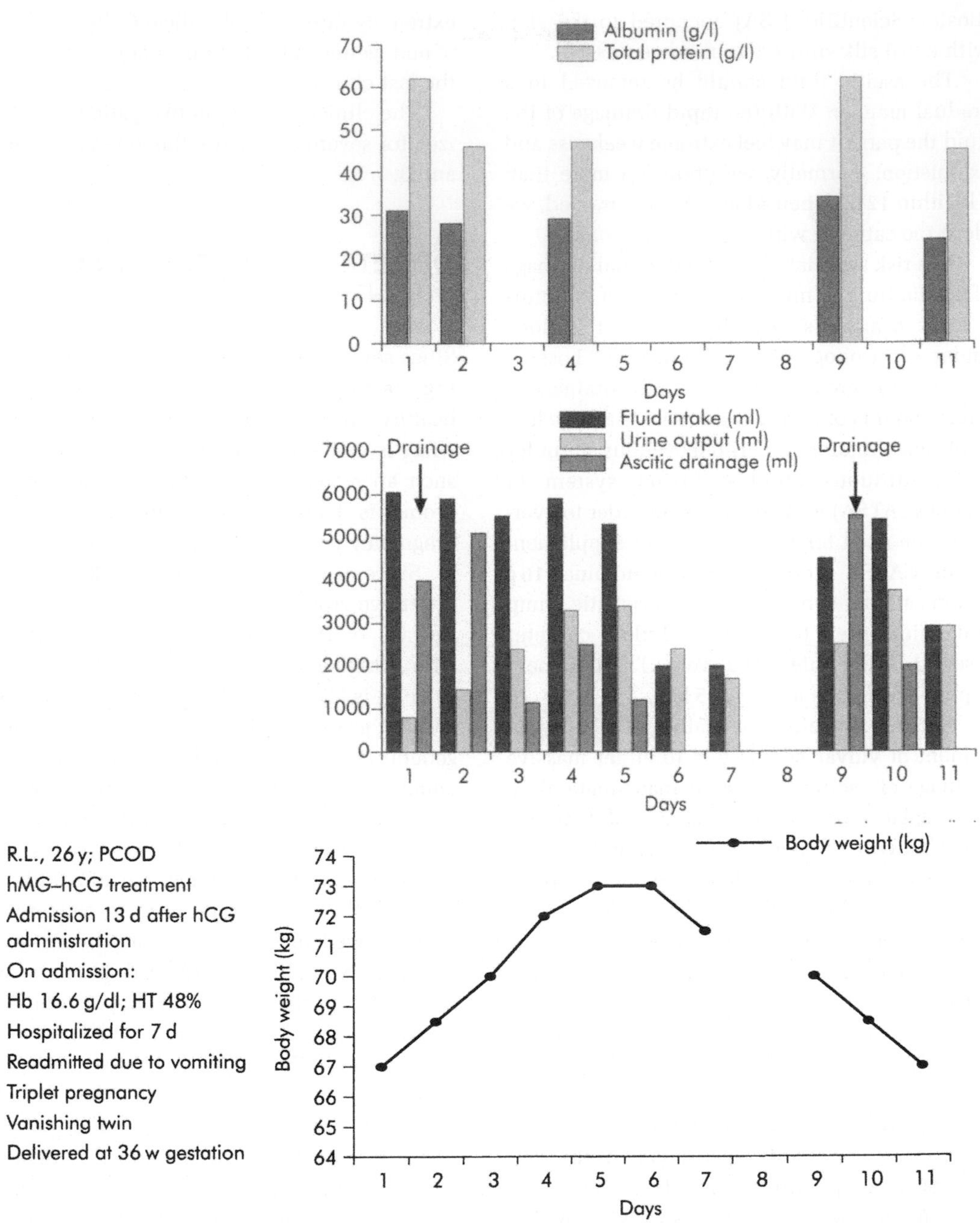

Figure 2 The management and clinical course of a polycystic ovarian disease (PCOD) patient post-ovulation induction, presenting with late onset of severe OHSS. y, years; hMG, human menopausal gonadotropin; hCG, human chorionic gonadotropin; d, days; Hb, hemoglobin; HT, hematocrit; w, weeks

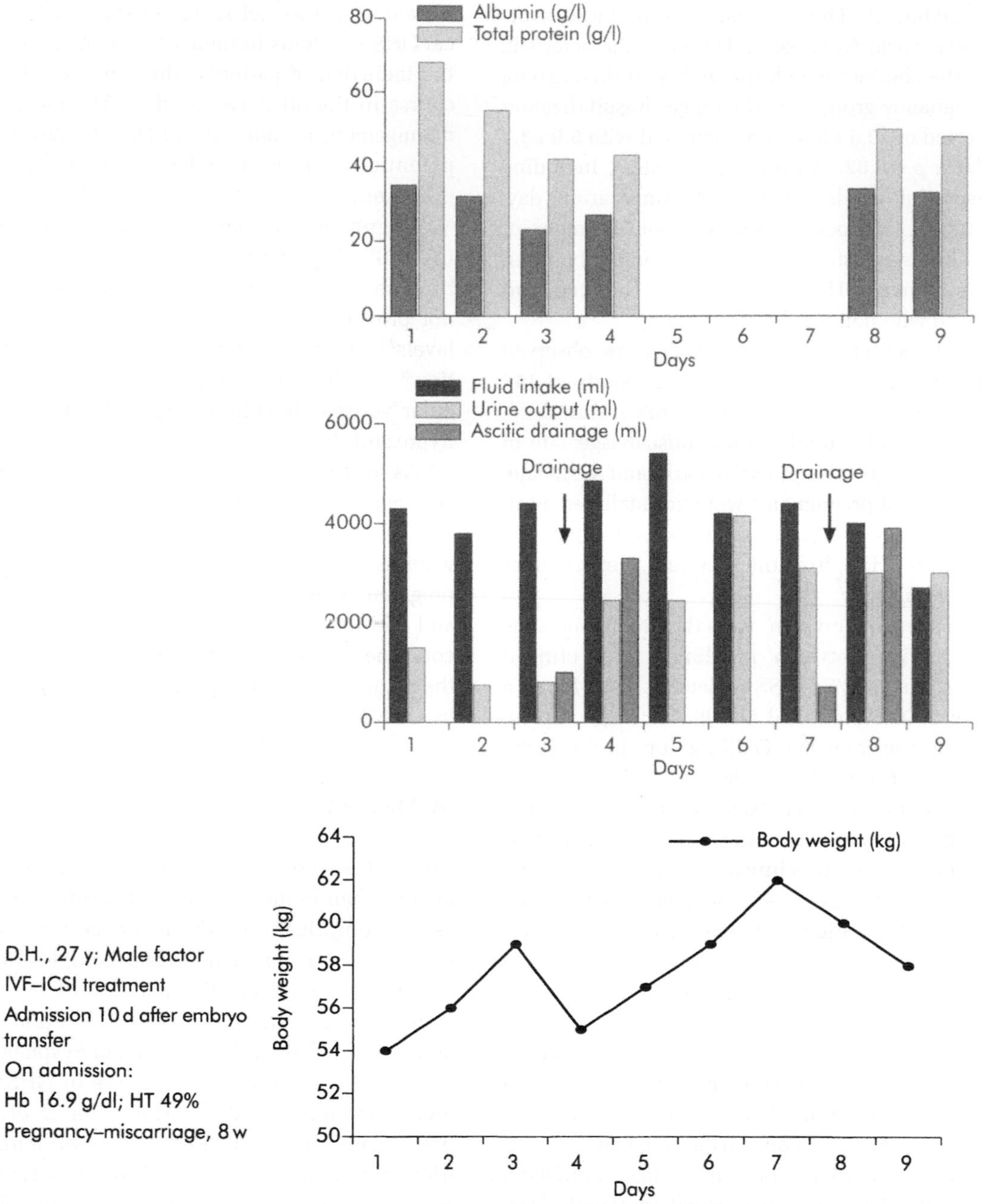

Figure 3 The management and clinical course of a patient who underwent *in vitro* fertilization–intracytoplasmic sperm injection (IVF–ICSI) treatment and was admitted with early onset of OHSS. She conceived; however, the pregnancy terminated with a missed abortion. See Figure 2 for definitions

$p < 0.001$)[19]. The vast majority of these abortions (83%) were early. The only characteristic of the aborters which differed from the ongoing pregnancy group was the longer hospitalization period of 10.5 ± 9.6 days compared with 5.9 ± 3.2 days; $p < 0.02$. All other parameters, including estradiol levels on hCG administration day, number of oocytes retrieved and number of embryos transferred, were comparable between the severe OHSS patients who aborted and those who delivered[19].

Higher rates of miscarriage were observed also by Abramov *et al.*, in a large study of 142 patients who underwent embryo transfer[21]. They found a total clinical miscarriage rate of 29.8%, of which 25% were early and 4.8% late. Preclinical pregnancies were not included as an outcome measure. Historical controls of patients with no OHSS, from the literature, were used for comparison.

Papanikolaou *et al.* were the first to make the distinction between preclinical and clinical abortions in IVF OHSS patients[23]. They found a rate of 91.8% clinical and 88.3% ongoing pregnancies in their late-OHSS group. In the early-OHSS group, they observed a biochemical pregnancy rate of 41.5% per cycle. Their clinical pregnancy rate was reduced to 28.3% per cycle due to a 31.8% preclinical pregnancy loss, compared with only 14.4% pregnancy loss in the non-OHSS patients. There was no difference between the incidence of miscarriage between their early- and late-OHSS patients (5.8% and 5.3%, respectively). These results of low miscarriage rate in OHSS patients compared with non-OHSS IVF patients were also found in a British study[24]. Mathur and Jenkins noted a total 12.2% miscarriage rate among OHSS pregnancies compared with 16.8% in the control non-OHSS patients. The study was small in sample size, and also did not report on preclinical abortion rates.

The discrepancy between the two pairs of studies (references 19, 21 and 23, 24) can be explained by different types of patients. Abramov and Raziel included severe and critical OHSS patients in their studies, in contrast to the inclusion of patients with a milder clinical course in the other two studies. The metabolic derangement in more severe OHSS cases might potentially directly affect the developing pregnancy.

It is unclear how any derangement occurring in OHSS may affect the early pregnancy. Is it because of higher estradiol levels, which were not proven in our study[20], abnormal cytokine levels[25] or excessive renin-angiotensin activation[26,27]? Or can it be attributed to intravascular volume depletion, hemoconcentration or hypoxemia?

As for the progress of pregnancies, maternal and neonatal complications during pregnancy and delivery among the severe OHSS patients were as frequent as the above in the general pregnant population when related to singleton and multiple pregnancies separately[21]. This was confirmed in a recent follow-up study beyond the second trimester of pregnancies complicated by OHSS[28].

SUMMARY

Although severe OHSS tends to occur less frequently than in the past, it is still a serious iatrogenic complication which demands active management to prevent further complications. Treatment should be directed toward replacement of the depleted vascular bed, and drainage of the ascitic fluid if discomfort and dyspnea are present. Since the miscarriage rate in OHSS is high, shortening of the unstable status of the patient may reduce it. Recently, some authors tried to maintain patients with severe OHSS in an out-patient regimen where close follow-up was performed, paracentesis was done if needed and albumin replacement was occasionally used[20,29,30]. Whether this is an adequately safe management has still to be tested. There is no doubt that the physician confronting patients with severe OHSS should be experienced enough to provide an efficacious treatment and to prevent complications and inconvenience for the patients.

REFERENCES

1. Mathur R, Akande A, Keay S, et al. Distinction between early and late ovarian hyperstimulation syndrome. Fertil Steril 2000; 73: 901–7.
2. Forman RG. Severe OHSS – an acceptable price? Hum Reprod 1999; 14: 2687–8.
3. Nyboe A, Andersen L, Gianaroli L, et al. The European IVF-monitoring programme (EIM) for the European Society of Human Reproduction and Embryology (ESHRE), Assisted reproductive technology in Europe, 2000. Results generated from European registers by ESHRE. Hum Reprod 2004; 19: 490–503.
4. Abramov Y, Elchalal U, Schenker J. An 'epidemic' of severe ovarian hyperstimulation syndrome: a price we have to pay? Hum Reprod 1999; 14: 2181–3.
5. Whelan JG III, Viahost NF. The ovarian hyperstimulation syndrome. Fertil Steril 2000; 73: 883–96.
6. Endo T, Kitajima Y, Hayashi T, et al. Low-molecular weight dextran infusion is more effective for the treatment of hemoconcentration due to severe ovarian hyperstimulation syndrome than human albumin infusion. Fertil Steril 2004; 82: 1449–51.
7. Ando H, Furugori K, Shibata D, et al. Dual renin–angiotensin blockage therapy in patients at high risk of early ovarian hyperstimulation syndrome receiving IVF and elective embryo cryopreservation: a case series. Hum Reprod 2003; 18: 1219–22.
8. Levin I, Almog B, Avni A, et al. Effect of paracentesis of ascitic fluids on urinary output and blood indices in patients with severe ovarian hyperstimulation syndrome. Fertil Steril 2002; 77: 986–8.
9. Padilla S, Zamaria S, Baramki T, et al. Abdominal paracentesis for ovarian hyperstimulation syndrome with severe pulmonary compromise. Fertil Steril 1990; 53: 365–7.
10. Rizk B, Aboulghar M. Modern management of ovarian hyperstimulation syndrome. Hum Reprod 1992; 6: 1082–7.
11. Al-Ramahi M, Leader A, Claman C, et al. A novel approach to the treatment of ascites associated with ovarian hyperstimulation syndrome. Hum Reprod 1997; 12: 2614–16.
12. Abuzeid MI, Nassar Z, Massaad Z, et al. Pigtail catheter for the treatment of ascites associated with ovarian hyperstimulation syndrome. Hum Reprod 2003; 18: 370–3.
13. Aboulghar M, Mansour R, Serour G, et al. Ultrasonically guided vaginal aspiration of ascites in the treatment of severe ovarian hyperstimulation syndrome. Fertil Steril 1990; 53: 933–5.
14. Raziel A, Friedler S, Schachter M, et al. Transvaginal drainage of ascites as an alternative to abdominal paracentesis in patients with severe ovarian hyperstimulation syndrome, obesity, and generalized edema. Fertil Steril 1998; 69: 780–3.
15. Al-Ramahi M. Severe OHSS: decreasing the risk of severe ovarian hyperstimulation syndrome. Hum Reprod 1999; 14: 2421–2.
16. Toshimitsu K, Shigeo A, Hisanori M, et al. Clinical efficacy of peritoneo-venous shunting for the treatment of severe ovarian hyperstimulation syndrome. Hum Reprod 2000; 15: 113–17.
17. Fakih H, Bello S. Ovarian cyst aspiration: a therapeutic approach to ovarian hyperstimulation syndrome. Fertil Steril 1992; 58: 829–32.
18. Amarin ZO. Bilateral partial oophorectomy in the management of severe ovarian hyperstimulation syndrome. Hum Reprod 2003; 18: 659–64.
19. Raziel A, Schachter M, Strassburger D, et al. Increased early pregnancy loss in IVF patients with severe ovarian hyperstimulation syndrome. Hum Reprod 2002; 17: 107–10.
20. Fluker MR, Copeland JE, Yuzpe AA. An ounce of prevention: outpatient management of the ovarian hyperstimulation syndrome. Fertil Steril 2000; 73: 821–4.

21. Abramov Y, Elchalal U, Schenker J. Obstetric outcome of in vitro fertilized pregnancies complicated by severe ovarian hyperstimulation syndrome: a multicenter study. Fertil Steril 1998; 70: 1070–5.

22. Enskog A, Henriksson M, Unander M, et al. Prospective study of the clinical and laboratory parameters of patients in whom ovarian hyperstimulation syndrome developed during controlled ovarian hyperstimulation for in vitro fertilization. Fertil Steril 1999; 71: 808–14.

23. Papanikolaou E, Tournaye H, Verpoest W, et al. Early and late ovarian hyperstimulation syndrome: early pregnancy outcome and profile. Hum Reprod 2005; 20: 636–41.

24. Mathur RS, Jenkins JM. Is ovarian hyperstimulation syndrome associated with a poor obstetric outcome? Br J Obstet Gynaecol 2000; 8: 943–6.

25. Abramov Y, Schenker JG, Lewin A, et al. Plasma inflammatory cytokines correlate to ovarian hyperstimulation syndrome. Hum Reprod 1996; 11: 1381–6.

26. Morris RS, Wong IL, Kirkman E, et al. Inhibition of ovarian-derived prorenin to angiotensin cascade in the treatment of ovarian hyperstimulation syndrome. Hum Reprod 1995; 10: 1355–8.

27. De Nuccio I, Salvati G, Genovesi G, et al. Physiopathology of the renin–angiotensin system in the ovary. Minerva Endocrinol 1999; 24: 77–81.

28. Wiser A, Levron J, Kreizer D et al. Outcome of pregnancies complicated by severe ovarian hyperstimulation syndrome (OHSS): a follow-up beyond the second trimester. Hum Reprod 2005; 20: 910–14.

29. Lincoln SR, Opsahi MS, Blauer SH, et al. Aggressive outpatient OHSS with ascites using transvaginal culdocentesis and intravenous albumin minimizes hospitalization. Fertil Steril 2000; 4: S165.

30. Esposito MA, Van Nest RL, Sagoskin AW, et al. Outpatient management of ovarian hyperstimulation syndrome (OHSS) without the use of albumin.Fertil Steril 2000; 78: S10–11.

CHAPTER 16

Management of ovarian hyperstimulation syndrome from an American perspective

Randy Morris

INTRODUCTION

Since ovarian hyperstimulation syndrome (OHSS) is a relatively uncommon complication, there is a paucity of data on methods to prevent or treat this complicated syndrome. The data that do exist are hampered by small numbers and lack of adequate control groups. This situation has led to a difference in methods of management between centers. In the United States, there are two primary methods for management of established OHSS. This chapter discusses these two methods and their underlying rationales. Methods to prevent or reduce the incidence of OHSS are also discussed.

It is described fully, elsewhere in this book, that the underlying pathophysiology of OHSS is increased capillary permeability with resultant third-space fluid accumulation. The third-space accumulation of fluid has been reported in the abdominal cavity[1], pleural cavity[2] and pericardial sac[3]. The presence of abnormal amounts of fluid in these cavities is responsible for specific problems. Many of the therapeutic modalities for OHSS have been directed toward reducing fluid in these locations in order to treat specific symptoms or, in some cases, induce remission of the syndrome entirely.

ABDOMINAL CAVITY FLUID (ASCITES)

The most common location for significant fluid accumulation is the abdominal cavity. Ascites causes the patient to have the physical sensations of abdominal distension, bloating, cramping and sometimes frank abdominal pain. From a physiological point of view, this fluid is suspected to be a cause of increased abdominal pressure, the net effect of which is compression of the vena cava resulting in decreased venous return to the heart. This, in turn, decreases cardiac output[4], reduces renal perfusion and causes further worsening of OHSS-associated oliguria[5]. Increased intra-abdominal pressure, in combination with enlarged ovaries, causes elevation of the diaphragm and restricts diaphragmatic movement, making inspiration more difficult and causing the patient to feel respiratory distress[6]. The supine position exacerbates this problem. The presence of ascitic fluid also poses a risk for secondary bacterial peritonitis[7].

PREVENTION OF ASCITES AND OHSS

Albumin prophylaxis

A small initial case series pointed to the possibility that intravenous infusion of salt-poor albumin might, through oncotic effect, prevent OHSS by causing the fluid to remain in the intravascular space[8]. However, this analysis was flawed. It has been reported that albumin, when administered intravenously, has a circulation half-life of approximately 19 days[9]. However, under circumstances of volume depletion such as that seen in OHSS, the oncotic actions of albumin last less than 36 h[10]. Thereafter, albumin leaves the intravascular space and resides in the insterstitium, where it can then act to draw fluid out of the intravascular space potentially worsening the course of OHSS. After the initial report, several small randomized controlled trials produced mixed results as to the efficacy of prophylactic albumin[11,12]. A 2002 Cochrane review of five randomized trials totaling 463 cases concluded that there was a mild beneficial effect, with an absolute risk reduction of 5.5%, with one case of OHSS prevented for every 18 women at risk of severe OHSS[13]. However, a subsequent randomized trial involving 976 women concluded that there was no beneficial effect[14]. At the current time, use of albumin for the prevention of OHSS or ascites cannot be recommended.

Cycle cancellation/avoidance of human chorionic gonadotropin

Since the first reports of OHSS, it is clear that the occurrence of pregnancy is a key risk factor in the development of OHSS. Patients who become pregnant are more likely to develop severe OHSS. Egg donors, for instance, have a very low risk for severe OHSS despite equivalent or greater levels of stimulation[15]. Patients with severe OHSS after *in vitro* fertilization are much more likely to be pregnant than *in vitro* fertilization patients who do not have OHSS. They are also much more likely to have a multiple pregnancy[16]. Furthermore, multiple pregnancies have a longer and more severe course than do singletons[17]. It is likely that the levels of human chorionic gonadotropin (hCG) exposure have a significant impact on the natural course of the syndrome.

Complete avoidance of pregnancy and hCG, therefore, are important methods to reduce the likelihood of development of (severe) OHSS. Withholding the hCG trigger injection has been offered as a means to reduce the incidence of (severe) OHSS. This method, while mostly effective, can still fail if the patient achieves pregnancy from a spontaneous luteinizing hormone surge[18].

In addition, most patients do not find this an acceptable option since it requires cancellation of the treatment cycle. This is seen as an inefficient route, which is costly from the standpoint of medication usage without a legitimate attempt at pregnancy.

Patients who use gonadotropins for ovulation induction or superovulation can have their cycles converted to an *in vitro* fertilization cycle[19]. Aspiration of the follicle load during egg retrieval has a protective effect on the development of OHSS[20].

Cryopreservation of all embryos

If an *in vitro* fertilization patient is thought to be at high risk, elective cryopreservation of all embryos can be performed. Several studies have indicated that elective cryopreservation of all embryos can reduce the incidence and severity of OHSS without compromising the chance for pregnancy in subsequent embryo thaw cycles[21,22]. However, a 2002 Cochrane database review did not find a benefit in terms of a reduced incidence of OHSS with elective cryopreservation when compared with either fresh transfer alone or fresh transfer and prophylactic albumin administration[23].

Modification of stimulation

'Coasting' is described as withholding or significantly reducing the dose of gonadotropins in patients thought to be at high risk for the development of severe OHSS. Coasting was first reported in 1995 in a small group of *in vitro* fertilization patients. In that report, no cycles were canceled, none of the patients developed severe OHSS and pregnancy rates were reported as high[24]. Other centers had similar experiences and did not find an adverse effect on *in vitro* fertilization cycle parameters[25].

Lee *et al.*, however, in a much larger study, did not find equivalent results[26]. Four out of 20 women treated by coasting still developed OHSS. Multiple regression analysis determined that other factors were more likely to be responsible for the better outcomes in those patients who did not develop OHSS.

One problem with these studies is the lack of uniformity in how coasting was performed. The time point in the cycle at which coasting was to be started and the duration of coasting varied significantly. A Cochrane review concluded that insufficient evidence existed to permit the recommondation of coasting as a valid means to reduce the risk of OHSS[27]. The most recent data also suggest that coasting is associated with a significant incidence of premature luteinization and, if needed for more than 4 days, that the implantation rate is reduced[28].

TREATMENT BY OVER-HYDRATION AND ASPIRATION

A number of authors have advocated the use of extensive fluid hydration combined with paracentesis for the treatment of OHSS and ascites. There are two underlying theories for the use of over-hydration. The first recognizes the fact that thromboembolic phenomena have been responsible for the majority of fatal complications of OHSS, and can be responsible for significant morbidity such as stroke or pulmonary embolus[29]. By hydrating the patient, it is hoped that this will maintain intravascular volume, reduce hemoconcentration and therefore lessen the chance for thrombosis. In addition, maintenance of intravascular volume may improve renal perfusion and assist with natural diuresis.

However, due to the increased vascular permeability, a significant amount of the fluid given for hydration will leave the intravascular space and worsen the ascites, thus necessitating paracentesis. Aspiration of the ascitic fluid by paracentesis provides some immediate relief to the patient. It is also hoped that decreasing the intra-abdominal pressure will increase venous return to the heart and improve renal perfusion and ultimately speed the resolution process.

Rabau *et al.* were the first to propose abdominal paracentesis for the treatment of OHSS[30]. Later, transvaginal ultrasound guided paracentesis was found to be an acceptable alternative[31].

Protocol for management of OHSS with over-hydration and paracentesis[32]

(1) Patients are advised to maintain a fluid intake of 1000–1500 ml daily;

(2) Patients are instructed to contact the nursing staff if they experience an increase in abdominal girth of more than 1–2 cm, weight gain of > 1 kg in 24 h, shortness of breath, nausea, vomiting, diarrhea or a subjective decrease in urine output;

(3) Patients reporting these signs or symptoms undergo blood evaluations and are instructed to increase fluid by 500 ml/day if hemoconcentration is observed;

(4) The patients then undergo transvaginal ultrasound-guided paracentesis with drainage of ascites fluid.

A typical hydration/aspiration protocol of the type used by many American infertility programs is given above. Many authors have published case series with various modifications of this protocol. In addition to vigorous oral hydration, Aboulghar *et al.* advocated intensive intravenous hydration to reduce hemoconcentration[33]. It was soon discovered that under this form of management many patients required repeat paracenteses due to reaccumulation of ascitic fluid[34]. Reports in the literature exist of patients having paracentesis five times[35]. Al-Ramahi and colleagues used an indwelling peritoneal catheter to decrease the need for repeated paracentesis[36]. Under ultrasound guidance a closed-system Dawson–Mueller catheter with 'simp-loc' locking design was inserted to allow continuous drainage of the ascitic fluid.

Risks of treatment

Massive hydration leads to worsening of tense ascites. Adverse consequences include the need for recurrent paracentesis as noted above. Other issues include the development of vulvar edema. Cases of massive vulvar edema have been reported during hydration therapy with albumin and lactated Ringer's solution[37,38].

A far more serious problem is the risk of pulmonary edema and/or adult respiratory distress syndrome (ARDS). In the multicenter study of Abramov *et al.*, ARDS was reported in five patients (2.4%), and all cases occurred after massive hydration (4800–7200 ml; mean 5780 ml/24 h)[6]. This fluid intake was significantly higher than that recorded in uncomplicated cases.

Although increased fluid intake is often stated as necessary for the prevention of thromboembolic phenomena, Abramov *et al.* showed that patients who developed pulmonary thromboembolism received similar volumes of fluids to those who did not[6].

Therefore, the main rationale for the use of this method of treatment is possibly in error.

Initially, the risks of paracentesis were thought to be due to the danger of puncture and laceration of enlarged ovarian cysts[39]. However, by using ultrasound guidance, the risk of puncturing a cyst seems minimal[40]. Damage to other intra-abdominal organs is likewise probably low with ultrasound guidance, but the cumulative risk increases with multiple aspirations. The risk for infection rises with each subsequent needle placement.

Another potential risk of paracentesis is the alteration of uterine blood flow. This is an especially important point when it is considered that the vast majority of patients who present with severe or critical OHSS have a clinical gestation[16]. However, Chen *et al.* measured uterine blood flow with color Doppler ultrasound and showed that drainage of 2500 ml of ascitic fluid within 30 min actually increased uterine perfusion in some, but not all cases. Furthermore, there was no significant difference in the pregnancy or miscarriage rate, although the numbers were small[41].

Concern has also arisen that rapid drainage of ascites may in itself cause volume depletion[42] and further reduction in intravasvular oncotic proteins by drainage of the protein-rich ascitic fluid. To counteract these effects, Aboulghar *et al.* reinfused the protein-rich ascitic fluid in three patients with OHSS, with no apparent adverse consequences[43]. Splendiani *et al.* performed ultrafiltration of the ascitic fluid with a common high-flow dialyzer (polyacrylonitrile membrane)[44]. The fluid was then reinfused intravenously in three patients. In all three patients, diuresis was initiated and subjective improvement was seen. Beck *et al.* used a continuous reinfusion system in one critically ill patient[45].

As noted above, vulvar edema can result from vigorous hydration of patients with OHSS. Performance of a paracentesis can increase that risk. Luxman *et al.* reported that abdominal paracentesis through lower-quadrant puncture sites was associated with the development of ipsilateral massive vulvar edema[46]. A literature search did not reveal any such reports with the use of transvaginal paracentesis, however.

CONSERVATIVE MEDICAL TREATMENT OF OHSS

Fluid restriction

As opposed to the hydration/aspiration method, another method of management is mild fluid restriction. In the past, a widely accepted view of OHSS has been that electrolyte losses into ascitic fluid along with increased capillary permeability are responsible for decreased plasma osmolality and lower plasma sodium levels. Because of this assumption, it has been believed that sodium and electrolyte replacement is necessary to correct the deficit. However, it has been demonstrated that decreased plasma osmolality occurs in most women undergoing superovulation for *in vitro* fertilization by 2–4 days after the hCG trigger injection[47]. Normally, these alterations last for only a few days. However, in women who develop OHSS, the reduction of osmolality persists for much longer despite the presence of intravascular volume depletion[48]. If these abnormalities were to occur in normal women, they would stop production of vasopressin, their thirst would decrease and they would initiate diuresis of dilute urine in an attempt to raise the serum osmolality. In patients with OHSS, however, these thresholds are altered so that the patient maintains a high level of thirst and does not initiate diuresis[48].

In this protocol, therefore, patients are encouraged to drink only moderate amounts. Only fluids with good diuretic properties are consumed. This includes those beverages with high sugar content such as juices and sodas. High-sodium fluids such as sport drinks and free water are avoided. By limiting fluid and sodium intake, the third-space fluid accumulation is kept to a minimum, especially in the abdominal compartment. Thus, the problems associated with increased intra-abdominal pressure are reduced.

Albumin volume expansion

A second component of this protocol involves fluid shifting from the third space back into the vasculature and subsequent diuresis. As noted above, albumin infusion is ineffective for preventing OHSS. However, it can be useful for the treatment of established OHSS.

Patients with established OHSS are often hypoproteinemic due to loss of albumin and other proteins into the ascitic fluid. Abramov *et al.* determined that proteins up to a molecular weight of 180 kDa are lost[49]. This lowers the osmotic pressure and promotes further third-space fluid loss. When albumin is infused intravenously, the osmotic pressure is increased, with return of some fluid into the intravascular space. The effect is temporary, however, as eventually the infused albumin will also leak out, drawing the fluid back into the third space[10].

We have used albumin followed immediately by diuretics to promote diuresis in OHSS[50]. The albumin draws the fluid into the vasculature. Immediately upon completion of the albumin infusion, diuretics are given. The first effect of the diuretic is to promote renal artery dilatation. The resulting large diuresis is achieved by using fluid from the third space. We and others have found that conservative management with salt-poor albumin and diuretics is an acceptable form of management, with rapid resolution of OHSS and maintenance of pregnancies[51].

Protocol for conservative management

Out-patient management

(1) Avoid food and beverages that are high in sodium;

(2) Do not force fluid intake;

(3) When drinking fluids, use those that are high in sugar and low in sodium;

(4) Narcotic pain medication as needed;

(5) Anti-emetics for nausea (Zofran ODT® 8 mg every 8 h as needed);

(6) If hemoglobin is > 15 g/dl, start Lovenox® 40 mg every day;

(7) Patient to measure input and output every day and phone the results to the office;

(8) Patient also to call the office if she has any of the following:

  (a) Sudden weight gain;

  (b) Shortness of breath;

  (c) Pain resistant to medication;

  (d) Nausea resistant to medication or emesis.

In-patient management

(1) Dextrose 5% in half normal saline (D5/0.45NS) + 10 mEq/l KCl to match urine output;

(2) 250 ml of salt-poor 25% albumin intravenously over 2 h;

(3) Upon completion of albumin drip, administer furosemide 20 mg intravenous push;

(4) If patient has persistent oliguria, start renal dose dopamine (2–3 μg/kg/min);

(5) Paracentesis reserved for refractory tense ascites or severe dyspnea.

Hydroxyethyl starch

Hydroxyethyl starch is a highly branched amylopectin that resembles glycogen. Its molecular weight ranges from 200 to 1000 kDa. At that size, it is potentially large enough to avoid leaking out of the vasculature. Abramov *et al.* compared the use of 6% hydroxyethyl starch solution with use of albumin in 16 patients with severe OHSS[52]. Eighty per cent of patients in the albumin group required paracentesis compared with only 33% in the starch group. Hospital stay averaged 3 days less in the starch group. Levin *et al.* used a 10% solution and also showed efficacy[53]. Dextran 40 has also been used as a plasma expander in the treatment of OHSS. Compared with 25% albumin, dextran 40-treated patients had less time to resolution of hemoconcentration without affecting the pregnancy or miscarriage rate[54]. The potential advantages of synthetic colloid expanders in the treatment of OHSS include lower cost and lower risk for infection compared with the blood-derived albumin. In theory, they may be more effective, since their size would limit their leakage out of the vasculature.

Dopamine

Dopamine is also an effective treatment for OHSS by virtue of its ability, at low doses, to effect dilatation of the renal vasculature, improve renal blood flow and thereby promote diuresis. Ferrareti *et al.* were the first to report the use of intravenous dopamine for the treatment of OHSS[55]. We also reported a series of patients successfully treated in this way[50].

One problem with dopamine is that it must be given intravenously. Although low-dose dopamine has a vasodilatory effect in selected tissues, high concentrations achieved locally as a result of intravenous (IV) site extravasation can still cause severe vasoconstriction and ischemic tissue injury. Because of this risk, most hospitals restrict by protocol the use of IV dopamine to an intensive-care setting with a higher nurse/patient ratio, so that the IV sites can be monitored more closely. This, of course, dramatically increases the cost of treatment. Treatment consists of the administration of subcutaneous phentolamine into the area of ischemia. Typically, dramatic resolution of ischemic changes rapidly follows phentolamine injection with no untoward effects.

Tsunoda *et al.* reported the use of a novel dopamine derivative for the treatment of OHSS[56]. Docarpamine is a synthetic, orally administered dopamine prodrug which is converted into dopamine. Twenty-seven patients received 750 mg of docarpamine every 8 h. Twenty were judged to have 'good' or 'fair' response based on the duration of time until hospital discharge. Mean daily urine output increased significantly by the first day of treatment, and remained high through 4 days. Symptoms of abdominal distension and pain and hemoconcentration all resolved in an average of 3–7 days.

The significant benefit of this therapy is the avoidance of IV administration and risk of extravasation, thus reducing the need for intensive-care monitoring. Unfortunately, this medication is not currently available in the United States.

PLEURAL EFFUSION

Increased pleural fluid can lead to decreased tidal volume and hypoxia[6]. This problem may be more common than is generally appreciated. Levin *et al.* found that in patients diagnosed with severe OHSS, 23% had evidence for pleural effusion[57].

Abramov *et al.* found that 4% of patients with severe OHSS had pulmonary infections, all of which consisted of lobar pneumonia (most commonly affecting the left lower lobe)[6].

Semba *et al.* reported a patient death from massive pulmonary edema during apparent improvement from other clinical signs of OHSS[58].

For those patients presenting with pleural effusion and respiratory compromise, thoracocentesis is an option. Rinaldi and Spirtos reported the use of a chest tube placed for treatment of pleural effusions[59]. They noted that placement of a chest tube corrected the pleural effusions and the accompanying abdominal ascites.

The best method to avoid pulmonary edema is to avoid extensive hydration. However, if it does occur, careful diuresis in an intensive-care setting is mandatory.

PERICARDIAL EFFUSION

There have been no specific studies that have addressed the issue of pericardial effusions directly. Fortunately, problems associated with pericardial effusion are rare. Tamponade with decreased cardiac output is the most serious possibility. There are no reported cases in the medical literature of cardiac tamponade being caused by OHSS.

Pericardiocentesis should be reserved for those emergency cases where tamponade is identified.

CONCLUSIONS

There are two favored methods for the treatment of OHSS in the United States. One method is characterized by *over-hydration* of the patient with repeated or continuous drainage of the ascitic fluid that is produced. The most serious risk associated with this method is the development of ARDS or pulmonary edema. Since it does not appear to reduce the risk of thromboembolism, additional prophylactic measures must not be forgotten.

Another method of treatment utilizes *mild fluid restriction* combined with medical diuresis. Diuresis is affected by the use of albumin or hydroxyethyl starch to shift fluid from the third space into the vasculature, followed by loop diuretics and/or the use of low-dose dopamine.

Unfortunately, no studies have compared these methods directly as to their efficacy, risks or pregnancy outcomes.

The most popular method to prevent the development of OHSS is conversion of superovulation cycles to *in vitro* fertilization cycles. Although this increases the expense of treatment, the pregnancy rates are expected to be higher, and other risks, such as multiple pregnancy, can be controlled. Patients at risk for OHSS from an *in vitro* fertilization cycle can be given the options of egg retrieval, fertilization and cryopreservation of all embryos. Avoidance of pregnancy will reduce the incidence of OHSS and the severity of cases that do occur.

REFERENCES

1. Roland M. Menotropin with HCG in ovulation induction. Results in 56 patients including a case of severe ovarian hyperstimulation. Fertil Steril 1969; 20: 1004–16.
2. Bassil S, Da Costa S, Toussaint-Demylle D, et al. A unilateral hydrothorax as the only manifestation of ovarian hyperstimulation syndrome: a case report. Fertil Steril 1996; 66: 1023–5.
3. Sovova E, Oborna I, Dostal J, et al. Ovarian hyperstimulation syndrome as a rare cause of pericardial effusion: 2 case reports. Vnitr Lek 1998; 44: 277–9.
4. Whelan JG III, Vlahos NF. The ovarian hyperstimulation syndrome. Fertil Steril 2000; 73: 883–96.
5. Levin I, Almog B, Avni A, et al. Effect of paracentesis of ascitic fluids on urinary output and blood indices in patients with severe ovarian hyperstimulation syndrome. Fertil Steril 2002; 77: 986–8.
6. Abramov Y, Elchalal U, Schenker JG. Pulmonary manifestations of severe ovarian hyperstimulation syndrome: a multicenter study. Fertil Steril 1999; 71: 645–51.
7. Laroche M, Harding G. Primary and secondary peritonitis: an update. Eur J Clin Microbiol Infect Dis 1998; 17: 542–50.
8. Asch RH, Ivery G, Goldsman M, et al. The use of intravenous albumin in patients at high risk for severe ovarian hyperstimulation syndrome. Hum Reprod 1993; 8: 1015–20.
9. Ben-Chetrit A, Eldar-Geva Y, Gal M, et al. The questionable use of albumin for the prevention of ovarian hyperstimulation syndrome in an IVF programme: a randomized placebo-controlled trial. Hum Reprod 2001; 16: 1880–4.
10. Rackw EC, Falk JL, Fein IA. Fluid resuscitation in circulatory shock: a comparison of the cardiorespiratory effects of albumin, hetastarch, and saline solutions in patients with hypovolemic and septic shock. Crit Care Med 1983; 11: 839–50.
11. Ng E, Leader A, Claman P, et al. Intravenous albumin does not prevent the development of severe ovarian hyperstimulation syndrome in an in-vitro fertilization programme. Hum Reprod 1995; 10: 807–10.
12. Shalev E, Giladi Y, Matilsky M, et al. Decreased incidence of ovarian hyperstimulation syndrome in high risk in-vitro fertilization patients receiving intravenous albumin: a prospective study. Hum Reprod 1995; 10: 1373–6.
13. Aboulghar M, Evers JH, Al-Inany H. Intravenous albumin for preventing severe ovarian hyperstimulation syndrome: a Cochrane review. Hum Reprod 2002; 17: 3027–32.
14. Jose B, Elkin A, Munoz A, et al. Intravenous albumin does not prevent moderate-severe ovarian hyperstimulation syndrome in high-risk IVF patients: a randomized controlled study. Hum Reprod 2003; 18: 2283–8.
15. Morris RS, Paulson RJ, Sauer MV, et al. Predictive value of serum oestradiol concentrations and oocyte number in severe ovarian hyperstimulation syndrome. Hum Reprod 1995; 10: 811–14.
16. Abramov Y, Elchalal U, Schenker JG. Obstetric outcome of in vitro fertilized pregnancies complicated by severe ovarian hyperstimulation syndrome: a multicenter study. Fertil Steril 1998; 70: 1070–6.
17. Koike T, Minakami H, Araki S, et al. Severity of ovarian hyperstimulation syndrome: its relation to number of conceptuses. Int J Fertil Womens Med 2004; 49: 36–42.
18. Lipitz S, Ben-Rafael Z, Bider D, et al. Quintuplet pregnancy and third degree ovarian hyperstimulation despite withholding human chorionic gonadotrophin. Hum Reprod 1991; 6: 1478–9.
19. Many A, Azem F, Lessing JB, et al. Pregnancy rate in IVF rescue in high responders to human

menopausal gonadotropin. Assist Reprod Genet 1999; 16: 520–2.

20. Lessing JB, Amit A, Libal Y, et al. Avoidance of cancellation of potential hyperstimulation cycles by conversion to in vitro fertilization-embryo transfer. Fertil Steril 1991; 56: 75–8.

21. Queenan JT Jr, Veeck LL, Toner JP, et al. Cryopreservation of all prezygotes in patients at risk of severe hyperstimulation does not eliminate the syndrome, but the chances of pregnancy are excellent with subsequent frozen–thaw transfers. Hum Reprod 1997; 12: 1573–6.

22. Amso NN, Ahuja KK, Morris N, et al. The management of predicted ovarian hyperstimulation involving gonadotropin-releasing hormone analog with elective cryopreservation of all pre-embryos. Fertil Steril 1990; 53: 1087–90.

23. D'Angelo A, Amso N. Embryo freezing for preventing Ovarian Hyperstimulation Syndrome. Cochrane Database Syst Rev 2002; 2: CD002806

24. Sher G, Zouves C, Feinman M, et al. 'Prolonged coasting': an effective method for preventing severe ovarian hyperstimulation syndrome in patients undergoing in-vitro fertilization. Hum Reprod 1995; 10: 3107–9.

25. Benadiva CA, Davis O, Kligman I, et al. Withholding gonadotropin administration is an effective alternative for the prevention of ovarian hyperstimulation syndrome. Fertil Steril 1997; 67: 724–7.

26. Lee C, Tummon I, Martin J, et al. Does withholding gonadotrophin administration prevent severe ovarian hyperstimulation syndrome? Hum Reprod 1998; 13: 1157–8.

27. D'Angelo A, Amso N. 'Coasting' (withholding gonadotrophins) for preventing ovarian hyperstimulation syndrome. Cochrane Database Syst Rev 2002; 3: CD002811.

28. Moreno L, Diaz I, Pacheco A, et al. Extended coasting duration exerts a negative impact on IVF cycle outcome due to premature luteinization. Reprod Biomed Online 2004; 9: 500–4.

29. Lamon D, Chang CK, Hruska L, et al. Superior vena cava thrombosis after in vitro fertilization: case report and review of the literature. Ann Vasc Surg 2000; 14: 283–5.

30. Rabau E, David A, Serr DM, et al. Human menopausal gonadotropins for anovulation and sterility. Am J Obstet Gynecol 1967; 98: 92–8.

31. Aboulghar MA, Mansour RT, Serour GI, et al. Ultrasonographic guided vaginal aspiration of ascites in the treatment of severe ovarian hyperstimulation syndrome. Fertil Steril 1990; 5: 933–5.

32. Fluker MR, Copeland JE, Yuzpe AA. An ounce of prevention: outpatient management of the ovarian hyperstimulation syndrome. Fertil Steril 2000; 73: 821–4.

33. Aboulghar MA, Mansour RT, Serour GI, et al. Management of severe ovarian hyperstimulation syndrome by ascetic fluid aspiration and intensive intravenous fluid therapy. Obstet Gynecol 1993; 81: 108–11.

34. Chen CD, Yang JH, Chao KH, et al. Effects of repeated abdominal paracentesis on uterine and intraovarian haemodynamics and pregnancy outcome in severe ovarian hyperstimulation syndrome. Hum Reprod 1998; 13: 2077–81.

35. Raziel A, Friedler S, Schachter M, et al. Transvaginal drainage of ascites as an alternative to abdominal paracentesis in patients with severe ovarian hyperstimulation syndrome, obesity, and generalized edema. Fertil Steril 1998; 69: 780–3.

36. Al-Ramahi M, Leader A, Claman P, et al. A novel approach to the treatment of ascites associated with ovarian hyperstimulation syndrome. Hum Reprod 1997; 12: 2614–16.

37. Coccia ME, Bracco GL, Cattaneo A, et al. Massive vulvar edema in ovarian hyperstimulation syndrome. A case report. J Reprod Med 1995; 40: 659–60.

38. Cline DL. Massive vulvar edema in ovarian hyperstimulation syndrome. Reprod Med 1996; 41: 780.

39. Schenker JG, Weinstein D. Ovarian hyperstimulation syndrome: a current survey. Fertil Steril 1978; 30: 255–68.

40. Runyon BA. Paracentesis of ascitic fluid: a safe procedure. Arch Intern Med 1986; 146: 2259–61.

CHAPTER 17

Life-threatening forms of ovarian hyperstimulation syndrome and intensive care of the ovarian hyperstimulation syndrome patient

Zalman Levine and Daniel Navot

INTRODUCTION

Ovarian hyperstimulation syndrome (OHSS) is an iatrogenic disease usually resulting from human chorionic gonadotropin (hCG) stimulation of ovarian granulosa cells in gonadotropin-stimulated ovaries. The syndrome exists in a clinical spectrum, with some patients exhibiting only mild disease, and other patients requiring intensive management. OHSS and the complications thereof have even resulted in reported fatalities[1–5]. In a widely used classification scheme, Navot *et al.* defined severe and critical forms of OHSS to help researchers and clinicians identify these serious and life-threatening conditions[6]. Clinicians managing patients with OHSS must be familiar with the syndrome and its diverse manifestations, and above all must be familiar with medical and surgical options in the treatment of the critically ill OHSS patient.

CRITICAL OHSS

Pathophysiology

The clinical manifestations of life-threatening OHSS are a cascade of pathophysiological events resulting from a global increase in vascular permeability due to ovarian overproduction of vasoactive substances[7]. This increased vascular permeability causes a change in extracellular fluid equilibrium, with fluid shifting into the extravascular or 'third' space, often causing ascites, pleural and pericardial effusions and hemoconcentration. Cardiac preload falls due to a combination of hypovolemia caused by the fluid shifts, and compression of the inferior vena cava from the increasing intraperitoneal ascitic pressure. Falling cardiac preload reduces cardiac output, which in turn leads to a decrease in renal perfusion. Decreasing renal perfusion increases proximal tubule reabsorption of salt and water, leading to decreased urinary sodium excretion and oliguria. The proximal sodium reabsorption, and consequently diminished exposure of the distal tubule to sodium, impaires sodium–hydrogen/potassium exchange in the distal tubule, causing hyperkalemic acidosis. A full prerenal azotemia can develop. OHSS also produces a hypercoagulable state, possibly due to a combination of hemoconcentration and high levels of ovarian steroids.

Symptomatology

The patient usually presents with initial symptoms of abdominal discomfort, bloating and anorexia, followed soon thereafter by the onset of nausea, and occasionally vomiting and diarrhea. Rapid progression of these symptoms, particularly within 48–72 h after administration of the hCG triggering injection, should alert the clinician to a significant risk for the development of severe or critical OHSS[8]. Enlarged ovaries, common in OHSS, are at risk for torsion as well, and acute abdominal pain must arouse suspicion for adnexal torsion.

Physical findings

Physical examination of the patient with severe or critical OHSS will reveal weight gain because of an increase in total body water, increased abdominal girth, shifting dullness and a fluid wave due to ascites, dullness to percussion over lung fields affected by hydrothorax and signs of hypovolemia including hypotension and oliguria. The ovaries are usually, but not always, palpable on abdominal examination, and are generally tender to palpation. Dyspnea, tachypnea and hypoxemia can be seen from hydrothorax, adult respiratory distress syndrome (ARDS) or thromboembolic events[9,10].

Laboratory findings

Laboratory evaluation of the patient with critical OHSS reveals severe hemoconcentration with a hematocrit greater than 55%, dramatic leukocytosis greater than 25 000/mm^3, serum creatinine at least 1.6 mg/dl, creatinine clearance 50 ml/min or less, hyperkalemic acidosis and dilutional hyponatremia with low serum osmolality. Low urinary sodium excretion can be measured. Liver function test abnormalities are often seen, including elevated transaminases and alkaline phosphatase, and hypoalbuminemia and hypogammaglobulinemia[11,12]. Plasma levels of measurable vasoactive substances are elevated, including plasma renin activity, aldosterone, atrial natriuretic peptide and antidiuretic hormone, prostaglandins, angiotensin II, vascular endothelial growth factor (VEGF), tumor necrosis factor-α and interleukins 1, 2 and 6. Ascitic, pleural and pericardial fluid is exudative, rich in protein exuded from plasma through hyperpermeable capillaries.

Pulmonary findings

OHSS leads to critical respiratory issues because of a combination of lung restriction due to abdominal pressure from enlarged ovaries and tense ascites, hydrothorax and pericardial effusions, thromboembolic occurrences leading to pulmonary embolus, and intrapulmonary increases in capillary permeability leading, in the extreme, to ARDS. Pleural effusions are almost universal in critical OHSS, and are usually but not always bilateral[13–15].

Renal findings

Because of the intravascular hypovolemia, renal blood flow and glomerular filtration are reduced, causing severe oliguria or anuria. A prerenal azotemia develops, with decreased creatinine clearance and elevated serum creatinine. Critical OHSS can feature the stigmata of acute renal failure, including hyperkalemia and metabolic acidosis occasionally necessitating dialysis. Volume overload, common in renal failure in other clinical settings, generally does not develop in OHSS because of the capillary hyperpermeability and consequent intravascular hypovolemia. Patients with critical OHSS often demonstrate an initial hypernatremia due to intravascular dehydration, but dilutional hyponatremia frequently develops as the syndrome begins to resolve and massive volumes of extravascular fluids are returned to the circulation.

Thromboembolic events

Thromboembolic disease is a known and potentially fatal feature of OHSS[16], thought to be caused by a combination of hemoconcentration, ovarian steroid oversecretion and intravascular hypovolemia. Intrinsic changes in blood clotting mechanisms may also occur in OHSS, as some have noted the presence of thrombocytosis as well as elevated coagulation factors and endogenous antifibrinolytics[17,18]. Patients developing OHSS who have other underlying coagulation abnormalities due to, for example, hereditary or autoimmune factors are at increased risk for the occurrence of thrombotic events. Such underlying coagulation abnormalities can coexist with OHSS, but do not seem to increase the risk of developing OHSS[19]. Most thrombotic events due to OHSS are venous, and most venous thromboses occur in the head, neck and upper limbs. Arterial thromboses, accounting for 25% of OHSS-associated thrombotic events, have been reported in carotid, subclavian, ulnar, iliac, mesenteric, femoral, popliteal, retinal and intracerebral arteries, as well as in the aorta itself.

Sepsis

Patients with critical OHSS have been found to have plasma deficiencies of immunoglobulins, particularly IgG and IgA; immunoglobulin levels in ascitic fluids are high, suggesting that the etiology of the plasma deficiency is transcapillary exudation of these proteins into the third space[12,20]. Presumably related to this immunodeficiency, febrile morbidity in patients with critical OHSS is high. The incidence of infections in such patients has been reported to be as high as 82%[21], and includes urinary tract infections, pneumonia and upper respiratory infections.

TREATMENT OF THE OHSS PATIENT

Medical approach

There are two possible approaches to the treatment of OHSS, one pathogenesis-oriented and one supportive. The former approach utilizes agents which specifically negate the putative causative factor(s) of OHSS. Indomethacin was hypothesized to be such an agent when prostaglandins were believed to play a role in OHSS. Angiotensin-converting enzyme (ACE) inhibitors are another group of specific pharmacological agents which were thought to have potential use in the treatment of OHSS because they inhibit the production of angiotensin II, a probable pathogenic factor for the syndrome. Unfortunately, indomethacin did not benefit the syndrome, and ACE inhibitors are teratogenic and thus contraindicated whenever a pregnancy is contemplated. Just as antagonists to VEGF may become useful for the prevention of OHSS, similar cytokine inhibitors are being studied for treatment of the syndrome. To date, such therapies remain investigational, largely preclinical and not yet compelling. One recent study found pentoxifylline, an inhibitor of the synthesis of tumor necrosis factor-α, to be ineffective in limiting ascites formation in an OHSS rabbit model, although it did decrease ovarian weight compared with controls[22]. However, until such interventions are validated in human trials, the treatment of OHSS remains largely supportive in nature, aiming to mitigate the potentially fatal threat of critical OHSS until the condition resolves on its own.

Individual treatment will depend on the severity of the syndrome. Mild forms of OHSS require little more than reassurance, since it is well established that mild symptoms usually resolve, in the absence of pregnancy, within 2 weeks after receiving hCG. If a pregnancy ensues, mild symptoms may progress, but rarely more than one degree in severity. In patients with moderate ascites and mild hemoconcentration (hematocrit < 45%), bedrest and abundant liquid intake should be prescribed. The tendency for intravascular volume depletion and hyponatremia may be treated with oral isotonic salt solutions; sports drinks, popular among athletes, are particularly suitable because they are engineered for optimal rehydration. The patient should be vigilant in noting any decreases in urine output, significant weight gain or abdominal bloating as self-assessed by daily abdominal girth measurement. These findings, if present, may be the first warning signals of accumulation of ascitic fluid and worsening hemoconcentration. A hematocrit > 45%, or 30% increased over baseline, indicates that the condition has entered the category of severe OHSS and that hospitalization is required.

Dramatic clinical deterioration is most likely to manifest 9–10 days after hCG administration, when endogenous, pregnancy-derived hCG becomes perceptible and the late form of OHSS sets in. Figure 1 outlines an algorithm for the management of the critically ill hospitalized OHSS patient. All fluid and electrolyte management of such a patient ought to be performed through frequent physical examinations, including vital signs and pulse oximetry, blood tests at least daily, abdominal ultrasound and chest radiographs. Strict monitoring of fluid intake and output should be performed through an indwelling transurethral urinary catheter and through large-bore intravenous lines, preferably a central venous line to measure central venous pressure.

The single most important variable that indicates the severity of the OHSS is hemoconcentration as reflected in the hematocrit. Because the hematocrit is actually the ratio between red cell volume and total blood volume where total blood volume = red cell volume + plasma volume, the change in plasma volume must always be larger than the change reflected by the hematocrit[23]. Thus, a change of 2 percentage points in the hematocrit from 42 to 44% is four times smaller than the actual 8% drop in plasma volume. This is extremely important to remember when managing patients with OHSS. Any increase in the hematocrit as it approaches 45% underestimates the magnitude of plasma volume depletion and thus the seriousness of the patient's condition. One should therefore not be lulled into a false sense of security when only a small incremental rise in hematocrit between 40 and 45% is observed. Similarly, in the face of hemoconcentration, small reductions in hematocrit may represent a significant improvement in plasma volume[6].

An additional measure of hemoconcentration is the magnitude of leukocytosis; white blood cell (WBC) counts higher than 25 000/mm^3, largely reflecting a granulocytosis, may be seen. This massive neutrophilia may be attributed to hemoconcentration and a generalized stress reaction. When oral isotonic fluid intake is insufficient to maintain plasma volume, intravenous fluid therapy becomes mandatory. Crystalloids alone, although seldom sufficient in restoring homeostasis because of massive protein loss through hyperpermeable capillaries, still remain the mainstay of intensive treatment of OHSS. Because of the tendency for hyponatremia, sodium chloride with or without glucose is the crystalloid of choice, and potassium-containing fluid should be avoided. The daily volume infused may vary from 1.5 l to greater than 3.0 l. Although some authors advocate fluid restriction to minimize the accumulation of ascites, one should rather deal with the discomfort of ascites than face the consequences of hypovolemia and hemoconcentration with the attendant risks of thromboembolism and renal shutdown. In order to maintain fluid balance, the patient's urine output, oral and intravenous fluid intake, body weight, abdominal girth, hematocrit and serum electrolytes must be monitored. In addition, coagulation parameters and liver enzymes should be periodically assessed. Intravenous volume replacement should aim to improve renal perfusion before fluid escapes into the peritoneal and/or pleural cavities; this transient hemodilution is achieved at the expense of increased third-spacing and increased total body water. Whenever adequate fluid balance cannot be restored by crystalloids alone, plasma expanders should be utilized. Since albumin is the main protein lost in OHSS, human albumin is physiological and thus the colloid of choice.

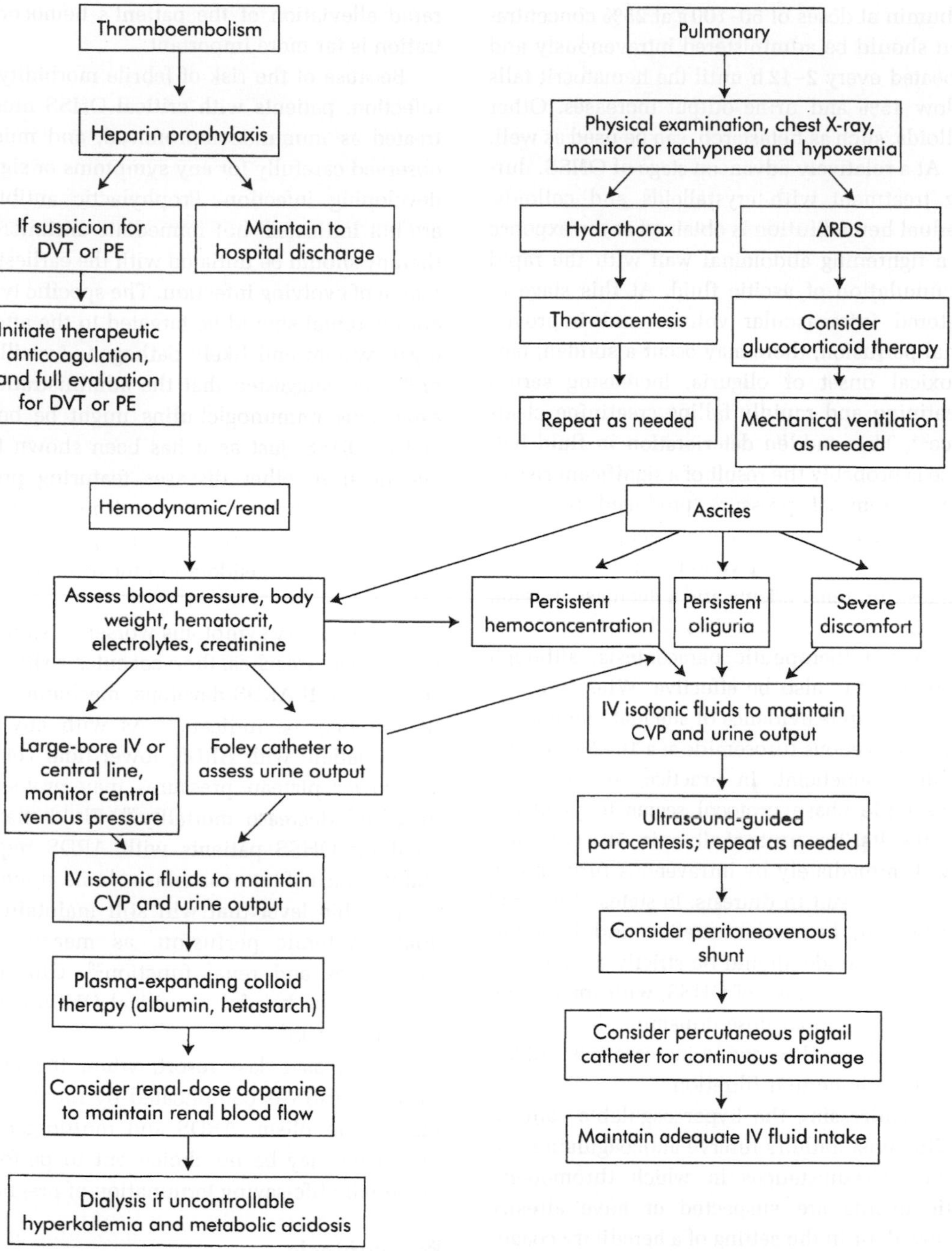

Figure 1 Algorithm for intensive care of the patient with critical OHSS. DVT, deep vein thrombosis; PE, pulmonary embolism; ARDS, adult respiratory distress syndrome; IV, intravenous; CVP, central venous pressure

Albumin at doses of 50–100 g at 25% concentration should be administered intravenously and repeated every 2–12 h until the hematocrit falls below 45% and urine output increases. Other colloids, such as hetastarch, can be used as well.

At a relatively advanced stage of OHSS, during treatment with crystalloids and colloids, gradual hemodilution is obtained at the expense of a tightening abdominal wall with the rapid accumulation of ascitic fluid. At this stage of restored intravascular volume and improved renal perfusion, there may occur a sudden, paradoxical onset of oliguria, increasing serum creatinine and rapidly falling creatinine clearance[24]. This sudden deterioration in fluid balance is probably the result of a significant rise in intra-abdominal pressure produced by tense ascites. Increased intra-abdominal pressure may in turn impede renal venous outflow, causing congestion, renal edema and a decrease in renal function. Such tense ascites is best treated surgically via therapeutic paracentesis, although diuretics may also be effective. When oliguria persists despite evidence of adequate hemodilution, intravenous furosemide at a 10–20-mg dose is often beneficial. In practice, an albumin–furosemide chase protocol seems to yield the best results. Two units of albumin, 50 g each, followed immediately by intravenous furosemide, will often result in diuresis. In states of volume contraction, hemoconcentration and hypotension, furosemide should be strictly avoided. In this precarious stage of OHSS, with impending renal failure, renal dose dopamine drip should be used for renal rescue to increase renal blood flow and glomerular filtration.

In addressing the hypercoagulable state of OHSS, most authors reserve anticoagulation for special circumstances in which thromboembolic events are suspected or have already occurred, or in the setting of a hereditary coagulopathy. Although prophylactic treatment with unfractionated or low-molecular-weight heparin is of some theoretical value and perhaps should be routine in all patients with critical OHSS[25], rapid alleviation of the patient's hemoconcentration is far more important.

Because of the risk of febrile morbidity and infection, patients with critical OHSS must be treated as immunocompromised, and must be observed carefully for any symptoms or signs of developing infection. Prophylactic antibiotics are not indicated, but immediate antimicrobial therapy should be initiated with the earliest suspicion of evolving infection. The specific type of antimicrobial should be targeted to the affected organ system and likely pathogen. Avecillas *et al.*[26] have suggested that the administration of exogenous immunoglobulins might be beneficial in OHSS, just as it has been shown to be beneficial in other diseases featuring protein loss such as the nephrotic syndrome[27], but this intervention for OHSS needs experimental validation prior to consideration for full-scale clinical use.

If pulmonary symptoms worsen despite conservative approaches, thoracocentesis should be considered. If ARDS develops, mechanical ventilation may be indicated. As with any non-OHSS patient with ARDS, lower tidal volumes and lower plateau pressures may protect the lung and decrease mortality[28]. Fluid management for OHSS patients with ARDS requires maintenance of intravascular volume at the lowest possible level that will still maintain adequate systemic perfusion, as measured by electrolytes and renal function[26]. Glucocorticoids may be helpful in critical OHSS complicated by ARDS[9].

Rarely, as a last resort, when the critical stage of OHSS is complicated by renal failure, thromboembolism, ARDS and multiorgan failure, there may be no choice but to perform a potentially life-saving termination of pregnancy.

Paracentesis

The single most important treatment modality for life-threatening OHSS unresponsive to medical therapy is paracentesis. Rabau *et al.* first proposed the use of paracentesis in the treatment of severe OHSS[29]. Paracentesis was temporarily discredited, but later regained popularity. Many investigators have promoted paracentesis as safe and exceptionally beneficial[24,30,31]. Dramatic improvements in the clinical symptoms of severe OHSS, with almost instantaneous diuresis, were reported. In a series of seven patients in whom paracentesis was performed, urine output rose from 780 ± 407 ml to 1670 ± 208 ml ($p < 0.05$), creatinine clearance rose from 75.4 ± 16 ml/min to 101 ± 15 ml/min ($p < 0.05$), hematocrit decreased from 46.3 ± 2.2% to 37.1 ± 2.5% ($p < 0.05$), and a mean weight loss of 5.3 kg was observed[32]. In the study by Forman *et al.*, 37 l of ascitic fluid with a protein content of 46–53 g/l (1.85 kg protein loss) was removed from a single patient, underscoring both the high protein content of ascitic fluid and the safety of the procedure[31].

The indications for paracentesis include the need for symptomatic relief, tense ascites, oliguria, rising creatinine or falling creatinine clearance and hemoconcentration unresponsive to medical treatment. Paracentesis should be performed aseptically under ultrasound guidance. Careful monitoring of hemodynamic stability is also mandatory. Rizk and Aboulghar advocated transvaginal ultrasonically guided aspiration of ascitic fluid as an effective and equally safe method[32], but a transabdominal approach can be used easily as well. Up to 4 l may be removed either by slow drainage to gravity[30] or with negative pressure using large evacuated containers. Paracentesis is contraindicated in patients who are hemodynamically unstable, or in the presence of suspected hemoperitoneum.

A new and innovative treatment for severe OHSS was suggested by Koike *et al.*[33]. These authors describe continuous peritoneovenous shunting in 18 patients with severe OHSS. This study group was compared with 36 control patients who had received intravenous albumin at a dose of 37.5 g/day. Recirculation of ascites fluid rich in proteins is not a novel idea[34]; however, the reliance on a continuous shunt from the peritoneal cavity into the antecubital vein is a logical way to replenish the vascular tree with the fluids, proteins and electrolytes that were lost from the vasculature. The study reports faster hemodilution, shorter hospital stay and prompt improvement in symptoms in the shunted patients due to diuresis and reduction in the amount of ascites. There are, however, some problems with the study, beside the complexity of the set-up. First, the reinfused ascites may contain the very substances which might be responsible for the profound hyperpermeability of OHSS, and thus may exacerbate the syndrome. Second, the group advocates fluid restriction, which may aggravate hemoconcentration and thus contribute to renal failure and thromboembolic phenomena.

Surgery

Because of the ovarian enlargement frequently present in OHSS, patients may present with ovarian cyst rupture or hemorrhage, or with ovarian torsion. Cyst rupture or hemorrhage can often be managed conservatively, but adnexal torsion is a surgical emergency in OHSS as it is in any other context. Successful laparoscopic detorsion for OHSS patients has been reported[35].

CONCLUSIONS

OHSS can present in a wide clinical spectrum, with some patients requiring nothing more than observation at home and others requiring intensive management. Critical OHSS is a life-threatening syndrome with multiorgan consequences. Familiarity with the pathophysiology of OHSS and with the manifestations of its critical form leads to a rational, supportive management scheme which can prevent further deterioration. With an understanding of the disease and with careful attention to fluid and electrolyte management, respiratory support, infection control and thromboembolism prophylaxis, clinicians can effectively protect the threatened lives of these critically ill patients.

REFERENCES

1. Moses M, Bogowsky H, Anteby E, et al. Thromboembolic phenomena after ovarian stimulation with menopausal gonadotrophins. Lancet 1965; 2: 1213.
2. Esteban-Altirriba J. Le syndrome d'hyperstimulation massive des ovaries. Rev Fr Gynecol Obstet 1961; 56: 555.
3. Figueroa-Casas P. Reaccion ovarica monstruosa a las gonadotrofinas a proposito de un caso fatal. Ann Cirug 1958; 23: 116.
4. Cluroe AD, Synek BJ. A fatal case of ovarian hyperstimulation syndrome with cerebral infarction. Pathology 1995; 27: 344–6.
5. Semba S, Moriya T, Youssef EM, et al. An autopsy case of ovarian hyperstimulation syndrome with massive pulmonary edema and pleural effusion. Pathol Int 2000; 50: 549–52.
6. Navot D, Bergh PA, Laufer N. Ovarian hyperstimulation syndrome in novel reproductive technologies: prevention and treatment. Fertil Steril 1992; 58: 249–61.
7. Navot D, Levine Z, Klein J. Severe ovarian hyperstimulation syndrome. In Gardner DK, ed. Textbook of Assisted Reproductive Techniques, 2nd edn. London: Taylor & Francis, 2004: 805–16.
8. Shanbhag S, Bhattacharya S. Current management of ovarian hyperstimulation syndrome. Hosp Med 2002; 63: 528–32.
9. Shigematsu T, Kubota E, Aman M. Adult respiratory distress syndrome as a manifestation of ovarian hyperstimulation syndrome. Int J Gynaecol Obstet 2000; 69: 169–70.
10. Rouzi AA. Life threatening ovarian hyperstimulation syndrome. Int J Gynaecol Obstet 2000; 68: 269–70.
11. Fabregues F, Balasch J, Gines P, et al. Ascites and liver test abnormalities during severe ovarian hyperstimulation syndrome. Am J Gastroenterol 1999; 94: 994–9.
12. Abramov Y, Naparstek Y, Elchalal U, et al. Plasma immunoglobulins in patients with severe ovarian hyperstimulation syndrome. Fertil Steril 1999; 71: 102–5.
13. Levin MF, Kaplan BR, Hutton LC. Thoracic manifestations of ovarian hyperstimulation syndrome. Can Assoc Radiol J 1995; 46: 23–6.
14. Daniel Y, Yaron Y, Oren M, et al. Ovarian hyperstimulation syndrome manifests as acute unilateral hydrothorax. Hum Reprod 1995; 10: 1684–5.
15. Cordani S, Bancalari L, Maggiani R, et al. Massive unilateral hydrothorax as the only clinical manifestation of ovarian hyperstimulation syndrome. Arch Chest Dis 2002; 57: 314–17.
16. Stewart JA, Hamilton PJ, Murdoch AP. Thromboembolic disease associated with ovarian stimulation and assisted conception techniques. Hum Reprod 1997; 12: 2167–73.
17. Tavmergen E, Ozeakir HT, Levi R, et al. Bilateral jugular venous thromboembolism and pulmonary emboli in a patient with severe ovarian hyperstimulation syndrome. J Obstet Gynaecol Res 2001; 27: 217–20.
18. Heinig J, Behre HM, Klockenbusch W. Occlusion of the ulnar artery in a patient with severe ovarian hyperstimulation syndrome. Eur J Obstet Gynecol Reprod Biol 2001; 96: 126–7.
19. Fabregues F, Tassies D, Reverter JC, et al. Prevalence of thrombophilia in women with severe ovarian hyperstimulation syndrome and cost-effectiveness of screening. Fertil Steril 2004; 81: 989–95.
20. Tukamizawa S, Shibahara H, Taneichi A, et al. Dynamic changes of the immunoglobulins in patients with severe ovarian hyperstimulation syndrome: efficacy of a novel treatment using peritoneo-venous shunt. Am J Reprod Immunol 2002; 47: 25–30.
21. Abramov Y, Elchalal U, Schenker JG. Febrile morbidity on severe and critical ovarian hyperstimulation syndrome: a multicentre study. Hum Reprod 1998; 13: 3128–31.

22. Serin IS, Ozcelik B, Bekyurek T, et al. Effects of pentoxifylline in the prevention of ovarian hyperstimulation syndrome in a rabbit model. Gynecol Endocrinol 2002; 16: 355–9.

23. Bergh PA, Navot D. Ovarian hyperstimulation syndrome – a review of pathophysiology. J Assist Reprod Genet 1992; 9: 429–38.

24. Borenstein R, Elchalal U, Lunenfeld B, et al. Severe OHSS; a reevaluated therapeutic approach. Fertil Steril 1989; 51: 791–5.

25. Whelan JG, Vlahos NF. The ovarian hyperstimulation syndrome. Fertil Steril 2000; 73: 883–96.

26. Avecillas JF, Falcone T, Arroliga AC. Ovarian hyperstimulation syndrome. Crit Care Clin 2004; 20: 679–95.

27. Ogi M, Yokoyama H, Tomosugi N, et al. Risk factors for infection and immunoglobulin replacement therapy in adult nephrotic syndrome. Am J Kidney Dis 1994; 24: 427–36.

28. Brower RG, Matthay MA, Morris A, et al. The acute respiratory distress syndrome network: ventilation with lower tidal volumes as compared with traditional tidal volumes for acute lung injury and the acute respiratory distress syndrome. N Engl J Med 2000; 342: 1301–8.

29. Rabau E, David A, Serr DM, et al. Human menopausal gonadotrophin for anovulation and sterility. Am J Obstet Gynecol 1967; 98: 92–8.

30. Thaler I, Yoffe M, Kaftory JK, et al. Treatment of OHSS; the physiologic basis for a modified approach. Fertil Steril 1981; 36: 110–13.

31. Forman RG, Frydman R, Egan D, et al. Severe OHSS using agonists of gonadotropin-releasing hormone for in vitro fertilization; a European series and a proposal for prevention. Fertil Steril 1990; 53: 502–9.

32. Rizk B, Aboulghar MA. Modern management of OHSS. Hum Reprod 1991; 6: 1082–7.

33. Koike T, Araki S, Minakami H, et al. Clinical efficacy of peritoneovenous shunting for the treatment of severe OHSS. Hum Reprod 2000; 15: 113–17.

34. Fukaya T, Funamaya Y, Chiba S, et al. Treatment of severe OHSS by ultrafiltration and reinfusion of ascitic fluid. Fertil Steril 1994; 61: 561–4.

35. Chew S, Ng SC. Laparoscopic treatment of a twisted hyperstimulated ovary after IVF. Singapore Med J 2001; 42: 228–9.

CHAPTER 18

Out-patient management of patients with ovarian hyperstimulation syndrome

Margo Fluker

INTRODUCTION

Ovarian hyperstimulation syndrome (OHSS) is potentially the most serious complication of exogenous gonadotropin administration. Various preventive measures have been proposed, as described in Chapters 19–24, yet none are completely effective. Thus, while prevention of the syndrome is intrinsically more desirable than treatment, unfortunately this goal has remained elusive.

In the absence of universally effective prevention strategies, many clinicians have sought methods to reduce the impact of OHSS. We previously developed a protocol for the proactive out-patient management of women with OHSS, aimed at avoiding hospitalization and minimizing the progression and complications of OHSS[1]. Traditional management of OHSS has involved bedrest and supportive measures at home until the clinical picture deteriorates sufficiently to require hospitalization. Once acutely ill and hospitalized, however, patients require intensive fluid and electrolyte management, often accompanied by colloid and/or diuretic administration, anticoagulation and paracentesis or thoracocentesis. In contrast, the out-patient management protocol utilizes vigilant fluid management at home, early out-patient paracentesis and judicious colloid replacement aimed at attenuating the course of the illness.

We have now used this out-patient protocol to monitor more than 4300 *in vitro* fertilization (IVF) cycles and manage 59 cases requiring paracentesis or thoracocentesis over the past 7 years. That approach for out-patient luteal phase management of OHSS is the focus of this chapter. Ultimately, however, the choice of out-patient versus in-patient management is best determined by the patient, her physician, the severity of the condition and the availability of facilities.

LUTEAL PHASE MONITORING

Although OHSS has a broad spectrum of clinical manifestations, the progression of symptoms often follows a predictable pattern through the luteal phase, affording the opportunity for close monitoring and early out-patient intervention. Various clinical risk factors can also be used to identify high-risk women who may benefit from more intensive monitoring (Chapters 2 and 3).

In our center, all patients are given written and verbal instructions about OHSS at the time of oocyte retrieval. High-risk patients receive similar instructions following human chorionic gonadotropin (hCG) administration in superovulation cycles. However, superovulation cycles that result in five or more preovulatory follicles are either canceled or converted to IVF in our center, so we rarely see the development of OHSS in this circumstance.

A patient hand-out describes the progression from mild to severe OHSS, instructions for monitoring and symptom relief at each stage, and a description of worsening signs and symptoms that necessitate contact with the clinic. Women are advised to limit their physical activities and to record their first-morning weight and abdominal girth at the umbilicus in order to obtain one or two baseline measurements in the early luteal phase. All women are encouraged to maintain an oral intake of at least 1000 ml daily. However, high-risk patients are also advised not to exceed an intake of 1500 ml per day during the luteal phase, based on the results of one small randomized trial[2].

Some programs advocate the use of prophylactic albumin infusions for high-risk patients at the time of oocyte retrieval. A meta-analysis of five randomized controlled trials initially indicated a small benefit from the prophylactic administration of human albumin at the time of oocyte retrieval in high-risk cases (odds ratio 0.28, 95% confidence interval 0.11–0.73)[3]. However, a subsequent single-center trial with a larger sample size than the entire meta-analysis revealed no effect[4]. In addition, controversy exists surrounding the effectiveness and safety of albumin administration in general, so the protocol has not achieved widespread support[5].

PROGRESSIVE SYMPTOMS

Women who experience progressive symptoms are instructed to contact the clinic if they experience a weight gain of ≥ 1 kg in 24 h, an increase in abdominal girth of more than 1–2 cm, shortness of breath, nausea, vomiting, diarrhea or a subjective decrease in urine output. Development of these symptoms prompts a standardized nursing-initiated assessment in which patients are advised to stay home from work (if applicable) and begin more intensive monitoring (Table 1), including baseline bloodwork within 24 h of symptom escalation and initiation of 24-h fluid intake and urine output measurements[1]. Daily contact with patients is summarized via key parameters recorded on an OHSS flow-sheet placed on the front of the chart (Figure 1).

OUT-PATIENT TREATMENT OF OHSS

The treatment for OHSS is generally conservative and supportive, dictated by the severity of the condition (Table 1). The syndrome is self-limited, although it may persist for several weeks, particularly in conception cycles[6,7]. In addition to medical interventions, substantial emotional support is also required to cope with the acute onset of distressing physical symptoms and the accompanying fears about the well-being of the woman and her early pregnancy.

Mild symptoms of ovarian hyperstimulation are a predictable consequence of hCG administration following stimulation with exogenous gonadotropins. Mild OHSS presents with bloating and weight gain; it responds to supportive measures including rest and analgesia.

The progression to moderate or severe OHSS involves the development of ascites, associated with hemoconcentration, increased thirst, marginal renal perfusion, oliguria and a tendency toward thromboembolic events[8]. Clinically, this is heralded by the triad of increasing symptoms: evidence of dehydration or hemoconcentration and low or declining serum albumin concentrations (Table 2). This constellation of signs and symptoms mandates assessment in the clinic and more intensive monitoring and/or therapy (Table 1).

Table 1 Out-patient management guidelines for progressive ovarian hyperstimulation syndrome (OHSS)

Mild–moderate OHSS	*Moderate–severe OHSS*
Advise bedrest at home	Continue bedrest, analgesics and antiemetics
Record daily weight and abdominal girth	Continue daily monitoring of weight, abdominal girth and 24-h fluid intake/urine output
Record daily 24-h fluid intake and urine output	Repeat baseline bloodwork every 1–3 days, or as clinically indicated: – Hb, Hct, sodium, potassium, serum albumin – as indicated: PT, PTT, BUN, creatinine and serial quantitative β-hCG
Provide analgesics and antiemetics as needed (e.g. acetaminophen and diphenhydramine)	Arrange transvaginal ultrasound to assess ascitic volume
Order baseline bloodwork (Hb, Hct, sodium, potassium, BUN, creatinine, PT, PTT, serum albumin and quantitative β-hCG)	Ensure appropriate rehydration and/or fluid resuscitation: – oral fluids or IV crystalloids, depending on severity – normalize hematocrit and electrolytes within 24 h, if possible – maintain urine output ≥ 20–25 ml/h in 24 h
Reinforce fluid intake of 1000–1500 ml daily	
Encourage intake of fluids rich in proteins, calories or electrolytes (e.g. fruit juices, soups, Popsicle®, Gator-Aid®, Ensure®, Boost®)	Consider paracentesis if: – ascitic fluid pocket ≥ 5–6 cm – abdominal distension increases daily – nausea and vomiting worsen daily – weight increases ≥ 1 kg/day – abdominal girth increases ≥ 1–2 cm/day – urine output drops below 20–25 ml/h in 24 h despite adequate rehydration – serum albumin falls below lower limit of normal
	Consider colloid replacement if: – urine output < 20–25 ml/h despite adequate crystalloid replacement – paracentesis is required – clinical edema develops
	Consider hospitalization if: – clinical condition does not stabilize quickly – patient cannot return rapidly for reassessment – symptoms are not manageable at home – fluid or electrolyte disturbances persist despite rehydration (e.g. Hb > 145 g/l, Hct > 45%) – other complications develop
	Consider heparinization if: – hospitalized and immobilized – coagulation parameters abnormal

Hb, hemoglobin; Hct, hematocrit; BUN, blood urea nitrogen; PT, prothrombin time; PTT, partial thromboplastin time; hCG, human chorionic gonadotropin

GENESIS FERTILITY CENTRE

Name ____________________ Home phone _______________

DOB ____________________ Cell phone _______________

		Date	Date	Date	Date
Patient data	Weight	57 kg	59.5 kg	57.5 kg	58 kg
	Abdominal girth	79 cm	84 cm	81 cm	81 cm
	24-h fluid intake	<< 1000 ml	1500 ml	1800 ml	1450 ml
	24-h urine output		450 ml	750 ml	725 ml
	Hourly output		19 ml/h	31 ml/h	30 ml/h
	Symptom summary	Bloated, nauseated, little oral intake	Very bloated, nauseated, diarrhea, short of breath	Feels much better. Still some diarrhea	Stable. Some nausea and diarrhea
Lab/clinic data	Hematocrit (%)	48		41	
	Albumin (35–50 g/l)	31		29	
	β-hCG (IU/l)	204		498	
	Paracentesis		1900 ml		
	IV fluids		500 ml HES, 250 ml Ringer's		
Rx		Do B/W. Increase oral intake. See in clinic tomorrow a.m	First paracentesis		

DOB, date of birth; Rx, treatment; hCG, human chorionic gonadotropin; IV, intravenous; B/W, blood work; HES, hydroxyethyl starch

Figure 1 Ovarian hyperstimulation syndrome (OHSS) out-patient monitoring flow-sheet

Table 2 Clinical triad heralding onset of ascites

1. Increasing symptoms
   - abdominal distension
   - shortness of breath
   - nausea, vomiting
   - diarrhea
2. Hemoconcentration
   - decreasing urine output (< 20 ml/h over 24 h)
   - elevated hematocrit
   - thirst
3. Subnormal serum albumin concentrations

Rehydration

Appropriate fluid management is the key initial intervention, and is probably critical in minimizing the risk of thromboembolic complications. Hemoconcentration requires prompt correction with oral or intravenous fluids, although rehydration will inevitably worsen the ascites because of the underlying increase in capillary permeability. The use of diuretics is generally counterproductive in this circumstance since it may aggravate the underlying hypovolemia without improving the extensive third-space losses.

In our experience, if promptly recognized, hemoconcentration can usually be rapidly corrected by increasing oral intake over a 24-h period. If oral intake is marginal secondary to nausea and abdominal distension, patients are reminded to consume frequent small amounts of calorie-, protein- or electrolyte-rich fluids such as soups, juices and commercial protein or sports drinks in order to achieve 1000–1500 ml of intake daily (Table 1). If urine output is marginal (< 20–25 ml/h) or hematocrit is elevated despite an intake of 1000–1500 ml, women are prompted to consume an additional 500–1000 ml daily. Antiemetics are often used orally or rectally to control nausea; their sedating side-effects may also facilitate rest.

Clinical assessment

If clinical symptoms continue to worsen over a 24-h period, patients are brought to the clinic for assessment and transvaginal ultrasonography the following morning. Most have been appropriately rehydrated over the preceding 24 h in response to advice from the nursing staff. However, they may have had substantial worsening of their abdominal distension in response to the increased oral intake. We occasionally administer an intravenous bolus of 500–1000 ml of Ringer's lactate or 5% dextrose in normal saline along with an intravenous antiemetic to women who are particularly nauseated or dehydrated when they attend the clinic for assessment.

Paracentesis

If ultrasonography demonstrates pockets of ascitic fluid greater than 5–6 cm in mean diameter, paracentesis should be considered. This is the single strategy that predictably produces clinical and biochemical improvement and hastens resolution of the process (Table 3)[9–13]. In an out-patient setting, our preference is for the transvaginal route, under paracervical block, in the same manner as oocyte collection. However, other centers have reported good success with abdominal paracentesis[13,14], and occasionally with an indwelling vaginal or abdominal catheter for ongoing drainage of large amounts of ascites[15–17]. Ultimately, the choice of paracentesis technique and setting will depend on the individual facility and operator experience.

Our transvaginal paracentesis procedure has previously been described in detail[1]. Briefly, an intravenous (IV) line is established with IV Ringer's lactate, the vaginal vault prepped with 0.05% chlorhexidine and a paracervical block inserted. Intravenous medications are given as needed based on clinical assessment and previous response during oocyte retrieval. These

Table 3 Improvement following first paracentesis in 53 women with late-onset ovarian hyperstimulation syndrome (OHSS) (July 1997–July 2004)

	0–24 h pre-paracentesis	*24–48 h post-paracentesis*	*Change*
Weight (kg)	63 ± 15	62 ± 15	−1 kg
Abdominal girth (cm)	89 ± 17	87.3 ± 17	−1.7 cm
Urine output (ml/h)	26 ± 15	35 ± 18	+9 ml/h
Albumin (g/l)	30 ± 4	27 ± 7	−3 g/l
Hematocrit (%)	45 ± 0.05	42 ± 0.1	−3%

include diphenhydramine 25 mg for nausea, fentanyl citrate 25–50 μg for analgesia and atropine 0.4 mg to minimize vasovagal reactions. We do not routinely use prophylactic antibiotics for paracentesis or oocyte collection.

There are no clear guidelines as to the amount or rate of fluid removal during paracentesis[18]. One recent report indicated that the majority of the reduction in intra-abdominal pressure and renal artery resistance occurred following withdrawal of the first 2000 ml of fluid[19]. In general, healthy young women without underlying medical conditions are unlikely to have difficulty with the compensatory fluid shift that accompanies paracentesis, unlike older patients with underlying hepatic disease or malignancy. It has been our practice to drain all ascitic fluid that is visible in the posterior cul de sac and can be safely accessed with a single puncture and without undue discomfort[1]. Between 2000 and 3000 ml can be drained in this fashion over 30–45 min using a 16-gauge single-lumen oocyte collection needle. We have not encountered bleeding, infection or other adverse sequelae in more than 100 such procedures. Patients report progressive resolution of distension, nausea and shortness of breath after the first 500 ml of ascitic fluid has been aspirated, usually followed by subjective reports of thirst and hunger. Women are generally discharged within 2 h after the procedure to continue with rest and monitoring at home.

In our experience, between one- and two-thirds of the patients who undergo each paracentesis will subsequently require another paracentesis (Table 4). However, both the interval between procedures and the volume drained increase progressively as the acuity of the illness decreases and the abdominal wall accommodates to the distension.

Pleural effusions may also occur, especially on the right, secondary to transfer of ascitic fluid through the thoracic duct. While they generally resolve following abdominal paracentesis, occasional cases require out-patient thoracocentesis, either alone or in addition to paracentesis, to alleviate persistent respiratory symptoms.

Colloid replacement

Serum albumin levels usually drop into the subnormal range in response to ascitic fluid accumulation, and may fall further after paracentesis and drainage of protein-rich ascitic fluid. Judicious colloid replacement may help to maintain urine output and prevent peripheral edema in these circumstances. Traditional therapy has involved 5 or 25% albumin, although recent concerns about the cost, efficacy and safety of albumin have prompted the use of synthetic

Table 4 Characteristics of repeated out-patient paracentesis in 53 women with late-onset ovarian hyperstimulation syndrome (OHSS) (July 1997–July 2004)

	Number	*Luteal day*	*Volume drained* (ml)	*Colloid administration* *
First paracentesis	53	17.6 ± 3.8 days post-hCG	1941 ± 709	38/53 (72%)
Second paracentesis	33	3.1 ± 1.7 days later	2245 ± 991	20/33 (61%)
Third paracentesis	11	4.2 ± 2.3 days later	2459 ± 1279	5/11 (45%)
Fourth or more	6	5.3 ± 2.9 days later	3110 ± 745	2/6 (33%)

*250 ml of 25% albumin or 500 ml of 10% hydroxyethyl starch

colloid products[5]. Preliminary evidence suggests that colloid alternatives such as hydroxyethyl starch may be equally effective[20–22]. Since late 2001, it has been our practice to administer 500 ml of 10% hydroxyethyl starch to most patients undergoing their first paracentesis, and as needed for subsequent procedures if urine output has been marginal despite appropriate fluid intake (Table 4). The administration of more than 1500 ml hydroxyethyl starch in a 24-h period has been associated with bleeding complications[23].

Anticoagulation

Correction of hemoconcentration is probably the single most important step in reducing the risk of thromboembolism[24]. Gentle mobilization, leg exercises and TED (antiembolic) stockings are also helpful, and are easy to incorporate in an out-patient management routine. The thromboembolic risks that accompany immobility are intuitively much higher in hospitalized patients confined to bed with an intravenous line and an indwelling urinary catheter than they are in women following a regimen of rest and limited activities at home.

The role of subcutaneous heparin remains controversial; some authors use it routinely in hospitalized patients, while others reserve it for those with abnormal coagulation parameters, or a suspicious personal or family history[25]. It has not been our practice to anticoagulate patients unless they have a positive history for thromboembolism. The sole thrombotic episode in the series described in Table 5 involved an axillary vein thrombosis more than 3 weeks after clinical resolution of the OHSS. The woman was subsequently found to have a thrombophilic disorder.

RESULTS OF OUT-PATIENT MANAGEMENT OF OHSS

During a 7-year period (July 1997–July 2004) we performed more than 4300 IVF cycles and identified 59 patients (1.4%) who developed moderate to severe OHSS and required drainage of ascitic fluid. Two of these 59 women were managed outside our standard protocol; one woman required a sole thoracocentesis in a local hospital out-patient clinic, and one woman was hospitalized at a distant center for albumin and paracentesis because it was not feasible for her to travel to us for management. Both were pregnant and delivered healthy singleton and triplet pregnancies, respectively.

The remaining 57 women underwent at least one out-patient paracentesis in our free-standing clinic and are summarized in Table 5. Of these, two women were hospitalized briefly to

Table 5 Outcome of OHSS out-patient management protocol (July 1997–July 2004)

	Characteristics	*Out-patient paracenteses*	*Pregnancies per embryo transfer*	*Fetal hearts at 7–8 week ultrasound*	*Delivery*
Late OHSS (> 10 days post-hCG)	$n = 53$ Age = 34 ± 4 years Oocytes = 13 ± 5	105* (range 1–7)	53/53	18 singletons 33 twins 2 triplets	22 singletons 24 twins‡ 1 triplet
Early OHSS (≤ 10 days post-hCG)	$n = 4$ Age = 33 ± 4 years Oocytes = 22 ± 5	6 (range 1–3)	2/3†	2 singletons	2 singletons
Total	$n = 57$		55/56		49/55 delivered 6/55 miscarried

*Including one woman who required thoracocentesis following paracentesis, and one woman hospitalized for unresponsive symptoms after two out-patient paracenteses; †the fourth woman had elective cryopreservation of all embryos; ‡including one dichorionic triplet pregnancy electively reduced to monozygotic twins

facilitate albumin administration in the first year of this protocol. All subsequent albumin or hydroxyethyl starch infusions were administered in our free-standing out-patient facility or in a hospital ambulatory clinic. One woman required hospital admission to manage severe symptoms and fluid balance issues that could not be controlled following two out-patient paracenteses. Her case appears to be the only true lack of success with out-patient management.

The most common presentation of OHSS is in the late luteal phase, generally 10–12 days or more following hCG administration. The condition is probably triggered by endogenous hCG concentrations, as the majority of cases are found to be pregnant around the time of symptom escalation and there is a high incidence of multiple pregnancy (Table 5)[1,6,26]. In keeping with these observations, 53/57 women in the current series presented with late-onset OHSS and all were pregnant following fresh embryo transfer. Of these, 41/53 (77%) had a multiple implantation and 35/53 (66%) had an ongoing multiple pregnancy with positive fetal hearts at 7–8 weeks' gestation.

In contrast, severe OHSS that develops in the early luteal phase, within 10 or 11 days after hCG administration, is less common and often follows a shorter clinical course. It is probably due to an excessive preovulatory response followed by sequelae of exogenous hCG administration, and is not necessarily accompanied by a pregnancy (Table 5)[6,26]. Indeed, only 4/59 cases in the current series presented with early-onset symptoms, but with an average of nearly nine more oocytes per patient than those with late OHSS. Two out of three conceived following fresh embryo transfer; the fourth woman did not have a fresh transfer, but still required paracentesis for early OHSS despite elective cryopreservation of all her embryos.

As most women learn that they are pregnant at the time they present with OHSS symptoms, concerns over the well-being of the pregnancy are often foremost in their thoughts. In the current series, only 6/55 pregnancies (10.9%) were lost in the first ($n = 2$ singletons) or second

($n = 3$ twins and 1 singleton) trimester. Nine additional twin pregnancies underwent spontaneous loss of one fetus after documentation of a positive fetal heartbeat, leaving ongoing singleton pregnancies.

Although follow-up data are sparse, the current series and previous published and anecdotal data about the outcome of pregnancies following OHSS are reassuring[6,8]. However, there are at least two reports of higher miscarriage rates and increased obstetric complications, particularly associated with higher-order multiple pregnancies, prolonged hospitalization and significant maternal complications of OHSS[27,28]. The current data emphasize the potential value of early intervention with aggressive attempts to attenuate the course of the disease, suggesting that early treatment may have a beneficial effect on both maternal and fetal outcome.

SUMMARY

In the absence of universally effective prevention strategies, we have developed and adhered to a protocol of active out-patient management of moderate to severe OHSS. Over the past 7 years and approximately 4300 IVF cycles, we have monitored 59 consecutive cases with symptomatic ascites or hydrothorax. Only one has required hospitalization related to true lack of success with the out-patient management protocol.

Our out-patient protocol encourages early paracentesis aimed at minimizing the progression of the disease, in contrast to late paracentesis aimed at hastening the recovery of critically ill hospitalized patients. We use oral rehydration and judicious colloid replacement in ambulatory patients in an attempt to circumvent the need for intensive parenteral fluid management in hospitalized patients. While OHSS remains a serious and potentially life-threatening disorder, our data suggest that vigilant monitoring and early out-patient intervention can serve as a safe and effective method of managing symptoms, attenuating the course of the illness and minimizing complications for both the affected women and their pregnancies.

ACKNOWLEDGMENTS

I am indebted to the nursing and medical staff at Genesis Fertility Centre for their excellent clinical care; to Geraldine Courtney RN and Cherri Huisman for assistance with data collection; and to Janice Copeland BSN and Stephanie Fisher MD for their helpful comments and discussion.

REFERENCES

1. Flukor MR, Copeland JE, Yuzpe AA. An ounce of prevention: out-patient management of the ovarian hyperstimulation syndrome. Fertil Steril 2000; 73: 821–4.

2. Bassil S, Verougstraete JC, Stallaert S, et al. Effects of preventive measures on the occurrence and the severity of ovarian hyperstimulation syndrome. J Assist Reprod Genet 1995; 12: 53S.

3. Aboulghar M, Evers JH, Al-Inany H. Intravenous albumin for preventing severe ovarian hyperstimulation syndrome: a Cochrane review. Hum Reprod 2002; 17: 3027–32.

4. Bellver J, Munoz EA, Ballesteros A, et al. Intravenous albumin does not prevent moderate–severe ovarian hyperstimulation syndrome in high-risk IVF patients: a randomized controlled study. Hum Reprod 2003; 18: 2283–8.

5. Cochrane Injuries Group Albumin Reviewers. Human albumin administration in critically ill patients: systematic review of randomised controlled trials. Br Med J 1998; 317: 235–40.

6. Richter KS, Van Nest RL, Stillman RJ. Late presentation with severe ovarian hyperstimulation syndrome is diagnostic of clinical in vitro fertilization pregnancy. Fertil Steril 2004; 82: 478–9.

7. Koike T, Minakami H, Araki S, et al. Severity of ovarian hyperstimulation syndrome: its relation to number of conceptuses. Int J Fertil Womens Med 2004; 49: 36–42.

8. Mathur RS, Jenkins JM. Is ovarian hyperstimulation syndrome associated with a poor obstetric outcome? Br J Obstet Gynaecol 2000; 107: 943–6.

9. Brinsden PR, Wada I, Tan SL, et al. Diagnosis, prevention and management of ovarian hyperstimulation syndrome. Br J Obstet Gynaecol 1995; 102: 767–72.

10. Aboulghar MA, Mansour RT, Serour GI, et al. Ultrasonically guided vaginal aspiration of ascites in the treatment of severe ovarian hyperstimulation syndrome. Fertil Steril 1990; 53: 933–5.

11. Aboulghar MA, Mansour RT, Serour GI, et al. Management of severe ovarian hyperstimulation syndrome by ascitic fluid aspiration and intensive intravenous fluid therapy. Obstet Gynecol 1993; 81: 108–11.

12. Borenstein R, Elhalah U, Lunenfeld B, et al. Severe ovarian hyperstimulation syndrome: a reevaluated therapeutic approach. Fertil Steril 1989; 51: 791–5.

13. Levin I, Almog B, Avni A, et al. Effect of paracentesis of ascitic fluids on urinary output and blood indices in patients with severe ovarian hyperstimulation syndrome. Fertil Steril 2002; 77: 986–8.

14. Shrivastav P, Nadkarni P, Craft I. Day care management of severe ovarian hyperstimulation syndrome avoids hospitalization and morbidity. Hum Reprod 1994; 9: 812–14.

15. Al-Ramahi M, Leader A, Claman P, et al. A novel approach to the treatment of ascites associated with ovarian hyperstimulation syndrome. Hum Reprod 1997; 12: 2614–16.

16. Raziel A, Friedler S, Schachter M, et al. Transvaginal drainage of ascites as an alternative to abdominal paracentesis in patients with severe ovarian hyperstimulation syndrome, obesity, and generalized edema. Fertil Steril 1998; 69: 780–3.

17. Abuzeid MI, Nassar Z, Massaad Z, et al. Pigtail catheter for the treatment of ascites associated with ovarian hyperstimulation syndrome [see Comment]. Hum Reprod 2003; 18: 370–3.

18. Practice Committee of the American Society for Reproductive Medicine. Ovarian hyperstimulation syndrome. Fertil Steril 2003; 80: 1309–14.

19. Maslovitz S, Jaffa A, Eytan O, et al. Renal blood flow alteration after paracentesis in women with ovarian hyperstimulation. Obstet Gynecol 2004; 104: 321–6.

20. Gokmen O, Ugur M, Ekin M, et al. Intravenous albumin versus hydroxyethyl starch for the prevention of ovarian hyperstimulation in an in-vitro fertilization programme: a prospective randomized placebo controlled study. Eur J Obstet Gynecol Reprod Biol 2001; 96: 187–92.

21. Chen D, Burmeister L, Goldschlag D, et al. Ovarian hyperstimulation syndrome: strategies for prevention. Reprod Biomed Online 2003; 7: 43–9.

22. Abramov Y, Fatum M, Abrahamov D, et al. Hydroxyethylstarch versus human albumin for the treatment of severe ovarian hyperstimulation syndrome: a preliminary report. Fertil Steril 2001; 75: 1228–30.

23. Treib J, Baron JF, Grauer MT, et al. An international view of hydroxyethyl starches. Intens Care Med 1999; 25: 258–68.

24. Stewart JA, Hamilton PJ, Murdoch AP. Thromboembolic disease associated with ovarian stimulation and assisted conception techniques. Hum Reprod 1997; 12: 2167–73.

25. Corrigan E. The management of ovarian hyperstimulation syndrome. http://www.ferti.net/fertimagazine/hottopic/1999_07_01.asp, cited October 26, 2002.

26. Mathur RS, Akande AV, Keay SD, et al. Distinction between early and late ovarian hyperstimulation syndrome. Fertil Steril 2000; 73: 901–7.

27. Raziel A, Friedler S, Schachter M, et al. Increased early pregnancy loss in IVF patients with severe ovarian hyperstimulation syndrome. Hum Reprod 2002; 17: 107–10.

28. Abramov Y, Elchalal U, Schenker JG. Obstetric outcome of in vitro fertilized pregnancies complicated by severe ovarian hyperstimulation syndrome: a multicenter study. Fertil Steril 1998; 70: 1070–6.

APPENDIX

Frequently asked questions

From patients

Q: Will this harm my pregnancy?

A: No, in our experience with out-patient management, the miscarriage rate is no higher than in other women of the same age group who have not developed OHSS. However, the chance of having a multiple pregnancy is higher than usual, occurring in about two-thirds of women who develop OHSS.

Q: How long will this last?

A: It is quite variable, but most women feel well enough to discontinue daily monitoring and contemplate returning to work within 1–2 weeks after the first paracentesis[1].

Q: Will I have to have another paracentesis?

A: Each time we do a paracentesis, approximately half of the women will require another procedure. If so, you will likely notice your symptoms becoming progressively worse over the next 3–5 days.

From other physicians

Q: I was taught during medical school not to drain more than about 1000 ml during a paracentesis. Why should this situation be any different?

A: Women with OHSS are generally young and healthy, and are unlikely to suffer cardiovascular compromise following a larger-volume paracentesis, in contrast to older individuals with a malignancy or hepatic failure. That said, it is still prudent to monitor clinical status and vital signs carefully during the paracentesis. Drainage of > 2000 ml at a time may not produce any additional improvement in renal or hemodynamic parameters, but may provide additional symptomatic relief and potentially diminish the need for repeat procedures[19].

Q: Can I use a colloid infusion to increase circulating oncotic pressure, followed by a diuretic to mobilize the ascites?

A: This has generally been an inefficient method of mobilizing ascites, and may even be counterproductive if it aggravates the underlying hypovolemia and marginal renal perfusion in an acutely ill patient. Drainage of the third-space fluid via paracentesis provides more immediate and predictable relief of symptoms and improvement in renal and hematological parameters. Diuretics may have some merit in a stable, recovering patient who still has residual peripheral edema that has not responded to other forms of therapy.

CHAPTER 19

Primary prevention of ovarian hyperstimulation syndrome: choice of ovulation induction and ovarian stimulation in IVF and non-IVF reproductive technologies

Juliette Guibert and François Olivennes

INTRODUCTION

Ovarian hyperstimulation syndrome (OHSS) is not frequent, its pathophysiology remains unclear and there are few criteria of reliable predictive value for its occurrence. For these reasons, its prevention remains an unresolved problem for reproductive specialists, who are without a sufficient scientific or clinical basis to develop methods to guarantee complete safety.

Nevertheless, primary prevention of OHSS should in principle be possible at different steps of the management of infertility, by recognizing high-risk situations and by respecting safety rules in choosing treatments and in conducting ovarian stimulation.

Before treatment, the known risk factors should be identified, in order to target a group of high-risk patients for specific preventive strategies. These include systematic interrogation about the necessity of ovarian stimulation and the duration of infertility, the timeliness of the treatment and the development of minimal-risk management procedures, with consideration for the alternative treatments of infertility, e.g. tubal surgery, ovarian drilling by electrocautery or laser vaporization, insulin-resistance-reducing drugs and natural-cycle *in vitro* fertilization (IVF).

During treatment, minimal safety rules of stimulation should be respected for all patients, and especially for those with an identified high risk. These rules concern the choice of stimulation regimen (drug, dose, protocol) and adjustment of the dose of gonadotropin according to the ovarian response (careful monitoring of the cycle).

PRIMARY PREVENTION BEFORE TREATMENT

Identification of factors influencing the incidence of OHSS

Patients with polycystic ovarian syndrome (PCOS) or showing isolated characteristics of PCOS (clinical, ultrasonographic or biological) should be considered at high risk of developing OHSS[1–5]. It appears to be the major predisposing factor in many studies: the proportion of patients showing ultrasonically diagnosed PCOS in severe OHSS is significantly higher than in patients who do not develop OHSS[4]. This is consistent with the fact that patients with PCOS produce more follicles than normo-ovulatory patients stimulated with the same protocols. Finding more than ten resting follicles on each ovary has been shown to be predictive of an excessive ovarian response and a risk factor for OHSS[6]. The baseline ovarian volume measured by three-dimensional ultrasonography has also been shown to be correlated with the risk of developing OHSS[7]. Furthermore, inversion of the luteinizing hormone (LH)/follicle stimulating hormone (FSH) ratio (LH > FSH), or increased ovarian androgen circulating levels observed separately or in patients with PCOS, could disturb the androgen conversion pathway and enhance the risk for OHSS[4,5]. Therefore, no stimulation should be performed without a day-3 evaluation of the LH/FSH ratio and of the number of resting follicles observed on ultrasound. The body mass index (BMI) is a paradoxical clue, since a lean BMI increases the risk of a high ovarian response and of OHSS, but a high BMI is often related to PCOS, which increases the risk of OHSS. Therefore, BMI does not appear to be a useful marker of increased risk of OHSS[8].

Young age appears to be a risk factor, since patients who develop OHSS are younger than those who do not[1,2].

It has also been reported that patients showing allergic dispositions may be more likely to develop OHSS. Because OHSS has many similarities to an exaggerated inflammatory response, it has been hypothesized that an individual tendency to develop pathological OHSS when the ovarian response is strong may have something to do with immunological sensitivity[1].

Apart from these known factors, the actual individual risk of developing OHSS remains mostly unpredictable in naive patients, who may show individual (hyper)sensitivity to gonadotropin stimulation. Previous ovarian response needs to be considered when available, as it is useful in predicting this sensitivity[9]. The previous occurrence of OHSS in a mild or severe form is highly predictive of a high-risk situation in subsequent treatment cycles[4]. A previous strong ovarian response with an estradiol level of over 1500 pg/l at day 8 or over 3000 pg/l at day 11, or with more than 15 oocytes retrieved, should be a warning, even though no OHSS has occurred[1].

All of these criteria should alert physicians to consider a preventive strategy for avoiding OHSS.

Initiation of treatment

First, the severity of the medical damage caused by OHSS has to be weighed against the necessity for ovarian stimulation. It is likely that most IVF procedures are initiated with good evidence for their medical justification. However, in many situations, IVF is not performed for any gynecological pathology. Examples are patients with intracytoplasmic sperm injection (ICSI) for male-related infertility, oocyte donors, human immunodeficiency virus (HIV)-serodifferent couples asking for virus-safe procreation, and those seeking prevention of transmission of known genetic abnormalities by preimplantation diagnosis. It is noteworthy that patients with these indications for treatment frequently undergo strong ovarian stimulation despite the fact that they do not show any reproductive disability. Complications following such treatments are particularly undesirable, and should be carefully explained to the women concerned.

In non-IVF procedures, the correct moment to initiate treatment is not easy to determine. It appears that OHSS does not occur in more severe forms in normo-ovulatory patients[8], but obviously the occurrence of a serious complication with no medical evidence of the necessity for such treatment is unjustifiable. This is particularly important for couples requiring donor sperm insemination if no gynecological abnormality is present, and for couples requiring assisted reproduction treatments despite a short duration of infertility, e.g. because of advanced female age or because of recurrent miscarriage. In these patients, the safety rules of ovarian stimulation have to be strictly followed, including giving information to patients about possible medical consequences and about the benefits of the particular choice of stimulation that has been made[10].

Development of minimal-risk procedures

With respect to non-IVF procedures, alternative approaches exist for the pharmacological induction of ovulation for patients with PCOS (Figure 1). The benefits and risks of such treatments have to be balanced against the risk of OHSS.

Diet and weight loss have been demonstrated to restore ovulation in some obese anovulatory women with PCOS, with beneficial effects on the incidence of diabetes mellitus and on cardiovascular risk[11]. Insulin-sensitizing drugs (e.g. metformin) have been shown to be beneficial in facilitating normal menses and pregnancy, and in preventing type 2 diabetes mellitus[12,13]. Ovarian drilling (either by laparoscopic electrocauterization or by laser vaporization) is also able to restore spontaneous menses and ovulation and induce pregnancy, with a very low risk of multiple pregnancy, OHSS and miscarriage, even though the procedure has still not been prospectively evaluated[14,15].

Preliminary weight loss prior to both non-IVF and IVF procedures and the administration of metformin or octreotide has been shown to normalize the ovarian response to exogenous gonadotropin in women with PCOS resistant to clomiphene citrate (CC), with a significant reduction of the serum estradiol level, the number of follicles and the cancellation rate, and with a similar pregnancy rate[16,17]. A statistically significant effect on prevention of OHSS could not be demonstrated in non-IVF patients, probably because of its very low incidence[16]. Ovarian drilling before stimulation for IVF in women with a high risk due to PCOS or with a previous experience of OHSS may help to avoid severe complications or cancellation of the cycle, but it has to be balanced against the risk of the operation[18,19].

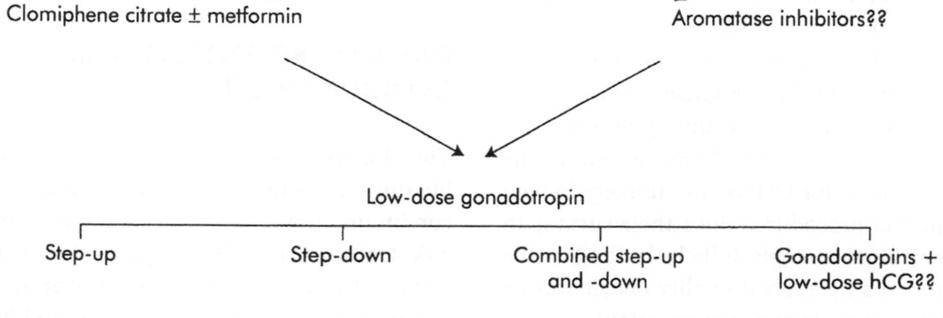

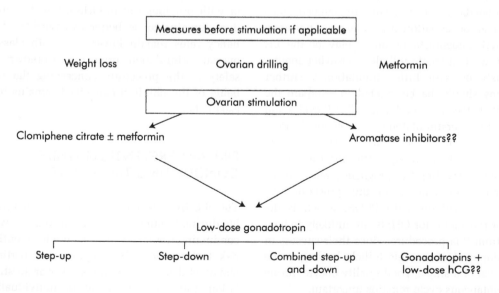

Figure 1 Stimulation regimen in non-*in vitro* fertilization (IVF) procedures. hCG, human chorionic gonadotropin; ??, treatment options which need to be confirmed by more studies

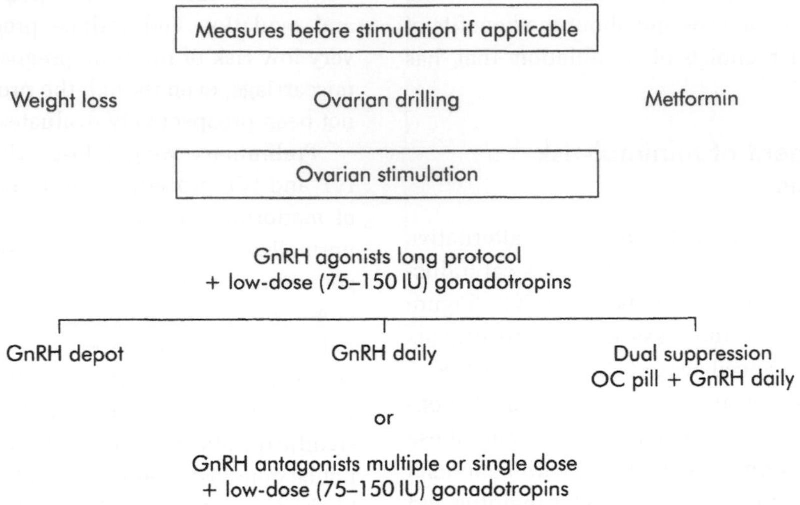

Figure 2 Stimulation regimen in *in vitro* fertilization (IVF) procedures. GnRH, gonadotropin-releasing hormone; OC, oral contraceptive

In high-risk patients, new approaches in IVF should be considered (Figure 2). The debate about natural IVF, conducted in a natural, non-stimulated cycle, has recently re-emerged, since the use of gonadotropin-releasing hormone (GnRH) antagonists permits delay of the LH surge while a single follicle is growing spontaneously or with little stimulation[20]. Further studies should be conducted to compare the results between several 'natural' IVF cycles and a single hyperstimulated cycle. Obviously, multiple pregnancy and OHSS rates would be reduced, but relatively little information is available regarding the pregnancy rate and the pregnancy outcome from this procedure[21,22]. Moreover, patients with PCOS, which is the major risk factor for OHSS, are unlikely to benefit from this procedure, since their success in development of a single follicle leading to the retrieval of a single, good-quality oocyte during a spontaneous cycle remains uncertain.

Culture development of immature oocytes could lead to the abandonment of ovarian controlled hyperstimulation and the administration of hCG in IVF procedures, at least in high-risk groups of patients, such as women with PCOS or with previous severe OHSS, but this procedure remains to be better assessed[23–27]. Pregnancy rates remain lower than with classical ovarian stimulation protocols. Moreover, the safety of the procedure concerning the well-being of the children conceived remains to be established.

PRIMARY PREVENTION WHILE CONDUCTING TREATMENT

The effective prevention of OHSS is also possible during treatment. Primary prevention while conducting treatment in women with identified risk factors for OHSS requires the pertinent choice of drug combinations for ovarian stimulation and the adjustment of individualized low-dose step-up regimens by very careful monitoring.

Choice of stimulation regimen

Clomiphene citrate

In non-IVF procedures, induction of ovulation by CC is rarely associated with severe OHSS[28]. Therefore, CC is the treatment of choice for induction of ovulation, rather than gonadotropins (urinary or recombinant), which increase the incidence of OHSS. However, in rare patients who have experienced OHSS after the use of CC, gonadotropin stimulation allows the modulation of therapy throughout the cycle, which is impossible with CC. In high-risk patients, the initial dose of CC must be increased carefully to find the ovulatory threshold, and gonadotropins are recommended for CC-resistant patients[29]. CC resistance is defined as failure to ovulate after a dose of 150 mg of CC for three cycles, even though higher doses have been proposed with variable success.

Gonadotropins

In non-IVF procedures, high-risk patients should undergo low-dose step-up regimens for ovulation induction, which have been shown to decrease considerably the risk of OHSS and multiple pregnancy. In strictly anovulatory patients, these regimens start with a daily dose of 50 or 75 IU of recombinant FSH (rFSH) or urinary human menopausal gonadotropin (hMG) during 7–14 days, and provide dose increments of 37.5 IU every 5 or 7 days until follicle development initiates. This allows the development of a single follicle, and reduces the occurrence of OHSS almost to nil[30]. An alternative protocol was proposed in which the gonadotropins were decreased in steps (step-down)[31]. A prospective randomized study concluded in favor of the step-up regimen[32]. A combination of step-up and step-down has also been proposed, and could warrant further study[33].

In IVF, the use of a low-dose stimulation regimen seems to reduce OHSS incidence[34]. To optimize the ovarian response without provoking OHSS is the best compromise that should be reached by an ideal regimen of stimulation, which is unfortunately still not consistently achievable. There is a fine balance between increasing oocyte recruitment to improve the success rate of IVF and preventing OHSS by promoting a small pool of granulosa cells, highly sensitive to the future luteinizing stimulus.

The starting dose for gonadotropin is based on age, body mass index (BMI) and existence of PCOS, as well as on previous history of OHSS or high response. A recent study found no reduction in the occurrence of OHSS in standard patients when reducing the initial dose from 200 to 100 IU[35]. But in high-risk patients, halving of the initial dosage of gonadotropins appears to prevent OHSS[36]. Likewise, the use of limited ovarian stimulation and ovulation triggering when the leading follicles reach 12 mm in PCOS patients with previous OHSS may reduce the recurrence of OHSS[37].

The choice of urinary or recombinant hMG or FSH does not seem to influence the incidence of OHSS[38].

More recently, Filicori *et al.* proposed conducting the end of stimulation using a treatment composed of low-dose hCG. Low-dose hCG as a source of LH activity was associated with FSH or was used alone in the second part of the follicular phase[39]. Furthermore, LH activity is capable of reducing the development of small ovarian follicles (< 10 mm) that may predispose patients to developing complications such as OHSS. This regimen was used in a small group of patients exposed to OHSS[40]. The absence of FSH stimulation reduced the amount of follicles and the estradiol value. This novel approach should be evaluated in prospective randomized studies. An excellent review exists that presents in detail all the studies available and the different therapeutic options summarized in this chapter[41].

GnRH agonists and antagonists

The use of the GnRH agonist long protocol, which consists of previous pituitary desensitization before the onset of ovarian stimulation by gonadotropins, is associated with a higher incidence of OHSS, mostly because it increases follicular recruitment. There is also a peripheral action of the GnRH agonist *per se* granulosa cells, which can explain why OHSS is more likely for the equivalent follicular recruitment. The type of GnRH agonist to be used in patients at risk of OHSS has not been extensively studied. It is obvious that the short protocol should not be proposed, as the initial flare-up effect could lead to an excessive ovarian response. In the long protocol, depot formulation versus daily injection and follicular versus luteal start have not been compared prospectively in patients at risk of OHSS. An interesting approach has been proposed by combining the suppression of the estrogen–progestogen pill with the GnRH agonist[42]. No comparative studies are available, but results appear to be very interesting and this protocol is the GnRH-agonist protocol of choice in many IVF centers.

The recent introduction of GnRH antagonists has been claimed to reduce the risk of OHSS, for several physiological reasons. First, follicular recruitment seems to be lower, and hence the granulosa cell pool undergoing the luteinizing stimulus. On the other hand, a possible ovarian action of GnRH antagonist could exist.

A reduction in the incidence of OHSS is observed in the majority of prospective randomized studies using GnRH antagonists[43–48]. Patients receiving antagonist treatment have lower estradiol serum levels at the time of hCG administration, mostly because of a lower number of follicles, which could explain the lower incidence of OHSS[49]. Recent meta-analyses failed to find a significant reduction in OHSS in unselected patients[50,51]. However, in the phase II and III studies analyzed in those meta-analyses, cancellation criteria were applied, and patients canceled in the agonist group introduced a bias into the OHSS data[45]. Only two small prospective randomized studies compared GnRH agonist and antagonist regimens[51,52]. They found similar IVF outcomes with reductions in lengths of treatment and estradiol levels, but they did not find a reduction in the incidence of OHSS; the study samples were not adequate to analyze OHSS.

The use of GnRH antagonists could further decrease the incidence of OHSS in high-risk patients when replacing hCG by a GnRH agonist to trigger ovulation. Several authors[53–56] have proposed triggering ovulation with a GnRH agonist to decrease the risk of OHSS. However, this approach cannot be proposed in a patient previously desensitized with a GnRH agonist, but GnRH agonists can be used to induce an endogenous LH surge during an ovarian stimulation cycle in which a GnRH antagonist is used to prevent LH surges[57]. A recent study carried out in a limited number of patients not at risk for OHSS, comparing the use of hCG, leuprolide (0.2 mg) and triptorelin (0.1 mg) to trigger ovulation in IVF patients treated with ganirelix (0.25 mg), found similar IVF–embryo transfer (ET) results between the three groups of patients[58]. A small group of high responders was treated with a combination of a GnRH antagonist and an agonist, and no OHSS was observed in this preliminary report[59]. The results should be evaluated, as pregnancy rates were found to be low by some authors (unpublished data). A recent prospective study, unfortunately unpublished, found a lower pregnancy rate in patients in whom GnRH agonists were used to trigger ovulation, despite luteal supplementation of estrogen and progesterone (Devroey *et al.*, unpublished). Overall, GnRH antagonists could offer a good alternative to current stimulation protocols, with a reduced incidence of OHSS[60,61].

Monitoring the cycle

Careful adaptation of the daily dose of gonadotropin administered for ovarian stimulation to the ovarian response results, in non-IVF and IVF procedures, leads to a decreased incidence of OHSS[62]. This necessary adaptation is possible by monitoring of the cycle, using a combination of frequent estradiol measurements and ultrasonographic assessments of follicular growth[63]. Some studies report a similar efficacy in preventing OHSS when using ultrasound assessment alone[64–66]. Whether or not the combination of serum estradiol measurement and ultrasound provides a better assessment of ovarian response than ultrasound assessment of follicular growth alone remains controversial for unselected patients. In high-risk patients, it is likely that as many clues as possible are necessary to warn physicians about the risk of OHSS: ultrasound can identify those at risk of early OHSS when a large number (more than 20) of follicles are present, and, moreover, are growing on day 8. At the least, such women with higher numbers of follicles are then advised to have serum estradiol measurement, which enables assessment of the size of the granulosa cell pool. Serum estradiol measurements have been shown to be positively correlated with OHSS. The incidence of OHSS in women with a high number of follicles (> 35) and high levels of serum estradiol (> 2500 pg/ml) has been estimated to be up to 80%, but the estradiol cut-off to distinguish those women at risk of OHSS from those who are not is still debatable[67,68]. The time at which a number of follicles and a serum level of estradiol are reached (slope of increment) may be more important than their absolute values. A recent case–control study showed that a serum estradiol level of 3300 pg/ml on day 11 of ovarian stimulation gave a sensitivity and specificity of 85% for the detection of women at risk for OHSS[69].

Nevertheless, *per se*, the strict observance of monitoring rules does not avoid all severe forms of OHSS. It merely allows tracking of the biological and ultrasonographic clues which compel the use of secondary preventive measures.

REFERENCES

1. Enskog A, Henriksson M, Unander M, et al. Prospective study of the clinical and laboratory parameters of patients in whom ovarian hyperstimulation syndrome developed during controlled ovarian hyperstimulation for in vitro fertilization. Fertil Steril 1999; 71: 808–14.
2. Delvigne A, Demoulin A, Smitz J, et al. The ovarian hyperstimulation syndrome in in-vitro fertilization: a Belgian multicentric study. I. Clinical and biological features. Hum Reprod 1993; 8: 1353–60.
3. Brinsden PR, Wada I, Tan SL, et al. Diagnosis, prevention and management of ovarian hyperstimulation syndrome. Br J Obstet Gynaecol 1995; 102: 767–72.
4. Delvigne A, Dubois M, Battheu B, et al. The ovarian hyperstimulation syndrome in in-vitro fertilization: a Belgian multicentric study. II. Multiple discriminant analysis for risk prediction. Hum Reprod 1993; 8: 1361–6.
5. Bodis J, Torok A, Tinneberg HR. LH/FSH ratio as a predictor of ovarian hyperstimulation syndrome. Hum Reprod 1997; 12: 869–70.
6. Tibi C, Alvarez S, Cornet D. Prédiction des hyperstimulations ovariennes. Contracept Fertil Sex 1989; 17: 751–2.
7. Danninger B, Brunner M, Obruca A, et al. Prediction of ovarian hyperstimulation syndrome by ultrasound volumetric assessment [corrected] of baseline ovarian volume prior to stimulation. Hum Reprod 1996; 11: 1597–9.
8. Navot D, Relou A, Birkenfeld A, et al. Risk factors and prognostic variables in the ovarian hyperstimulation syndrome. Am J Obstet Gynecol 1988; 159: 210–15.
9. Fauser BC, Van Heusden AM. Manipulation of human ovarian function: physiological concepts and clinical consequences. Endocr Rev 1997; 18: 71–106.
10. Mathur RS, Jenkins JM. Severe OHSS: patients should be allowed to weigh the morbidity of OHSS against the benefits of parenthood. Hum Reprod 1999; 14: 2183–5.

11. Velazquez E, Acosta A, Mendoza SG. Menstrual cyclicity after metformin therapy in polycystic ovary syndrome. Obstet Gynecol 1997; 90: 392–5.

12. Glueck CJ, Wang P, Fontaine R, et al. Metformin-induced resumption of normal menses in 39 of 43 (91%) previously amenorrheic women with the polycystic ovary syndrome. Metabolism 1999; 48: 511–19.

13. Knowler WC, Barrett-Connor E, Fowler SE, et al. Reduction in the incidence of type 2 diabetes with lifestyle intervention or metformin. N Engl J Med 2002; 346: 393–403.

14. Amer SA, Gopalan V, Li TC, et al. Long term follow-up of patients with polycystic ovarian syndrome after laparoscopic ovarian drilling: clinical outcome. Hum Reprod 2002; 17: 2035–42.

15. Fernandez H, Watrelot A, Alby JD, et al. Fertility after ovarian drilling by transvaginal fertiloscopy for treatment of polycystic ovary syndrome. J Am Assoc Gynecol Laparosc 2004; 11: 374–8.

16. De Leo V, la Marca A, Ditto A, et al. Effects of metformin on gonadotropin-induced ovulation in women with polycystic ovary syndrome. Fertil Steril 1999; 72: 282–5.

17. Morris RS, Karande VC, Dudkiewicz A, et al. Octreotide is not useful for clomiphene citrate resistance in patients with polycystic ovary syndrome but may reduce the likelihood of ovarian hyperstimulation syndrome. Fertil Steril 1999; 71: 452–6.

18. Rimington MR, Walker SM, Shaw RW. The use of laparoscopic ovarian electrocautery in preventing cancellation of in-vitro fertilization treatment cycles due to risk of ovarian hyperstimulation syndrome in women with polycystic ovaries. Hum Reprod 1997; 12: 1443–7.

19. Homburg R. Management of infertility and prevention of ovarian hyperstimulation in women with polycystic ovary syndrome. Best Pract Res Clin Obstet Gynaecol 2004; 18: 773–88.

20. Rongieres-Bertrand C, Olivennes F, Righini C, et al. Revival of the natural cycles in in-vitro fertilization with the use of a new gonadotrophin-releasing hormone antagonist (Cetrorelix): a pilot study with minimal stimulation. Hum Reprod 1999; 14: 683–8.

21. Pelinck MJ, Hoek A, Simons AH, et al. Efficacy of natural cycle IVF: a review of the literature. Hum Reprod Update 2002; 8: 129–39.

22. Olivennes F. Patient-friendly ovarian stimulation. Reprod Biomed Online 2003; 7: 30–4.

23. Tan SL, Child TJ. In-vitro maturation of oocytes from unstimulated polycystic ovaries. Reprod Biomed Online 2002; 4: 18–23.

24. Jaroudi KA, Hollanders JM, Sieck UV, et al. Pregnancy after transfer of embryos which were generated from in-vitro matured oocytes. Hum Reprod 1997; 12: 857–9.

25. Le Du A, Kadoch IJ, Bourcigaux N, et al. In vitro oocyte maturation for the treatment of infertility associated with polycystic ovarian syndrome: the French experience. Hum Reprod 2005; 20: 420–4.

26. Cha KY, Chung HM, Lee DR, et al. Obstetric outcome of patients with polycystic ovary syndrome treated by in vitro maturation and in vitro fertilization-embryo transfer. Fertil Steril 2005; 83: 1461–5.

27. Söderström-Anttila V, Makinen S, Tuuri T, et al. Favourable pregnancy results with insemination of in vitro matured oocytes from unstimulated patients. Hum Reprod 2005; 20: 1534–40.

28. Kistner RW. Induction of ovulation with clomiphene citrate (Clomid). Obstet Gynecol Surv 1965; 20: 873–900.

29. Hughes E, Collins J, Vandekerckhove P. Ovulation induction with urinary follicle stimulating hormone versus human menopausal gonadotropin for clomiphene-resistant polycystic ovary syndrome. Cochrane Database Syst Rev 2000; (2): CD000087.

30. Homburg R, Howles CM. Low-dose FSH therapy for anovulatory infertility associated with polycystic ovary syndrome: rationale, results, reflections and refinements. Hum Reprod Update 1999; 5: 493–9.

31. Eijkemans MJ, Imani B, Mulders AG, et al. High singleton live birth rate following classical ovulation induction in normogonadotrophic anovu-

latory infertility (WHO 2). Hum Reprod 2003; 18: 2357–62.

32. Christin-Maitre S, Hugues JN. Recombinant FSH Study Group. A comparative randomized multicentric study comparing the step-up versus step-down protocol in polycystic ovary syndrome. Hum Reprod 2003; 18: 1626–31.

33. Hugues JN, Cedrin-Durnerin I, Avril C, et al. Sequential step-up and step-down dose regimen: an alternative method for ovulation induction with follicle-stimulating hormone in polycystic ovarian syndrome. Hum Reprod 1996; 11: 2581–4.

34. Marci R, Senn A, Dessole S, et al. A low-dose stimulation protocol using highly purified follicle-stimulating hormone can lead to high pregnancy rates in in vitro fertilization patients with polycystic ovaries who are at risk of a high ovarian response to gonadotropins. Fertil Steril 2001; 75: 1131–5.

35. Tan SL, Child TJ, Cheung AP, et al. A randomized, double-blind, multicenter study comparing a starting dose of 100 IU or 200 IU of recombinant follicle stimulating hormone (Puregon) in women undergoing controlled ovarian hyperstimulation for IVF treatment. J Assist Reprod Genet 2005; 22: 81–8.

36. Forman RG, Frydman R, Egan D, et al. Severe ovarian hyperstimulation syndrome using agonists of gonadotropin-releasing hormone for in vitro fertilization: a European series and a proposal for prevention. Fertil Steril 1990; 53: 502–9.

37. El-Sheikh MM, Hussein M, Fouad S, et al. Limited ovarian stimulation (LOS), prevents the recurrence of severe forms of ovarian hyperstimulation syndrome in polycystic ovarian disease. Eur J Obstet Gynecol Reprod Biol 2001; 94: 245–9.

38. Daya S. Updated meta-analysis of recombinant follicle-stimulating hormone (FSH) versus urinary FSH for ovarian stimulation in assisted reproduction. Fertil Steril 2002; 77: 711–14.

39. Filicori M, Cognigni GE, Samara A, et al. The use of LH activity to drive folliculogenesis: exploring uncharted territories in ovulation induction. Hum Reprod Update 2002; 8: 543–57.

40. Lee KL, Couchman GM, Walmer DK. Successful pregnancies in patients with estrogenic anovulation after low-dose human chorionic gonadotropin therapy alone following hMG for controlled ovarian hyperstimulation. J Assist Reprod Genet 2005; 22: 37–40.

41. Homburg R. The management of infertility associated with polycystic ovary syndrome. Reprod Biol Endocrinol 2003; 1: 109.

42. Damario MA, Barmat L, Liu HC, et al. Dual suppression with oral contraceptives and gonadotrophin releasing-hormone agonists improves in-vitro fertilization outcome in high responder patients. Hum Reprod 1997; 12: 2359–65.

43. The Ganirelix dose-finding study group. A double-blind, randomized, dose-finding study to assess the efficacy of the gonadotrophin releasing hormone antagonist ganirelix (Org 37462) to prevent premature luteinizing hormone surges in women undergoing ovarian stimulation with recombinant follicle stimulating hormone (Puregon). Hum Reprod 1998; 13: 3023–31.

44. Albano C, Felberbaum RE, Smitz J. Ovarian stimulation with HMG: results of a prospective randomized phase III European study comparing the luteinizing hormone-releasing hormone (LHRH)-antagonist cetrorelix and the LHRH-agonist buserelin. Hum Reprod 2000; 15: 526–31.

45. Olivennes F, Belaisch-Allart J, Emperaire JC. A prospective randomized controlled study in IVF–ET with a single dose of a LH-RH antagonist (cetrorelix) or a depot formula of a LH-RH agonist (triptorelin). Fertil Steril 2000; 73: 314–20.

46. The European Orgalutran Study Group. Treatment with the gonadotrophin-releasing hormone antagonist ganirelix in women undergoing ovarian stimulation with recombinant follicle stimulating hormone is effective, safe and convenient: results of a controlled, randomized, multicentre trial. Hum Reprod 2000; 15: 1490–8.

47. The European and Middle East Orgalutran Study Group. Comparable clinical outcome using the GnRH antagonist ganirelix or a long protocol of the GnRH agonist triptorelin for the

prevention of premature LH surges in women undergoing ovarian stimulation. Hum Reprod 2001; 16: 644–51.

48. Ragni G, Vegetti W, Riccaboni A, et al. Comparison of GnRH agonists and antagonists in assisted reproduction cycles of patients at high risk of ovarian hyperstimulation syndrome. Hum Reprod 2005; 20: 2421–5.

49. Ludwig M, Felberbaum RE, Devroey P, et al. Significant reduction of the incidence of ovarian hyperstimulation syndrome (OHSS) by using the LHRH antagonist Cetrorelix (Cetrotide) in controlled ovarian stimulation for assisted reproduction. Arch Gynecol Obstet 2000; 264: 29–32.

50. Al-Inany H, Aboulghar M. GnRH antagonist in assisted reproduction: a Cochrane review. Hum Reprod 2002; 17: 874–85.

51. Ludwig M, Katalanic A, Diedrich K. Use of GnRH antagonists in ovarian stimulation for assisted reproductive technologies compared to the long protocol. Meta-analysis. Arch Gynecol Obstet 2001; 265: 175–82.

52. Hwang JL, Seow KM, Lin YH, et al. Ovarian stimulation by concomitant administration of cetrorelix acetate and HMG following Diane-35 pre-treatment for patients with polycystic ovary syndrome: a prospective randomized study. Hum Reprod 2004; 19: 1993–2000.

53. Gonen Y, Balakier H, Powell W, et al. Use of gonadotropin-releasing hormone agonist to trigger follicular maturation for in vitro fertilization. J Clin Endocrinol Metab 1990; 71: 918–22.

54. Emperaire JC, Ruffie A. Triggering ovulation with endogenous luteinizing hormone may prevent the ovarian hyperstimulation syndrome. Hum Reprod 1991; 6: 506–10.

55. Itskovitz J, Boldes R, Levron J, et al. Induction of preovulatory luteinizing hormone surge and prevention of ovarian hyperstimulation syndrome by gonadotropin-releasing hormone agonist. Fertil Steril 1991; 56: 213–20.

56. Lewit N, Kol S, Manor D, et al. Comparison of gonadotrophin-releasing hormone analogues and human chorionic gonadotrophin for the induction of ovulation and prevention of ovarian hyperstimulation syndrome: a case-control study. Hum Reprod 1996; 11: 1399–402.

57. Olivennes F, Fanchin R, Bouchard P, et al. Triggering of ovulation by a gonadotropin-releasing hormone (GnRH) agonist in patients pretreated with a GnRH antagonist. Fertil Steril 1996; 66: 151–3.

58. Fauser BC, de Jong D, Olivennes F, et al. Endocrine profiles after triggering of final oocyte maturation with GnRH agonist after cotreatment with the GnRH antagonist ganirelix during ovarian hyperstimulation for in vitro fertilization. J Clin Endocrinol Metab 2002; 87: 709–15.

59. Itskovitz J, Kol S, Mannaerts B. Use a single bolus of GnRH agonist triptorelin to trigger ovulation after GnRH antagonist ganirelix treatment in women undergoing ovarian stimulation for assisted reproduction, with special reference to the prevention of ovarian hyperstimulation syndrome: preliminary report. Hum Reprod 2000; 15: 1965–68.

60. Kolibianakis EM, Schultze-Mosgau A, Schroer A, et al. A lower ongoing pregnancy rate can be expected when GnRH agonist is used for triggering final oocyte maturation instead of HCG in patients undergoing IVF with GnRH antagonists. Hum Reprod 2005; 20: 2887–92.

61. Olivennes F, Cunha-Filho JS, Fanchin R, et al. The use of GnRH antagonists in ovarian stimulation. Hum Reprod Update 2002; 8: 279–90.

62. Franks S. Polycystic ovary syndrome: a changing perspective. Clin Endocrinol (Oxf) 1989; 31: 87–120.

63. Karam KS, Taymor ML, Berger MJ. Estrogen monitoring and the prevention of ovarian overstimulation during gonadotropin therapy. Am J Obstet Gynecol 1973; 115: 972–7.

64. Murad NM. Ultrasound or ultrasound and hormonal determinations for in vitro fertilization monitoring. Int J Gynaecol Obstet 1998; 63: 271–6.

65. Ben-Shlomo I, Geslevich J, Shalev E. Can we abandon routine evaluation of serum estradiol levels during controlled ovarian hyperstimulation for assisted reproduction? Fertil Steril 2001; 76: 300–3.

66. Thomas K, Searle T, Quinn A, et al. The value of routine estradiol monitoring in assisted conception cycles. Acta Obstet Gynecol Scand 2002; 81: 551–4.

67. Aboulghar M. Prediction of ovarian hyperstimulation syndrome (OHSS). Estradiol level has an important role in the prediction of OHSS. Hum Reprod 2003; 18: 1140–1.

68. The ESHRE Capri Workshop. Infertility revisited: the state of the art today and tomorrow. Hum Reprod 1996; 11: 1779–807.

69. D'Angelo A, Davies R, Salah E, et al. Value of the serum estradiol level for preventing ovarian hyperstimulation syndrome: a retrospective case control study. Fertil Steril 2004; 81: 332–6.

APPENDIX

Strategic considerations to limit the incidence of OHSS

Primary prevention of OHSS

- To identify the known risk factors;
- To initiate specific preventive strategies:
  - Is stimulation really necessary?
  - Are there alternative treatments (diet, life-style, laparoscopic surgery)?
- To respect the minimal safety rules of stimulation:
  - Choice of proper stimulation regimen: drug, dose, protocol;
  - Careful monitoring of the cycle: estradiol (E_2) plasma level, number of follicles;
  - Activation of secondary prevention measures.

Risk factors for OHSS

- **Polycystic ovarian syndrome (PCOS);**
- High number of resting follicles at day 3 (> 10/ovary);
- Isolated characteristics of PCOS:
  - Enlarged ovary volume;
  - Inversion of LH/FSH;
  - Increased ovarian androgen circulating levels;
- Young age;
- Allergic dispositions;
- Previous occurrence of OHSS;
- Previous strong ovarian response to stimulation:
  - $E_2 > 1500$ pg/l day 8;
  - $E_2 > 3000$ pg/l day 11;
  - > 15 oocytes retrieved.

Primary prevention during treatment

- Choice of proper stimulation regimen:
  - Clomiphene citrate in first line of non-IVF procedures;
  - Reducing the dose of gonadotropins in IVF;
  - Use of GnRH antagonist: no previous ovarian desensitization with GnRH agonist;
- Careful monitoring of the cycle:
  - E_2 measurements:
    - Threshold of 2500 pg/l?
  - Ultrasound assessment of number of follicles:
    - > 20 growing follicles on day 8?
    - > 35 measurable follicles?
  - Combination to identify high-risk situations;
- Activation of secondary prevention measures:
  - Reduction of the dose of gonadotropins;
  - Coasting.

CHAPTER 20

Does ovulation triggering influence the risk for ovarian hyperstimulation syndrome?

Shahar Kol

INTRODUCTION

Ovarian hyperstimulation syndrome (OHSS) is the price patients pay for our attempt to override nature's delicate balances that were created to assure a single oocyte ovulation. Spontaneous OHSS does occur, as we delineate later. It is, however, very rare. Indeed, natural-cycle-based assisted reproductive technologies (ART) were responsible for the birth of the first IVF baby; however, this method was abandoned because it is cumbersome and, more important, yields poor results in terms of pregnancy rate. Therefore, human menopausal gonadotropin (hMG) has been used for decades in ovulation induction cycles, particularly in the context of *in vitro* fertilization (IVF). In recent years, recombinant follicle stimulating hormone (FSH) preparations have replaced hMG in most centers. Typically, in these cycles, human chorionic gonadotropin (hCG) is used as a surrogate to luteinizing hormone (LH) for the purpose of oocyte maturation and induction and ovulation. Given its significantly longer half-life (> 24 h versus 60 min for LH[1,2]), hCG administration results in a prolonged luteotrophic effect, characterized by the development of multiple corpora lutea and supraphysiological levels of estradiol (E_2) and progesterone (P). This sustained luteotrophic effect may result in the development of OHSS, still the most frequent and severe complication of ovarian stimulation treatments as described in other chapters of this volume. Although hCG (recombinant or urinary-derived in different doses) is used routinely, other modes of ovulation trigger are also available, namely, recombinant LH, native gonadotropin-releasing hormone (GnRH) and GnRH agonists. The aim of this chapter is to explore the association between the mode of trigger and the risk of OHSS. This association culminates in an OHSS risk-free clinical protocol that is available at the end of the chapter.

THE SPONTANEOUS LH/FSH SURGE: NATURAL-CYCLE OHSS

The mid-cycle spontaneous LH surge is characterized by three phases: a rapidly ascending limb of 14-h duration, a plateau of 14 h and a descending phase of 20 h[3]. The parallel FSH surge is of lower amplitude. Serum E_2 levels reach a peak at the time of onset of the LH surge and then decline rapidly. Serum levels of P begin to rise 12 h before the LH surge, continue to rise for an additional 12 h and then plateau until follicular rupture (36 h after the LH surge onset). Follicular rupture is associated with a second rise in P and a fall in E_2, as the luteal pattern of ovarian steroidogenesis is attained.

The human natural cycle is designed to allow the recruitment of a single dominant follicle, from which a fertilizable oocyte emerges. Antral follicles that failed to reach dominance are destined to atresia, which occurs before the mid-cycle LH surge. This mechanism assures that only a single corpus luteum is formed in each cycle, explaining the rarity of spontaneous OHSS.

Spontaneous OHSS is typically associated with high hCG levels, i.e. multiple pregnancy or hydatidiform mole. Recurrent OHSS suggests a genetic predisposition. Indeed, an FSH receptor gene mutation was identified in a woman who developed spontaneous OHSS during each of her four pregnancies[3].

The corpus luteum originating from the dominant follicle is not 'responsible' for the development of spontaneous OHSS, but rather secondary corpora lutea that emerge while pregnancy is established.

OVULATION TRIGGERING WITH hCG

hCG is routinely used to trigger ovulation in ovarian stimulation cycles. Given its long half-life and luteotrophic activity, it is blamed for the initiation of the OHSS process. If pregnancy is achieved, the endogenous hCG production replaces and augments the trigger dose, leading to enhancement of the OHSS pathology. In the non-IVF patient, a low-dose stimulation protocol, resulting in monofollicular ovulation, will completely prevent OHSS[4] regardless of the hCG dose used. When multifolliculogenesis is required for ART, the risk of OHSS is a concern. Although there appears to be some degree of correlation with the degree of ovarian response, individual cases tend to be unpredictable. Withholding the hCG trigger (e.g. aborting the cycle) completely prevents OHSS, if measures are taken to prevent spontaneous ovulation. For the purpose of inducing ovulation and minimizing OHSS risk, reducing the hCG dose seems to be a logical step to take. While a dose of 10 000 IU is routinely used, reducing the trigger dose may be beneficial in terms of reducing OHSS risk. The comparison of single intramuscular doses of 2000, 5000 and 10 000 IU of hCG resulted in poor oocyte yield with the lowest dose[5]. Indeed, most clinicians administer the lower effective dose of hCG (5000 IU) in an effort to reduce OHSS risk. A retrospective review of IVF clinical data regarding high responders (defined as $E_2 \geq 2500$ but < 4000 pg/ml on the day of hCG trigger) tried to confirm that hCG in a dose of 3300 IU is sufficient to provide adequate oocyte maturation and fertilization. While the above was indeed confirmed, as the lower dose resulted in a similar proportion of mature eggs, similar fertilization rate and similar pregnancy rate compared with 5000 IU, reducing the dose did not eliminate the risk of OHSS[6]. Although a randomized controlled study that compares the two hCG doses has not been carried out, available data suggest that the practice of relying on the minimal hCG dose as a safeguard against OHSS should be discouraged.

Recombinant hCG (rhCG) has largely replaced the urinary product. Subcutaneous rhCG (250 μg) is superior to urinary hCG (5000 IU) in terms of luteal-phase progesterone and serum hCG levels post-administration (Figures 1 and 2)[7]. However, in the context of OHSS it seems that there is no advantage. Although recombinant hCG (250 μg = 6500 IU) is as effective as 10 000 IU urinary hCG in terms of triggering, the rate of OHSS is similar[8,9].

Any discussion about triggering ovulation should include the type of protocol used for ovarian stimulation. Currently, ovarian stimulation for ART relies on GnRH analogs to prevent a premature LH surge. Long GnRH agonist-based protocols are associated with an increased incidence of OHSS, reflecting the recruitment of a large number of follicles[10]. GnRH antagonist-based protocols may reduce the incidence of

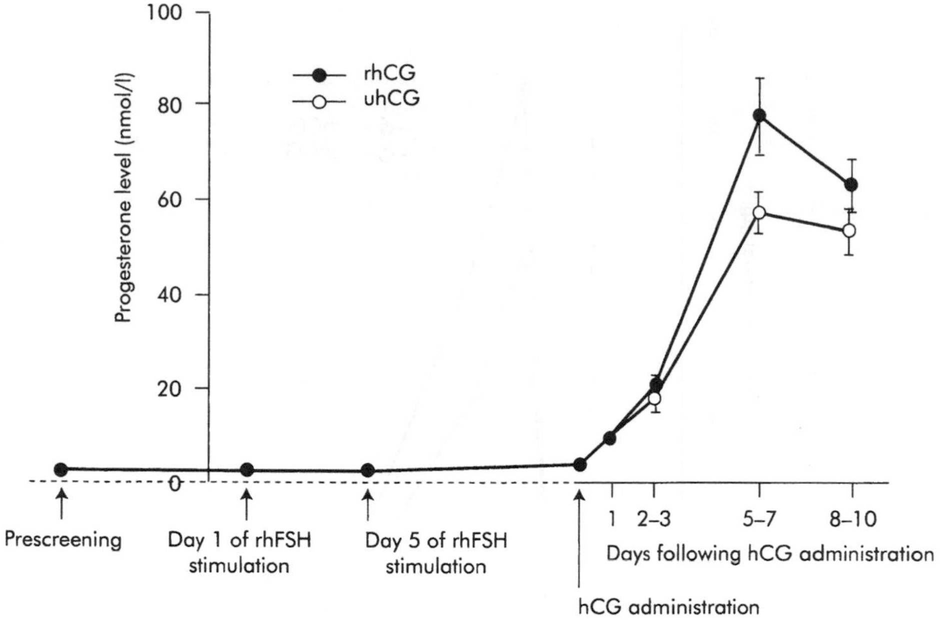

Figure 1 Mean progesterone levels (± SEM) before and during recombinant human follicle stimulating hormone (rhFSH) stimulation and after human chorionic gonadotropin (hCG) administration. Closed circles represent mean values in the group receiving recombinant rhCG 250 μg ($n = 85$); open circles represent mean values in the group receiving urinary uhCG 5000 IU ($n = 92$). The difference in values at days 5–7 after hCG administration is statistically significant ($p = 0.0361$; analysis of variance (ANOVA), ranked data). From reference 7, by permission of the American Society for Reproductive Medicine

OHSS[11]. However, conflicting publications[12] suggest that the difference, if it exists, is minimal. The significant advantage of GnRH antagonist-based protocols, as discussed herein, lies in the ability to trigger ovulation with a GnRH agonist, and prevent OHSS altogether.

In summary, triggering ovulation with hCG is always associated with some risk of OHSS, depending primarily on the magnitude of the ovarian response. When the prolonged luteotrophic effect of hCG merges with endogenous hCG (if pregnancy is achieved), the continuous overstimulation of the corpora lutea may give rise to OHSS.

OVULATION TRIGGERING WITH LH

The availability of recombinant LH was met with hopes to replace hCG as trigger. After all, it makes sense to imitate nature. A prospective, comparative, dose-finding study was conducted to determine the minimal effective dose of recombinant LH[13]. In a long agonist protocol, recombinant LH was used in doses of 5000, 15 000 or 30 000 IU, or two doses of 15 000 and 10 000 IU 3 days apart. A control group was triggered with hCG 5000 IU. Moderate OHSS was reported in 12.4% of patients who received hCG and in 12% of patients who received the

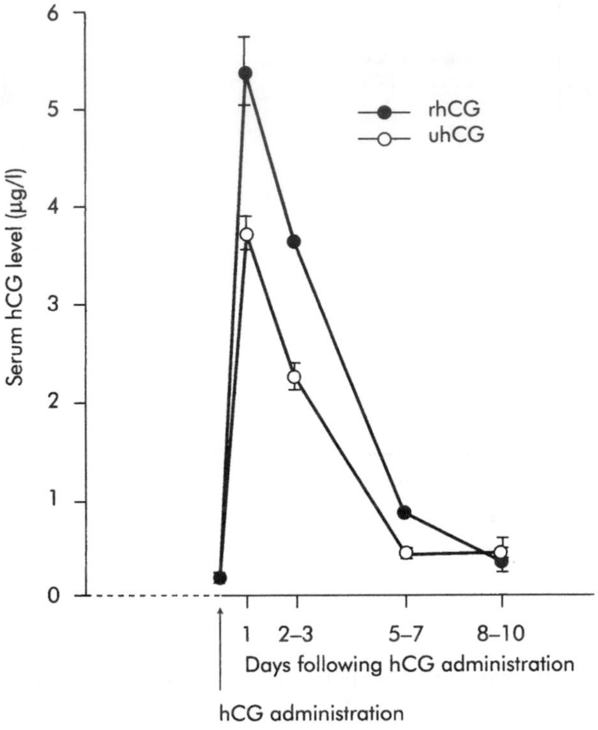

Figure 2 Mean human chorionic gonadotropin (hCG) levels (± SEM) at and after hCG administration. Closed circles represent mean values in the group receiving recombinant rhCG 250 µg ($n = 85$); open circles represent mean values in the group receiving urinary uhCG 5000 IU ($n = 92$). Serum hCG levels on days 1, 2–3 and 5–7 after hCG administration were significantly higher in the rhCG group ($p = 0.0001$ for all time points; ANOVA, ranked data). From reference 7, by permission of the American Society for Reproductive Medicine

recombinant LH double dose. However, no OHSS was reported in patients who received a single dose of recombinant LH (up to 30 000 IU). The conclusion of this study was that a single dose of recombinant LH results in a significant reduction in OHSS, compared with hCG. Unfortunately, the sponsoring company, Serono International, chose not to pursue this project further, and hence recombinant LH is not commercially available for ovulation triggering.

OVULATION TRIGGERING WITH NATIVE GnRH

In an effort to mimic the endogenous LH/FSH surges, native GnRH was used as trigger[14] in 32 OHSS high-risk patients with polycystic ovaries undergoing hMG ovulation induction. Late-follicular E_2 of > 6000 pmol/l was chosen as high-risk cut-off. Ten patients became pregnant, of whom two experienced OHSS. Evidently, native GnRH lacks the luteolytic effect of GnRH agonist as trigger, and hence its failure to prevent OHSS. Native GnRH trigger in the context of OHSS prevention was not pursued further to the above-cited study; therefore, there is no evidence to recommend its use.

OVULATION TRIGGERING WITH GnRH AGONIST

The GnRH agonist-induced LH/FSH surge

A GnRH agonist (GnRH-a) elicits pituitary secretion of gonadotropins, which can be utilized for triggering oocyte maturation and ovulation, if given at the right time of the cycle. Numerous compounds, administered in different regimens, have been successfully used for that purpose[15–22]. Based on these studies, it appears that the single administration of a GnRH-a in a dose of 200–500 μg effectively and reliably triggers the required gonadotropin surge[21,22]. However, the minimal effective dose of GnRH-a required to trigger an endogenous mid-cycle LH surge sufficient to induce oocyte maturation and ovulation remains to be established. Preliminary experience[23] suggests that a single dose of 50 μg intranasal buserelin is the minimal effective dose to trigger ovulation.

The pituitary and ovarian responses to mid-cycle GnRH-a injections in stimulated cycles have been described previously[18]. The injection of GnRH-a results in an acute release of LH and FSH. Serum LH and FSH levels rise during 4 and 12 h, respectively, and are elevated for 24–36 h. The amplitude of the surge is similar to that seen in the normal menstrual cycle, but in contrast with the natural cycle, the surge consists of only two phases: a short ascending limb (> 4 h) and a long descending limb (> 20 h). This has no bearing on the ovarian hormone secretion pattern, which is qualitatively similar to the pattern observed in a natural cycle. The LH surge is associated with a rapid rise of P and the attainment of peak E_2 levels during the first 12 h after GnRH-a administration. This is followed by a transient suppression of P biosynthesis and a gradual decline in E_2 levels during the 24 h preceding follicle aspiration. After oocyte retrieval, a second rapid rise in P and a continuous fall in E_2 are observed, reflecting normal transition from the follicular to the luteal phase in ovarian steroidogenesis.

The luteal phase

While the endogenous LH surge triggered by GnRH-a is associated with a normal early follicular–luteal shift in ovarian steroidogenesis, serum levels of E_2 and P during the luteal phase are lower compared with those achieved after hCG administration[18]. This may be related to the longer duration of plasma hCG activity compared with the shorter GnRH-a-induced LH elevation. Normal function of the corpus luteum is dependent on pituitary pulsatile LH[24]. It is possible, therefore, that the presumed down-regulation of pituitary GnRH receptors after a mid-cycle injection of GnRH-a results in reduced LH support for the developing corpora lutea, reduced steroidogenesis and early luteolysis. Based on these considerations, it is prudent to support the luteal phase with P (and possibly E_2) in patients treated with mid-cycle GnRH-a. Continued support during early pregnancy (until the luteal–placental shift) is probably required.

Prevention of OHSS

The most important benefit emerging from the use of GnRH-a, rather than hCG, for ovulation induction, is the ability of this regimen to eliminate completely the threat of clinically significant OHSS. It should be emphasized that the clinical findings attributable to mild[25] OHSS (e.g. ovarian enlargement, abdominal discomfort and excessive steroid production) are an integral part of most cases of ovulation induction in IVF, and hence are meaningless in this context. As mentioned above, clinical experience with mid-cycle administration of GnRH-a in the context of OHSS prevention is very encouraging. Effective ovulation is triggered with no risk of OHSS even in patients with extremely high E_2 levels during the late follicular phase[20].

Previous reports described cases in which OHSS developed despite the use of GnRH-a to induce ovulation. Three cases were reported by van der Meer *et al.*[26]. The clinical details of these cases are in line with mild to moderate OHSS. Severe ascites, hypovolemia or electrolyte imbalance did not occur, nor were the patients hospitalized. Of note, the three patients received nasal GnRH-a preparations (buserelin; Suprefact®; Hoechst, Germany). In one of them, a very weak response to GnRH-a was noted, with an LH-surge peak of 15.9 mIU/ml, suggesting that the dose used or the route of administration was less than optimal. The possibility of incomplete absorption using nasal administration cannot be ignored. In addition, the three patients were stimulated in preparation for intrauterine insemination (IU). Gerris *et al.*[27] have also reported OHSS following this approach; however, in this case, use was made of *native* GnRH (and not *GnRH-a*), resulting in successful ovulation triggering, but without the critical gonadotropin suppression, which is the key element in preventing OHSS. Shoham *et al.*[28] reported a personal communication of two OHSS cases. However, the complete details of the treatment protocols, symptoms and signs leading to the diagnosis of OHSS, severity of the syndrome and clinical outcome were not available. Last, a group from Saudi Arabia has presented its large and impressive experience with this strategy[29]. Of 708 polycystic ovarian syndrome (PCOS), high-responder IVF patients (mean E_2 on the day of ovulation triggering 7817 pg/ml!), ovulation was effectively triggered with GnRH-a in 682 (96%). One patient (0.1%) developed severe OHSS. Significantly, this patient was treated with hCG-based luteal support, probably by mistake, as the protocol dictated progesterone-only luteal support. Also of note is that in 26 patients a GnRH-a-induced LH surge was judged as 'inadequate'. In 18 of these patients, hCG was used, resulting in 11 (61%) cases of severe OHSS. This last figure may reflect the large number of severe OHSS cases in this series that were prevented by this strategy. The reason(s) for an inadequate LH surge may have to do with the dose (too low) or route (intranasal) of GnRH-a administration. A key point in this strategy is the ability of an adequate single dose of GnRH-a to bring about an effective LH surge, and subsequently to induce early luteal-phase relative pituitary down-regulation. Luteolysis could be induced by diminished early luteal-phase LH pulsatility, leading to the prevention of OHSS. Our protocol calls for a single subcutaneous. injection of 0.2 mg triptorelin (Decapeptyl®; Ferring, Malmö, Sweden). We recorded no LH surge failures with this protocol, and of course, no clinically significant OHSS thus far (thousands of patients, some of which have been published).

Benefits and limitations

As discussed above, GnRH-a is an effective alternative to hCG in ART, particularly when the threat of OHSS is imminent. In addition, it offers a more physiological stimulus for ovulation, combining both LH and FSH surges. Apparently, the presence of a mid-cycle FSH surge is not obligatory for successful ovulation, given the widespread use of hCG, and hence it is not known whether the FSH surge associated with GnRH-a is of any advantage.

Although a large body of evidence supports the role of this approach in OHSS prevention, none of the published papers reports the results of a bone fide prospective, randomized, study comparing GnRH-a and hCG in terms of OHSS occurrence. Admittedly, without such a study, rapid dissemination of this approach cannot be anticipated. The applicability of such a study at this time is questionable owing to ethical considerations ('Catch 22' situation).

A practical, major, limitation of GnRH-a-induced ovulation is that it would not be effective in women with a low gonadotropin reserve. Therefore, it is not applicable in IVF stimulation cycles during which pituitary down-regulation with a GnRH agonist is used. This protocol renders the pituitary unresponsive for induction of an endogenous LH surge. Since GnRH agonist-based protocols have been used routinely by most IVF programs until the year 2000, GnRH-a-induced ovulation for OHSS prevention has not gained much popularity.

GnRH antagonists: new opportunities

The introduction of GnRH antagonists in controlled ovarian hyperstimulation (COH) protocols[22,23], has opened up opportunities for novel stimulation protocols. A large (730 subjects) prospective randomized study[30] was carried out to compare long GnRH-a (buserelin) and GnRH antagonist (ganirelix; Orgalutran®) protocols. The results suggest that ganirelix introduces a new treatment option for patients undergoing ovarian stimulation for IVF or intracytoplasmic sperm injection (ICSI) which is safe, short and simple. The clinical outcome was good, and the ongoing pregnancy rate was acceptable. This novel protocol also introduces new opportunities in the context of OHSS prevention. One possibility is to prevent spontaneous LH surges in high-risk patients safely with a high-dose GnRH antagonist, waiting for follicular demise and ovarian quiescence[31]. In order to prevent OHSS effectively, and to rescue the cycle at the same time, the quick reversibility of antagonist-induced pituitary suppression can be of advantage by allowing the use of GnRH-a for the purpose of ovulation triggering. This possibility was assessed in a randomized prospective multicenter study[32]. Two different GnRH agonists (0.2 mg triptorelin and 0.5 mg leuprorelin) were compared with hCG for triggering ovulation in a GnRH antagonist-based (Orgalutran® or Antagon®) protocol for IVF. High responders (> 25 follicles beyond 11 mm) were considered drop-outs from the study; hence, agonist trigger in the context of OHSS prevention was not assessed. Luteal support was given by daily progesterone administration. Both agonists kick-started a successful LH surge (peak LH 4 h post-trigger). Interestingly, LH dynamics post-trigger was similar to that reported without GnRH antagonist pretreatment[18]. In other words, the routine daily dose of a GnRH antagonist (ganirelix 0.25 mg) does not blunt the effect of an agonist (given about 12 h apart) at the pituitary level. The three treatment groups (two agonists and hCG) had comparable numbers of oocytes retrieved, percentages of mature oocytes, fertilization rates and implantation rates. The authors summarized the results stating, 'corpus luteum formation is induced by GnRH agonists with luteal phase steroid level closer to the physiological range compared with hCG'. This statement merits a deeper look. Since progesterone was given as luteal support, the estradiol level may represent endogenous luteal activity. Mid-luteal levels of estradiol were 46 pg/ml and 45 pg/ml in the agonist trigger groups vs. 490 pg/ml in the hCG group. These levels reflect the sum of E_2 production by all the corpora lutea, the number of which can be drawn from the number of oocytes retrieved (8.3 in the hCG group, 8.7 and 9.8 in the agonist groups). When the estradiol levels are plotted against the natural cycle (Figure 3), it becomes apparent that the agonist triggers resulted in extremely low mid-luteal E_2 levels that cannot be considered as 'physiological'. In fact, the natural-cycle mid-luteal estradiol levels from a single corpus luteum (around 600 pmol/l, or 160 pg/ml[33]) is > 3-fold higher than the mid-luteal estradiol levels produced by 8–9 corpora lutea post-agonist triggers. These low levels can only be interpreted as a result of complete luteolysis, far from the 'physiological range'.

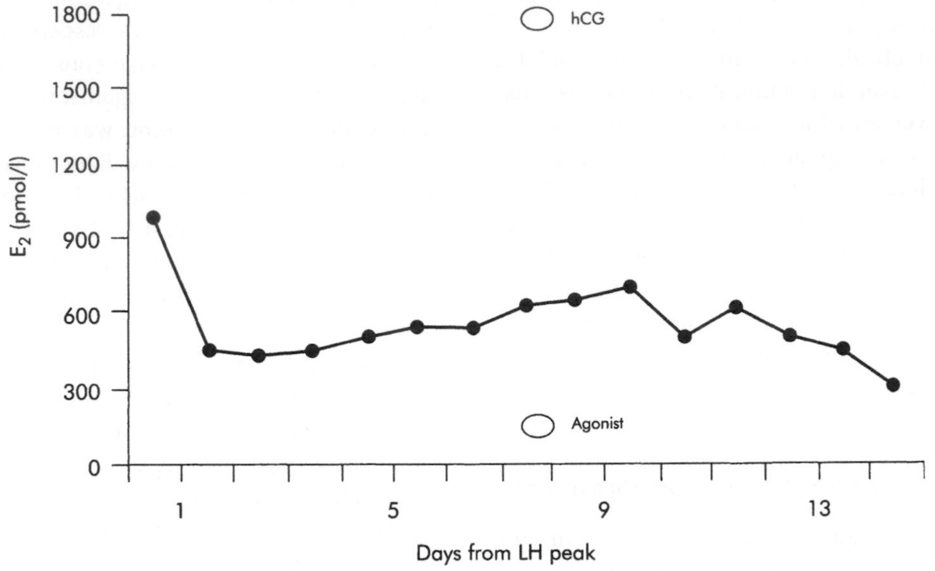

Figure 3 Luteal phase estradiol (E_2) (reflecting total luteolysis) after triggering ovulation with gonadotropin-releasing hormone (GnRH) agonist. Natural-cycle luteal phase estradiol is depicted by gray circles (based on reference 33). Mean mid-luteal serum concentrations of E_2 after triggering of final oocyte maturation with GnRH agonist or human chorionic gonadotropin (hCG) after ovarian stimulation for *in vitro* fertilization (IVF) (based on reference 32) are plotted against the natural-cycle levels. In agonist- and hCG-triggered cycles, 9 and 8 (mean) oocytes were retrieved, respectively (reference 32). LH, luteinizing hormone

Another randomized controlled study was performed to compare unsupplemented luteal phase characteristics after three different triggers: recombinant hCG, recombinant LH and GnRH agonist[34]. This approach allows assessment of progesterone levels to reflect luteal activity. Indeed, the 'area under the curve' progesterone secretion post-agonist trigger was practically zero. This remarkable phenomenon again attests for complete luteolysis post-agonist trigger. The concept of luteolysis post-agonist was first put forward by Casper and Yen[35], in 1979. They gave mid-luteal agonist to five normal volunteers. Luteolysis occurred as indicated by a fall in E_2 and P levels, followed by a shortened luteal phase.

To characterize further the presumed luteolytic process induced by mid-cycle injection of GnRH-a, and to avoid confusion between endogenous biosynthesis and exogenous luteal support, we have measured non-steroidal luteal function markers, inhibin A and pro-αC[36]. Agonist trigger caused a sharp decrease in these markers compared with patients who were treated with hCG (Figure 4). Pregnancy was not associated with a rise in the levels of luteal markers. This is the most important message arising from this chapter: GnRH-agonist trigger results in complete and dramatic luteolysis. By the time endogenous hCG appears (if pregnancy is achieved), the corpora lutea are beyond the point of 'resuscitation'; therefore, endogenous

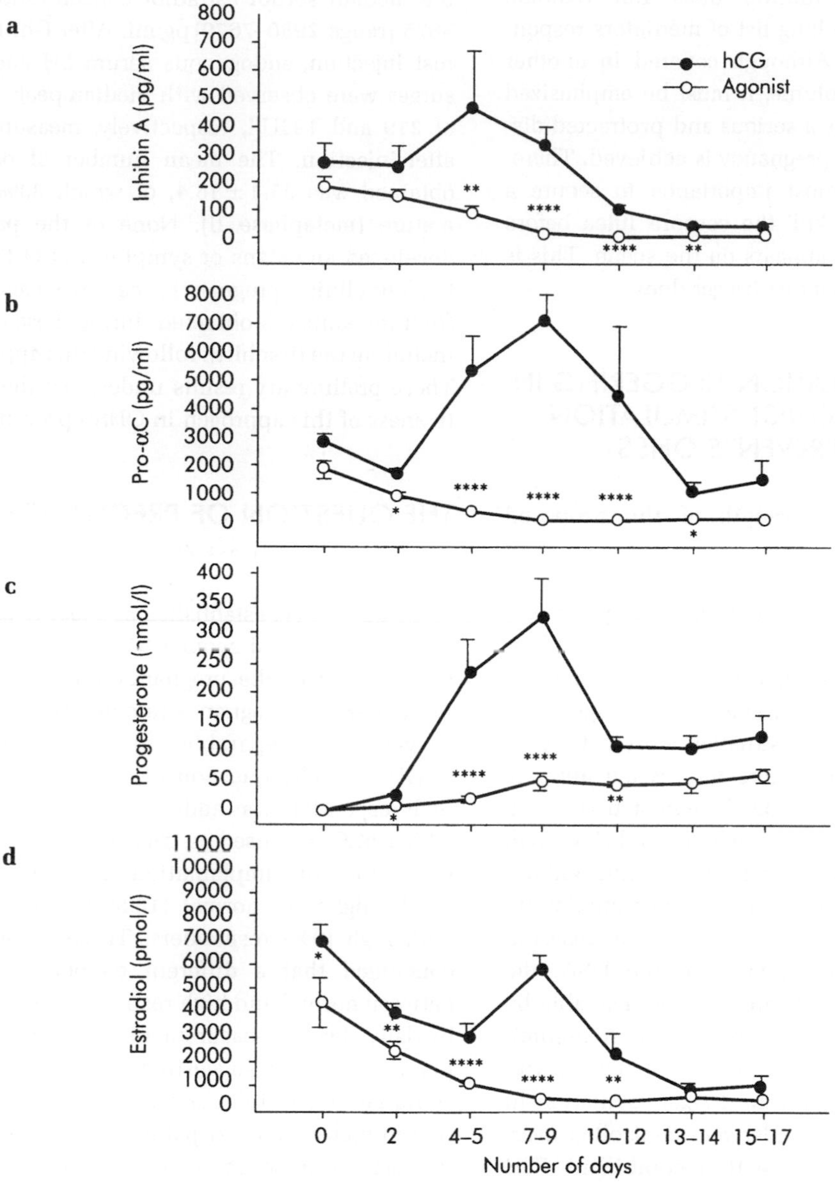

Figure 4 Luteal-phase serum concentrations (mean ± SE) of inhibin A (a), pro-αC (b), progesterone (c) and estradiol (d) in two *in vitro* fertilization (IVF) protocols: GnRH antagonist for ovulation prevention and hCG (hCG group) or GnRH-a (agonist group) for oocyte maturation triggering. Time is represented as days relative to oocyte maturation triggering day (day 0). Changes in levels of all four hormones in both groups were significant over time ($p < 0.0001$) (Friedman test). $^{*}p < 0.05$; $^{**}p < 0.01$; $^{***}p < 0.001$; $^{****}p < 0.0001$. From reference 36, by permission of the American Society for Reproductive Medicine

sex steroid production does not resume, together with the long list of mediators responsible for OHSS. Although covered in another chapter in this volume, it must be emphasized here that OHSS is a serious and protracted disease especially if pregnancy is achieved. Therefore, it is of utmost importance to secure a trigger that will 'kill' the corpora lutea before endogenous hCG appears on the scene. This is exactly what an agonist trigger does.

GnRH-a OVULATION TRIGGERING IN GnRH ANTAGONIST STIMULATION PROTOCOLS PREVENTS OHSS

The tremendous strength of the proposed approach is also its weakness in terms of 'evidence-based medicine'. It is very difficult to conduct a randomized controlled study comparing hCG and agonist trigger in high responders. Ethics committees might find it problematic to administer hCG to extremely high responders. One can compare the situation with a study on the merit of using a parachute when jumping from an airplane[37]. Indeed, agonist trigger can be looked on as a parachute to bring high responders safely down to the ground without an OHSS crash. Consequently, such studies are not available, although an unpublished research effort is currently ongoing in the USA, the results of which will probably be available by the time this volume is published. A preliminary report[38] describes the use of 0.2 mg triptorelin (Decapeptyl®) to trigger ovulation in eight patients who underwent controlled ovarian hyperstimulation with recombinant FSH (Puregon®) and concomitant treatment with the GnRH antagonist ganirelix (Orgalutran®) for the prevention of a premature LH surge. All patients were considered to have an increased risk for developing OHSS (at least 20 follicles ≥ 11 mm and/or serum estradiol at least 3000 pg/ml). On the day of triggering the LH surge, the mean number of follicles ≥ 11 mm was 25.1 ± 4.5, and the median serum estradiol concentration was 3675 (range 2980–7670) pg/ml. After GnRH agonist injection, endogenous serum LH and FSH surges were observed with median peak values of 219 and 19 IU/l, respectively, measured 4 h after injection. The mean number of oocytes obtained was 23.4 ± 15.4, of which 83% were mature (metaphase II). None of the patients developed any signs or symptoms of OHSS. So far, four clinical pregnancies have been achieved from the embryos obtained during these cycles, including the first birth following this approach. These preliminary results underlined the effectiveness of this approach in OHSS prevention.

THE QUESTION OF PREGNANCY RATE FOLLOWING AGONIST TRIGGER

Although not yet established as a tool to prevent OHSS, criticism of agonist trigger arose around the question of the pregnancy rate. In normal responders the pregnancy rate following agonist trigger is comparable to that following hCG[19,21,39]. The question of pregnancy rate in high responders was addressed in cycles during which hCG was used as trigger. Pellicer *et al.*[40] found that the implantation rate was significantly higher in normal (18.5%) as compared with high (0%) responders. These researchers concluded that a different endocrine milieu between normal and high responders is detected by daily steroid measurements up to the preimplantation period, suggesting that this difference could be responsible for an impaired implantation in high-responder patients undergoing IVF. An increase in serum E_2 levels seems to be the cause of this difference. Simon *et al.*[41] reached similar conclusions, stating that their clinical results demonstrate that high serum estradiol concentrations on the day of hCG injection in high- and normal-responder patients, regardless of the number of oocytes retrieved and the serum progesterone concentration, are detrimental to uterine receptivity without affecting embryo quality. These results led to an effort to increase uterine receptivity by decreasing estradiol levels in high responders with the use of a follicle stimulating hormone step-down regimen. Simon *et al.*[42] were successful in that regard, although the step-down regimen resulted in a 17% cancellation rate, i.e. patients in whom FSH support to the growing follicles was too low, leading to a sharp decrease in estradiol level. At the 2004 annual European Society of Human Reproduction and Embryology (ESHRE) meeting in Berlin, Bankowski *et al.*[43] presented their experience with agonist trigger in high responders. Apparently, they have adopted a routine to trigger high responders (E_2 > 3000 pg/ml) with an agonist. From May 2000 to July 2003, a total of 317 patients were triggered with hCG (normal responders) while 97 patients were triggered with an agonist (high responders). Peak E_2 levels were 2050 vs. 4800 pg/ml, number of oocytes 10 vs. 21 and number of embryos 5.6 vs. 12.5, respectively. The pregnancy rate was 21.5% in the normal responders vs. 11.3% in the high responders. Importantly, they had three cases of severe OHSS, *all in the hCG group*. These results demonstrate again the tremendous efficacy of agonist trigger in terms of OHSS prevention. In addition, given the large number of oocytes and embryos obtained (with no risk of OHSS), the clinical rate per oocyte retrieval (fresh and thaw cycles combined) is more relevant to the patient. It may be argued that a decrease in fresh-cycle pregnancy rate is a reasonable price to pay for total OHSS prevention (patient safety) and a large number of embryos obtained (subsequent thaw cycles).

TAKE-HOME MESSAGES

A single mid-cycle dose of GnRH-a is able to trigger a preovulatory LH/FSH surge, leading to oocyte maturation in women undergoing ovarian stimulation for IVF, or induction of ovulation *in vivo*. The main advantage of this approach is the complete elimination of clinically significant OHSS. The application of this trigger in high responders requires a responsive pituitary. Therefore, it is not applicable in GnRH agonist-based cycles during which pituitary down-regulation is achieved. GnRH antagonist-induced competitive inhibition of the pituitary GnRH receptors is easily reversible with a GnRH agonist. In fact, a major reason to use GnRH antagonists in ovarian stimulation is to keep the option of agonist trigger if needed. A clinical protocol for the high responder is as follows:

(1) Start stimulation with 150–225 IU recombinant FSH.

(2) Start antagonist on day 6 of stimulation. Consider adding 1 ampoule of recombinant LH (75 IU) daily.

(3) Ignore E_2 levels! There is no need to step down! Give the growing follicles *full* FSH support!

(4) Trigger with 0.2 mg triptorelin or 0.5 mg leuprorelin (at least 12 h after the last antagonist injection).

(5) Start luteal support with E_2 and progesterone on the day of oocyte retrieval.

In our experience, this protocol will eliminate OHSS.

REFERENCES

1. Yen SSC, Lenera G, Little B, et al. Disappearance rate of endogenous luteinizing hormone and chorionic gonadotropin in man. J Clin Endocrinol Metab 1968; 28: 1763–7.
2. Damewood MD, Shen W, Zacur HA, et al. Disappearance of exogenously administered human chorionic gonadotropin. Fertil Steril 1989; 52: 398–400.
3. Smits G, Olatunbosun OA, Delbaere A, et al. Spontaneous ovarian hyperstimulation syn-

drome caused by a mutant follitropin receptor. N Engl J Med 2003; 349: 760–6.

4. Homburg R, Howles CM. Low dose FSH therapy for anovulatory infertility associated with polycystic ovary syndrome: rationale, reflections and refinements. Hum Reprod Update 1999; 5: 493–9.
5. Abdalla HI, Ah-Moye M, Brinsden P, et al. The effect of the dose of hCG and the type of gonadotropin stimulation on oocyte recovery rates in an IVF program. Fertil Steril 1987; 48: 958–63.
6. Schmidt DW, Maier DB, Nulsen JC, et al. Reducing the dose of human chorionic gonadotropin in high responders does not affect the outcomes of in vitro fertilization. Fertil Steril 2004; 82: 841–6.
7. International Recombinant Human Chorionic Gonadotropin Study Group. Induction of ovulation in World Health Organization group II anovulatory women undergoing follicular stimulation with recombinant human follicle-stimulating hormone: a comparison of recombinant human chorionic gonadotropin (rhCG) and urinary hCG. Fertil Steril 2001; 75: 111–18.
8. Driscoll GL, Tyler JP, Hangan JT, et al. A prospective randomized controlled, double-blind, double-dummy comparison of recombinant and urinary HCG for inducing oocyte maturation and follicular luteinization in ovarian stimulation. Hum Reprod 2000; 15: 1305–10.
9. Chang P, Kenley S, Burns T, et al. Recombinant human chorionic gonadotropin (rhCG) in assisted reproductive technology: results of a clinical trial comparing two doses of rhCG (Ovidrel) to urinary hCG (Profasi) for induction of final follicular maturation in in vitro fertilization–embryo transfer. Fertil Steril 2001; 76: 67–74 .
10. Smitz J, Camus M, Devroey P, et al. Incidence of severe ovarian hyperstimulation syndrome after GnRH agonist/HMG superovulation for in-vitro fertilization. Hum Reprod 1990; 5: 933–7.
11. Ludwig M, Katalinic A, Diedrich K. Use of GnRH antagonists in ovarian stimulation for assisted reproductive technologies compared to the long protocol. Meta-analysis. Arch Gynecol Obstet 2001; 265: 175–82.
12. Al-Inany H, Aboulghar M. GnRH antagonist in assisted reproduction: a Cochrane review. Hum Reprod 2002; 17: 874–85.
13. European Recombinant LH Study Group. Human recombinant luteinizing hormone is as effective as, but safer than, urinary human chorionic gonadotropin in inducing final follicular maturation and ovulation in in vitro fertilization procedures: results of a multicenter double-blind study. J Clin Endocrinol Metab 2001; 86: 2607–18.
14. Blumenfeld Z, Lang N, Amit A, et al. Native gonadotropin-releasing hormone for triggering follicular maturation in polycystic ovary syndrome patients undergoing human menopausal gonadotropin ovulation induction. Fertil Steril 1994; 62: 456–60.
15. Emperaire JC, Ruffie A. Triggering ovulation with endogenous luteinizing hormone may prevent the ovarian hyperstimulation syndrome. Hum Reprod 1991; 6: 506–10.
16. Imoedemhe DAG, Chan RCW. Sigue AB, et al. A new approach to the management of patients at risk of ovarian hyperstimulation in an in-vitro fertilization programme. Hum Reprod 1991; 6: 1088–91.
17. Itskovitz J, Boldes R, Barlev A, et al. The induction of LH surge and oocyte maturation by GnRH analogue (buserelin) in women undergoing ovarian stimulation for in vitro fertilization. Gynecol Endocrinol 1988; 2: 165.
18. Itskovitz J, Boldes R, Levron J, et al. Induction of preovulatory luteinizing hormone surge and prevention of ovarian hyperstimulation syndrome by gonadotropin-releasing hormone agonist. Fertil Steril 1991; 56: 213–20.
19. Lanzone A, Fulghesu AM, Villa P, et al. Gonadotropin-releasing hormone agonist versus human chorionic gonadotropin as a trigger of ovulation in polycystic ovarian disease gonadotropin hyperstimulated cycles. Fertil Steril 1994; 62: 35–41.
20. Lewit N, Kol S, Manor D, et al. The use of GnRH analogs for induction of the preovulatory gonadotropin surge in assisted reproduction

and prevention of the ovarian hyperstimulation syndrome. Gynecol Endocrinol 1995; 4: 13–17.

21. Segal S, Casper RF. Gonadotropin-releasing hormone agonist versus human chorionic gonadotropin for triggering follicular maturation in in vitro fertilization. Fertil Steril 1992; 57: 1254–8.

22. Lewit N, Kol S, Manor D, et al. Comparison of GnRH analogs and hCG for the induction of ovulation and prevention of ovarian hyperstimulation syndrome (OHSS): a case–control study. Hum Reprod 1996; 11: 1399–402.

23. Buckett WM, Bentick B, Shaw RW. Induction of the endogenous gonadotrophin surge for oocyte maturation with intra-nasal gonadotrophin-releasing hormone analogue (buserelin): effective minimal dose. Hum Reprod 1998; 13: 811–14.

24. Mais V, Kazar RR, Cetel NS, et al. The dependency of folliculogenesis and corpus luteum function on pulsatile gonadotropin secretion in cycling women using a gonadotropin-releasing hormone antagonist as a probe. J Clin Endocrinol Metab 1986; 62: 1250–5.

25. Schenker JG, Weinstein D. Ovarian hyperstimulation syndrome: a current survey. Fertil Steril 1978; 30: 255–68.

26. van der Meer S, Gerris J, Joostens M, et al. Triggering of ovulation using a gonadotropin-releasing hormone agonist does not prevent ovarian hyperstimulation syndrome. Hum Reprod 1993; 8: 1628–31.

27. Gerris J, De Vits A, Joostens M, et al. Triggering of ovulation in human menopausal gonadotropin-stimulated cycles: comparison between intravenous administered gonadotrophin-releasing hormone (100 and 500 μg), GnRH agonist (buserelin, 500 μg) and human chorionic gonadotrophin (10,000 IU). Hum Reprod 1995; 10: 56–62.

28. Shoham Z, Schachter M, Loumaye E, et al. The luteinizing hormone surge – the final stage in ovulation induction: modern aspects of ovulation triggering. Fertil Steril 1995; 64: 237–51.

29. Imoedemhe D, Chan R, Pacpaco E, et al. Preventing OHSS in at-risk patients: evidence from a long-term prospective study. Hum Reprod 1999; 14: 102–3.

30. The European Orgalutran Study Group. Treatment with the gonadotrophin-releasing hormone antagonist ganirelix in women undergoing ovarian stimulation with recombinant follicle stimulating hormone is effective, safe and convenient: results of a controlled, randomized, multicentre trial. Hum Reprod 2000; 15: 1490–8.

31. de Jong D, Macklon NS, Mannaerts BMJL, et al. High dose gonadotrophin-releasing hormone antagonist (ganirelix) may prevent ovarian hyperstimulation syndrome caused by ovarian stimulation for in-vitro fertilization. Hum Reprod 1998; 13: 573–5.

32. Fauser BC, de Jong D, Olivennes F, et al. Endocrine profiles after triggering of final oocyte maturation with GnRH agonist after cotreatment with the GnRH antagonist ganirelix during ovarian hyperstimulation for in vitro fertilization. J Clin Endocrinol Metab 2002; 87: 709–15.

33. Yen SSC. The human menstrual cycle: neuroendocrine regulation. In Yen SSC, Jaffe RB, eds. Reproductive Endocrinology, 3rd edn. Philadelphia, PA: WB Saunders Co, 1991: 273–308.

34. Beckers NG, Macklon NS, Eijkemans MJ, et al. Nonsupplemented luteal phase characteristics after the administration of recombinant human chorionic gonadotropin, recombinant luteinizing hormone, or gonadotropin-releasing hormone (GnRH) agonist to induce final oocyte maturation in in vitro fertilization patients after ovarian stimulation with recombinant follicle-stimulating hormone and GnRH antagonist cotreatment. J Clin Endocrinol Metab 2003; 88: 4186–92.

35. Casper RF, Yen SSC. Induction of luteolysis in the human with a long acting analog of luteinizing hormone releasing factor. Science 1979; 205: 408–10.

36. Nevo O, Eldar-Geva T, Kol S, et al. Lower levels of inhibin A and pro-alphaC during the luteal phase after triggering oocyte maturation with a gonadotropin-releasing hormone agonist versus human chorionic gonadotropin. Fertil Steril 2003; 79: 1123–8.

37. Smith GC, Pell JP. Parachute use to prevent death and major trauma related to gravitational challenge: systematic review of randomised controlled trials. Br Med J 2003; 327: 1459–61.

38. Itskovitz-Eldor J, Kol S, Mannaerts B. Use of a single bolus of GnRH agonist triptorelin to trigger ovulation after GnRH antagonist ganirelix treatment in women undergoing ovarian stimulation for assisted reproduction, with special reference to the prevention of ovarian hyperstimulation syndrome: preliminary report: Short communication. Hum Reprod 2000; 15: 1965–8.

39. Gonen Y, Balakier H, Powell W, et al. Use of gonadotropin-releasing hormone agonist to trigger follicular maturation for in vitro fertilization. J Clin Endocrinol Metab 1990; 71: 918–22.

40. Pellicer A, Valbuena D, Cano F, et al. Lower implantation rates in high responders: evidence for an altered endocrine milieu during the preimplantation period. Fertil Steril 1996; 65: 1190–5.

41. Simon C, Cano F, Valbuena D, et al. Clinical evidence for a detrimental effect on uterine receptivity of high serum oestradiol concentrations in high and normal responder patients. Hum Reprod 1995; 10: 2432–7.

42. Simon C, Garcia Velasco JJ, Valbuena D, et al. Increasing uterine receptivity by decreasing estradiol levels during the preimplantation period in high responders with the use of a follicle-stimulating hormone step-down regimen. Fertil Steril 1998; 70: 234–9.

43. Bankowski B, Bracero N, King J, et al. Triggering ovulation with leuprolide acetate is associated with lower pregnancy rate. Hum Reprod 2004; 19 (Suppl 1): i103.

CHAPTER 21

Secondary prevention of threatening ovarian hyperstimulation syndrome

Annick Delvigne

Primary prevention and early recognition of ovarian hyperstimulation syndrome (OHSS) are important in order to ensure the patient's safety. The first step of primary prevention is the identification of risk factors, to individualize the patient's stimulation regimen. Second, it is mandatory to monitor the ovarian response to gonadotropins strictly in order to adapt the stimulation to this response. For this purpose, monitoring ovulation using ultrasound and serum estradiol (E_2) assays constitutes the 'gold standard'. Several studies have evaluated the impact of follow-up by either technique alone or in combination, and concluded that the combination of both methods provides the best results[1]. Nevertheless, while it is believed that both E_2 and ultrasound monitoring is necessary, it is insufficient, as most *in vitro* fertilization (IVF) centers still report the occurrence of severe forms of OHSS, even though such monitoring is practiced[2].

Strict monitoring, however, allows the application of a number of preventive methods to minimize the probability and/or severity of OHSS for high-risk patients, defined by their exaggerated ovarian response.

The preventive measures that have been described are the following:

(1) Canceling the cycle;

(2) Coasting;

(3) Early unilateral ovarian follicular aspiration (EUFA);

(4) Modifying the methods of ovulation triggering;

(5) Administration of glucocorticoids;

(6) Macromolecules and progesterone;

(7) Cryopreservation of all embryos;

(8) Electrocautery or laser vaporization of one or both ovaries;

(9) Reduction of the number of transferred embryos.

CANCELING THE CYCLE

Some authors suggest canceling the cycle by not giving human chorionic gonadotropin (hCG) when several risk factors of OHSS are present, because hCG triggers the development of OHSS.

As early as 1970, preliminary data indicated that the complications of superovulation could be totally avoided if the ovulation trigger by hCG stimulus was withheld[3]. Others confirmed that canceling cycles at risk by withholding hCG when estrogen levels were too high prevented severe OHSS[4,5]. Spontaneous OHSS is very rare indeed.

In ovulation-induction cycles, when gonadotropin-releasing hormone (GnRH) agonists (GnRH-a) or antagonists are not used, one should remain vigilant, since a spontaneous LH peak may still occur, resulting in a pregnancy that is sometimes associated with OHSS complications induced by endogenous hCG. In a situation where natural conception is possible, the couple should be advised to avoid intercourse or to use condoms, as spontaneous ovulation may occur up to 11 days after discontinuing gonadotropin treatment.

This attitude is much more difficult to apply in an *in vitro* fertilization (IVF) program, since the goal here is, by definition, to increase the number of oocytes. Therefore, it is much more difficult to establish a danger threshold. Furthermore, physicians may also feel more reluctant to propose cancellation to patients, as IVF implies a great commitment on the patients' part in terms of procedures, time and money. Moreover, the physicians are also under pressure to obtain a 'successful' outcome when there is no coverage of costs by insurance[6]. On the other hand, as luteinizing hormone (LH) surge inhibitors (such as GnRH-a and antagonists) are almost always used, canceling results in an absolute prevention in these much more dangerous situations. It has been suggested that, after stopping human menopausal gonadotropin (hMG), the GnRH-a treatment should be continued until the ovaries recover to a normal size and then they are restimulated using lower doses of gonadotropins[7]. Unfortunately, such lower doses may lead to an inadequate ovarian response[8–10].

The necessity to maintain the administration of GnRH-a, after taking the decision to cancel the cycle, is discussed later in the section concerning embryo cryopreservation.

In the future, *in vitro* maturation of human oocytes, with and without stimulation, will be available and yield several oocytes, thereby avoiding hCG administration.

Summary

Canceling the cycle and withholding hCG is the only method that totally avoids the risk of OHSS in ovarian induction cycles or in IVF.

All other procedures usually succeed in decreasing either the risk or the severity of OHSS, rather than totally preventing it.

COASTING

This technique was first described in hyperstimulated cycles[11,12] and first applied in IVF cycles by Sher *et al.* in 1993[13]. The method is based on the assumption that E_2 levels reached at the time of hCG administration are predictive of the risk for OHSS. When a patient considered at risk has a high E_2 level, exogenous gonadotropins are stopped, while GnRH-a are maintained. hCG administration is then postponed until the patient's serum E_2 level decreases to 'a safer zone', attesting to the atresia of granulosa cells. Coasting acts probably by apoptosis of granulosa cells and a reduction of their functional capacity to produce vasoactive factors, such as vascular endothelial growth factor (VEGF)[14,15].

In a recent survey conducted among gynecologists specialized in infertility treatment, 'coasting' appeared to be the most popular method used to prevent OHSS[16]. There are many advantages in using this technique: the cycle is not abandoned, it enables the transfer of fresh embryos and, finally, no supplementary procedure or medical therapy is involved. It is therefore not surprising that some two-thirds of physicians who chose to apply a preventive method advocated the use of coasting[16].

A systematic review, aimed at deciding whether there was sufficient evidence to justify *the general acceptance of coasting,* was also performed[17,18]. It involved 493 patients in 12 studies and showed the data to be highly heterogeneous in terms of characteristics and number of patients, stimulation schemes and coasting procedures. In most studies, either a threshold value of serum E_2 was used (often a value of 3000 pg/ml), and/or the number of follicles was considered. Fertilization rates (36.7–71%) and pregnancy rates (20–57%) were acceptable in terms of IVF results, in comparison with those of large IVF databanks. In 16% of cycles, ascites was described; in 2.8%, hemoconcentration was recorded; and 2.5% of patients required hospitalization. While coasting does not totally avoid the risk of OHSS, it certainly decreases its incidence in high-risk patients.

In practice, different types of coasting protocols have been proposed: early coasting is initiated on the basis of a large number of follicles; and late coasting is initiated later in the cycle when high E_2 levels are observed[19].

A relevant problem is to decide *how coasting should be managed,* to obtain the best results in terms of oocyte quality and IVF outcome. Indeed, some investigators have suggested that oocyte quality deteriorates when using coasting under certain conditions. Aboulghar *et al.*[20] reported a low number of good-quality oocytes when classical coasting was applied, and recommended using a 'modified form of coasting', by decreasing the dose of hMG before withholding it completely.

Whelan and Vlahos[21] also reported poor oocyte quality when E_2 fell, and suggested monitoring daily follicle size and E_2 levels and administering hCG when E_2 levels had plateaued for 2–3 days.

Two retrospective studies of 207 and 157 coasted patients, respectively, analyzed the implications of E_2 drop and coasting duration on IVF outcome[17,22].

According to Ulug *et al.*[22], coasting for more than 3 days appeared to reduce the implantation and pregnancy rates, while oocyte and embryo qualities did not appear to be affected. This suggests that endometrial receptivity may be hampered. Still, in another study conducted in an oocyte donation program, the implantation and pregnancy rates of recipient patients coasted for more than 4 days were significantly lower, indicating that oocyte quality decreases after coasting[23]. Nevertheless, in our study, no significant relationship was found between the number of coasting days, the E_2 level on the day of hCG or the fall in E_2 and outcome, whether measured in terms of oocyte quality, pregnancy rate or incidence of OHSS[24].

According to these conflicting results, Egbase *et al.*[25] applied early coasting with a fixed period of 3 days in 102 obese polycystic ovarian syndrome (PCOS) patients in order to avoid a possible reduction of quality. These authors obtained a clinical pregnancy rate of 45.1% without the occurrence of severe OHSS.

The discrepancy between studies may be due to the heterogeneous criteria for initiating and ending the coasting process. For example, in early coasting, starting when the follicles are still small, the E_2 drop could have a greater impact on oocyte quality, whereas coasting beginning later in the cycle when larger follicles and higher E_2 already exist could have less implication for oocyte quality. Furthermore, in these latter conditions, the length of coasting may have a more pronounced effect on endometrial receptivity.

Reviewing ten relevant studies, Levinsohn-Tavor *et al.*[26] recommended stopping gonadotropins only when the leading follicles reached 15 mm, and administering hCG only when E_2 fell below 3000 pg/ml, to ensure effective prevention of OHSS. The authors underlined the lack of prospective randomized studies which would allow them to give recommendations.

Summary

Coasting is a popular and effective method for reducing OHSS rates, but it does not totally eliminate the condition. The procedure seems to be associated with a reduced oocyte collection rate and especially so when the coasting period is prolonged. The quality of oocytes after coasting is still the subject of debate, as is endometrial receptivity after E_2 lowering. Available data are reassuring in terms of pregnancy rates.

EARLY UNILATERAL OVARIAN FOLLICULAR ASPIRATION

Gonen *et al.*[27] observed that follicular aspiration induces intrafollicular hemorrhage which has a negative impact on corpus luteum function. It has therefore been suggested that growing follicles be punctured, with the hope that the withdrawal of follicular contents may significantly interfere with follicular maturation and modify the intraovarian mechanisms responsible for OHSS.

Contradictory results have been reported for the protective effect against OHSS of follicular aspiration during oocyte pick-up[28,29].

The timing of the trigger dose of hCG in relation to the expected protective effect of follicular aspiration may be of importance for preventing OHSS.

In 1995, early unilateral ovarian follicular aspiration (EUFA) was first applied to 17 patients at risk of OHSS (excessive E_2 values, multiple follicles) *12 h after hCG* administration, followed by regular oocyte retrieval 36 h later[30]. The method of post-hCG aspiration in one ovary was effective, leading to the withdrawal of all signs of OHSS within 6 days after the second aspiration post-hCG. For these authors, this is a quick, simple and effective method that prevents the development of OHSS and allows pregnancy in the treated cycles.

In 1997, a prospective randomized study was performed to evaluate unilateral ovarian aspiration *6–8 h before hCG* administration[31]. In an IVF program, 31 patients at risk (E_2 levels > 3269 pg/ml and > 12 follicles of 12 mm size per ovary) were randomized between EUFA ($n = 16$) or no pretreatment ($n = 15$). Fewer oocytes were recovered in the pretreated group, but fertilization, embryonic cleavage and pregnancy rates were similar. OHSS was recorded in 25% of the EUFA group and in 33.3% of the control group (12.5% and 6.6% of severe forms, respectively). The authors concluded that unilateral ovarian aspiration before hCG administration failed to prevent or diminish the occurrence of severe OHSS.

Two years later, the same group performed a prospective randomized study comparing EUFA *10–12 h after hCG* administration with the coasting method for high-risk patients (defined as an E_2 level > 6000 pg/ml and > 15 follicles of > 18 mm per ovary). Oocyte retrieval was carried out in the contralateral ovary at 35–36 h after hCG administration. Fewer oocytes were recovered in the coasted group, but fertilization, embryonic cleavage and pregnancy rates were similar. Neither method completely prevented the occurrence of severe OHSS, as 26.6% in the EUFA group and 20.0% in the coasted group developed the severe condition. This may be explained by the rather loose criteria used to identify high risk[32].

More recently, EUFA before hCG was tested again by Schröder *et al.*[33], who performed unilateral follicular aspiration *at variable times before hCG* administration according to the degree of follicular maturation. EUFA was programmed for five high-risk patients when ≥ 15 follicles of 12–15 mm in each ovary with ≥ 2500 pg/ml E_2 was reached. *In vitro* maturation of this first cohort of oocytes was carried out and these embryos were cryopreserved. Regular oocyte retrieval was performed for the contralateral ovary, 36 h after the administration of hCG. No pregnancy was obtained in this study, while the rate of severe OHSS remained high (80%).

Summary

It was expected that intraovarian bleeding induced by aspiration of granulosa cells from one ovary would limit the production of ovarian mediators of OHSS and thus reduce the risk of developing severe OHSS. Clinical data are, however, contradictory, with only one out of four studies in favor of EUFA. The number of cases is insufficient to establish the efficacy of this method. Moreover, the invasive nature of the method, necessitating two oocyte retrievals (sometimes under anesthesia), explains why it has been attempted less often than coasting.

MODIFICATION OF METHODS TO TRIGGER OVULATION

In most stimulation schemes for fertility treatment, ovulation is induced using hCG of urinary origin, and this has been chosen for its LH-like effect. hCG is a well-known promoter of OHSS. hCG seems to initiate the complex cascade that leads to the development of symptomatic hyperstimulation, whereas an endogenous LH surge rarely causes OHSS.

Reduction of the hCG dose or triggering ovulation with recombinant human (rh)LH or an endogenously induced LH surge are different approaches to reduce the OHSS incidence. This approach is treated in more depth in the preceding chapter.

hCG is characterized by a longer half-life than that of LH (> 24 h versus 60 min for LH), a higher receptor affinity and a longer duration of intracellular effect, compared with endogenous LH. Consequently, the duration of hCG activity lasts for up to 6 days. Urinary hCG is not only able to separate the cumulus–oophorus complex from the follicular wall and induce final maturation of the oocytes, but it also has a certain FSH-like effect which contributes to ovarian stimulation, as demonstrated by Gerris *et al.*[34].

The regularly used *dose of hCG* is 10 000 IU, but the pregnancy rate seems not to vary for doses above 5000 IU[35]. Schenker and Weinstein[4] reported, in an uncontrolled study, fewer cases of OHSS when using 1000–5000 IU. Hence, it has been suggested that a dose of 5000 IU, rather than 10 000 IU, be used in the presence of risk factors for OHSS[21]. In high-responder patients, 3300 IU versus 5000 IU was tested (and analyzed retrospectively), and no difference was observed in terms of oocyte maturation[36]. There is a need for a large prospective study to evaluate the efficacy of a reduced dose of hCG in preventing OHSS.

Some *alternatives to hCG* have been suggested. As LH activity is characterized by a shorter duration compared with hCG, LH administration may reduce stimulation of the luteal ovary. Some authors have proposed using the *flare-up effect of the GnRH-a* to produce ovulation. Indeed, the rise of LH and follicle stimulating hormone (FSH) lasts for only 34 h following a GnRH-a flare-up (200–500 μg). This combination of initial gonadotropin 'flare-up' followed by pituitary down-regulation with complete luteolysis offers a unique advantage to minimize the risk of OHSS[37–42].

This alternative can be applied when no down-regulation is used for stimulation. The recent development of giving a GnRH antagonist to avoid a spontaneous LH surge also permits the use of a GnRH-a to induce the LH peak.

GnRH-a flare-up to trigger ovulation of women with extremely high levels of E_2 (> 4000 pg/ml) was tested, and no patients developed OHSS[18]. Imoedemhe *et al.*[43] used this approach in a large group ($n = 682$) of very-high-risk patients (PCOS with mean $E_2 = 7817$ pg/ml) and observed a prevalence of only 0.1% of severe OHSS. Among OHSS cases that still occurred using this method of ovulation induction, none developed severe ascites, whereas luteal supplementation was indeed performed with hCG[40].

Finally, an adequate dose and route of GnRH-a administration has to be defined. The dosage that is necessary to induce ovulation (triptorelin 0.1 mg) seems to be lower than that necessary to prevent OHSS (triptorelin 0.5 mg), and the nasal route seems to be less efficient in inducing ovulation. Kol[44] recommended using subcutaneous triptorelin (0.2 mg).

In all cases, luteal supplementation with exogenous progesterone and probably estradiol is necessary to compensate the complete luteolysis induced by GnRH-a. Unfortunately, insufficient controlled studies have been carried out to validate this practice, and a small controlled series did not permit any definitive conclusions to be made[38]. Nevertheless, the physiological basis and preliminary clinical applications are promising.

Native GnRH also constitutes an alternative, but its efficiency in reducing OHSS incidence still needs to be assessed. Gerris *et al.*[34] observed one case of OHSS after the use of native GnRH (500 μg) in a controlled study. These results can be interpreted as a consequence of successful ovulation triggering, without critical gonadotropin suppression and luteolysis, which is one of the elements that prevents OHSS by the use of GnRH-a.

Finally, a recent European prospective, randomized, double-blind ($n = 259$) multicenter study assessed the safety and the minimal effective dose of *rhLH* in patients undergoing IVF, in comparison with 5000 IU of urinary hCG. This study concluded that single doses of 5000–15 000 IU of rhLH induced significantly fewer moderate cases of OHSS and ascites as compared with a 5000-IU dose of hCG (respectively, 18% and 21% vs. 45%)[18].

Summary

Alternatives to hCG have a strong theoretical basis and initial clinical experience, but further clinical studies are needed to establish the value of these approaches. Moreover, efforts have been hampered by lack of interest from the pharmaceuticals industry.

ADMINISTRATION OF GLUCOCORTICOIDS

The use of steroids in patients at high risk of OHSS has been evaluated in two studies. The first randomized study discredited the use of corticoids[45]. More recently, a retrospective controlled study has brought renewed attention to the use of corticosteroids[46]. Tan *et al.*[45] randomized high-risk patients, of whom 17 were receiving corticoids and 14 were controls. Treatment began with 100 mg intravenous hydrocortisone immediately after oocyte recovery, followed by decreasing oral doses of prednisolone from the day of oocyte recovery for 5 days. Ovarian response was similar in both groups: 41.2% of treated patients developed OHSS compared with 42.9% in the control group. Even when considering only the moderate or severe forms, the incidence of OHSS remained high in all groups (11% and 6% in the corticoid-treated group and 7% and 7% for the control group, respectively). The authors concluded that glucocorticoids did not reduce the incidence of OHSS.

In contrast, oral methylprednisolone administration (16 mg/day) from day 6 of stimulation to the first pregnancy test appeared to reduce the risk of OHSS from 43.9 to 10.0% in a retrospective, clinical, controlled study of 91 high-risk patients[46].

However, the preventive protocols, identification of at risk patients and design and number of patients tested were largely different in the two studies, and therefore definitive conclusions cannot be drawn based on these studies.

Nevertheless, recent theories suggesting an inflammatory etiopathology of OHSS will bring about a reconsideration of the use of corticosteroids and other anti-inflammatory drugs in this context.

Summary

There is insufficient proof to consider glucocorticoids as a useful treatment for the prevention of OHSS, but future trials are warranted.

MACROMOLECULES AND PROGESTERONE

Albumin

Albumin is thought to prevent the development of OHSS by increasing plasma oncotic pressure and binding of OHSS mediators of ovarian origin. In contrast, however, because capillary permeability is compromised, the duration of the oncotic effect would be insufficient to prevent OHSS.

A pilot study was performed in rabbits, with and without bovine serum albumin (BSA) pretreatment. Despite an increase in serum protein levels, the BSA-treated group showed a comparable increase in body weight and degree of ascites formation. The authors concluded that albumin did not prevent severe OHSS, despite its oncotic or carrier protein properties, in this model[47].

Doldi *et al.*[48] evaluated the possible effect of albumin on vascular endothelial growth factor (VEGF), one of the etiological factors of OHSS. These authors reported that in cultured human luteinizing granulosa cells, VEGF mRNA expression was increased after human albumin administration, with maximal expression being observed in cultured cells from patients with high E_2.

A series of clinical studies have evaluated the efficacy of albumin in preventing OHSS. The dose varied from 10 to 125 g in one or five administrations, also with a variable duration from 1 day before until 5 days after oocyte pick-up. For these reasons, it is impossible to pool all results, although the principal observations of these studies are summarized in Tables 1 and 2.

Studies have also been limited by the low sensitivities and predictive values of the criteria used to define high-risk patients.

Because most cases of severe OHSS, after albumin treatment, seem to be associated with pregnancy, it is possible that intravenous albumin might be more effective in preventing the occurrence of early OHSS than of late OHSS.

In two studies, the pregnancy rate was significantly lower after intravenous (IV) albumin infusions, although this may be the consequence of prolonged infusion[49,50]. Indeed, albumin administration close to the implantation period may have bound some factors necessary for implantation.

When considering data from prospective randomized studies and a single retrospective study which included a control group, a total of 39 OHSS cases have been recorded among 468 high-risk treated patients (8.3%) and 89 OHSS cases in a control group comprising a total of 611 high-risk patients (14.6%)[17,18]. An extensive statistical analysis cannot be achieved because of the disparity of protocols mentioned earlier.

Nevertheless, the Cochrane review by Aboulghar *et al.*[67] shows that the administration of IV albumin at the time of oocyte retrieval has a beneficial preventive effect in high-risk cases of severe OHSS.

Finally, according to a more recent and large ($n = 988$) single-center randomized controlled study, there is no use in administering albumin on the day of oocyte retrieval[68]. Indeed, after the administration of 40 mg of albumin immediately after the retrieval of more than 20 oocytes, the incidence of moderate–severe and severe–only OHSS was not statistically different from that in the control group (6.8% vs. 4.7%).

The possible *adverse effects* of albumin should not be underestimated:

Table 1 Design of study, population characteristics, selection criteria and *in vitro* fertilization (IVF) data for cycles treated with albumin

Author	*Study design (n)*	*Control group*	*At-risk patients*	*OHSS incidence with albumin use*	*OHSS incidence in controls*	*Comment*
Asch[51]	Not controlled (36)	Historical high-risk patients	$E_2 > 6000$ pg/ml and > 30 oocytes	0%	80% OHSS	In 21 patients no transfer occurred
Shoham[52]	Prospective randomized controlled (31)	Placebo (NaCl)	$E_2 > 1906$ pg/ml and multiple follicular development	0/16	4/15 severe OHSS ($p < 0.05$)	No information about moderate forms
Shahata[53]	Retrospective (200)	Historical whole IVF population	$E_2 > 2997$ pg/ml and > 20 oocytes or > 30 follicles	0/104	8/96	Only 18% of controls had $E_2 > 2997$ pg/ml
Ng[54]	Prospective controlled (207)	Placebo versus Ringer's solution	$E_2 > 2724$ pg/ml and > 15 follicles	2/49	10/158 (NS)	Albumin blunted the severity of OHSS
Mukherjee[55]	Case report (2)	—	$E_2 > 4500$ pg/ml and > 20 oocytes	2 severe OHSS (1 early, 1 late)	—	
Orvieto[56]	Case report (1)	—	$E_2 = 2293$ pg/ml and 46 oocytes	Early severe OHSS	—	
Ben-Rafael[57]	Case report (1)	—	Patient with $E_2 > 2293$ pg/ml, > 35 oocytes	Early severe OHSS	—	
Halme[58]	Case report (1)	—	1 oocyte donor, $E_2 = 2400$ pg/ml, 15 oocytes	Early severe OHSS	—	

continued

Table 1 *Continued*

Author	*Study design (n)*	*Control group*	*At-risk patients*	*OHSS incidence with albumin use*	*OHSS incidence in controls*	*Comment*
Shalev[59]	Prospective randomized (40)	No treatment	$E_2 > 2500$ pg/ml and > 20 follicles	0/22	4/18	No transfer in 5.5% of control and 13.6% of study group
Shaker[49]	Prospective randomized controlled (26)	Cryopreservation	$E_2 > 3540$ pg/ml or > 2745 and > 15 oocytes	4/13 moderate OHSS (no severe)	3/13 moderate OHSS (not severe) (NS)	Pregnancy significantly higher in controls
Isik[60]	Prospective randomized controlled (55)	No treatment	$E_2 > 3000$ pg/ml	0/27	1 severe and 4 moderate/28 ($p < 0.05$)	
Lewit[40]	Retrospective cases review (5)	—	Previous OHSS, $E_2 > 3600$ pg/ml and large number of follicles	2/5 early severe, 2/5 moderate	—	The most severe received 75 g, and had no transfer
Orvieto[61]	Retrospective review (30)	—		2/30 early severe OHSS	—	
Chen[62]	Prospective (72)	Historical controls	$E_2 > 3600$ pg/ml and > 20 oocytes)	4/30, 0/16 non-pregnant, 4/14 pregnant	14/42 ($p = 0.047$), 5/23 non-pregnant, 9/19 pregnant	Prevention is effective in non-pregnant and singleton pregnancies

E_2, estradiol; NS, not significant

Table 2 Design of study, population characteristics, selection criteria and *in vitro* fertilization (IVF) data for cycles treated with albumin

Author	*Study design (n)*	*Control group*	*At-risk patients*	*OHSS incidence with albumin use*	*OHSS incidence in controls*	*Comment*
Egbase[31]	Uncontrolled (31)	—	$E_2 > 3269$ pg/ml and > 12 follicles > 12 mm per ovary	9.7% severe	—	Early follicular aspiration before hCG was also performed ($n = 16$)
Ndukwe[63]	Retrospective (60)	—	> 4086 pg/ml and > 20 follicles	5/60 severe, 1 early, 4 late, 8/60 moderate	—	No preventive effect especially in pregnant patients
Koike[64]	Prospective randomized controlled (98)	No treatment	> 20 oocytes	11 early, 2 late severe OHSS/43	15 early, 6 late severe OHSS/55 (NS)	
Panay[65]	Prospective randomized (86)	No treatment	$E_2 > 3541$ pg/ml or > 20 follicles	2 mild, 2 moderate/37	4 mild/49	Pregnancy rate per cycle significantly higher in controls
Costabile[50]	Prospective randomized controlled (96)	200 mg/day progesterone from day post-retrieval	$E_2 > 2452$ pg/ml and > 20 follicles	4/42 moderate (no severe)	0/54 moderate (no severe)	High progesterone dose is effective in preventing OHSS and better for pregnancy rate
Gökmen[66]	Prospective randomized placebo (168)	Placebo	$E_2 > 3000$ pg/ml or > 20 follicles	0 severe and 4 moderate/85	4 severe and 12 moderate/83 ($p < 0.05$)	

E_2, estradiol; NS, not significant; hCG, human chorionic gonadotropin

(1) Albumin may leave blood vessels and enter the interstitium, whereby it may draw fluid from the intravascular space;

(2) Albumin is a human product, and the transmission of infections by blood-borne viruses can never be entirely excluded.

Other side-effects include nausea, vomiting, febrile reactions and allergic reactions.

Summary

Current published clinical studies, as well as fundamental and animal studies, do not support a role for albumin in preventing late-severe OHSS. At most, albumin may improve, but not eliminate, early-severe OHSS in certain types of protocols. The large prospective randomized study of Bellver *et al.*[68] seems to bring to an end the controversy concerning the inefficiency of albumin administered on the day of oocyte retrieval.

Prophylactic infusion of hydroxyethyl starch solution

In view of the potential transmission of infective viruses when administering human albumin, some groups have tested a safe non-biological substitute with comparable physical properties, namely hydroxyethyl starch solution (HES). HES has a molecular weight of 200–1000 kDa, and significantly increases intravascular volume, therefore raising osmotic pressure. HAES has a serum half-life of 10 h, and also inhibits platelet aggregation.

One prospective study investigated the effect of HES, involving 100 high-risk patients (E_2 levels > 3000 pg/ml and/or > 20 oocytes)[69]. These patients received 1000 ml of 6% HES at the time of oocyte retrieval and 500 ml 48 h later. A historical control group of 82 high-risk patients who had not been treated with HES was included. A significantly lower rate of moderate OHSS using HES was seen, but there was no reduction in severe OHSS.

Another group evaluated a regimen of 1000 ml of 6% HES given shortly after embryo transfer, in a prospective, randomized, placebo-controlled study, involving a total of 101 high-risk patients ($E_2 > 1500$ pg/ml or > 10 follicles)[70]. One case of moderate OHSS developed in the HES group, whereas one severe and six moderate cases occurred in the placebo group ($p = 0.031$).

Subsequently, others performed a prospective randomized study to compare the efficacy of 500 ml of 6% HES ($n = 85$), and of 50 ml of 20% human albumin ($n = 85$) or placebo ($n = 83$) in at-risk patients ($E_2 > 3000$ pg/ml or > 20 follicles)[66]. All treatments were administered during oocyte retrieval. No severe OHSS case was observed in the albumin and HES groups, while four were seen in the placebo group. Moderate OHSS was encountered in four and five patients in the albumin and HES groups, respectively, and in 12 patients receiving placebo ($p < 0.05$).

The authors recommended preventing OHSS by using HES, since it is as efficient as but safer and cheaper than human albumin.

These three studies provide concordant results, thereby suggesting a beneficial effect of HES in decreasing OHSS incidence. Although the patient cohort was too small to draw definitive conclusions, these preliminary results suggested that HES rather than albumin should be further evaluated.

Summary

Although the trials are small, existing results seem to warrant further clinical research with the use of HES.

High doses of intramuscular progesterone

Three different mechanisms of action of the prophylactic use of progesterone to prevent OHSS have been hypothesized:

(1) A general antiestrogenic effect of progesterone mediated by the down-regulation of estrogen receptors, for example on the vascular endothelium;

(2) A direct inhibition of ovarian hormone secretion, such as prorenin;

(3) An antagonistic effect toward aldosterone.

In a prospective randomized controlled study[50], the effectiveness of intramuscular progesterone was compared with IV albumin in preventing OHSS. High-risk patients ($E_2 > 2452$ pg/ml and > 20 follicles) received either 200 mg progesterone per day ($n = 54$), intramuscularly, for 14 days starting immediately after oocyte retrieval, or 100 ml of a 20% albumin suspension, intravenously ($n = 42$).

Progesterone prevention was significantly more efficient, with fewer moderate OHSS cases (0% vs. 5%). No severe forms were observed in these two groups, but a higher pregnancy rate was observed in the progesterone group (68% vs. 52.3%). This isolated and limited study has to be confirmed.

However, progesterone is the best choice for luteal supplementation, because it is associated with a lower incidence of OHSS[71].

CRYOPRESERVATION OF ALL EMBRYOS

Instead of canceling the cycle, it is possible to administer hCG, retrieve the oocytes and then cryopreserve all embryos. Using this preventive strategy, patients are still exposed to exogenous hCG, and early OHSS is not totally avoided. Nevertheless, the risk of secondary exacerbation of early OHSS is avoided as well as late OHSS, since this is induced by endogenous hCG[72–74].

Moreover, endometrial biopsies were performed during the luteal phase of such canceled cycles in 33 patients who presented biological risk signs of OHSS ($E_2 = 4722 \pm 1190$ pg/ml)[74]. Half of these biopsies showed glandular stromal asynchrony, suggesting that patients who have very high E_2 levels may have a reduced chance of conception, and therefore reinforcing the idea that cryopreservation constitutes a valid alternative.

This treatment has the advantage of maintaining many of the benefits of the IVF cycle, since it is hoped that in a later cycle, thawed embryos may be successfully replaced[75].

Pattinson *et al.*[76] recorded in these conditions a pregnancy rate significantly higher than that obtained with 'normal' frozen transfer, and equivalent to that following fresh transfer in the same center, also encouraging cryopreservation. On the other hand, Awonuga *et al.*[77] were the only ones to observe a decrease in pregnancy rate after cryopreservation as compared with controls, while OHSS incidence was similar in both groups. A review summarizing the several studies and reporting their conflicting results is presented in Table 3[18].

Among these studies, only Ferraretti *et al.*[78] conducted a prospective randomized study, although the selection criteria in this group of 58 patients in whom cryopreservation was undertaken were much more loose than those generally applied. Women with E_2 levels > 1500 pg/ml and > 15 oocytes were selected. The control group comprised 67 patients who presented the same criteria and in whom fresh embryos were transferred. The pregnancy rates were comparable (46.3% vs. 48.3%); no cases of OHSS occurred in the 58 cycles with cryopreservation, but four cycles were complicated by OHSS in the control group (0% vs. 6%).

The Cochrane review by D'Angelo and Amso[67] has shown that there is insufficient evidence to support routine cryopreservation.

These controversies may be explained by the different criteria that were used to define patients at risk, the different freezing procedures adopted and the lack, for ethical reasons, of a prospective randomized study in two very-high-risk groups.

One question that remains to be solved is *whether GnRH-a should be continued* when embryos are cryopreserved, in order to reduce the risk of OHSS. One group showed that LH levels remained low for at least 14 days during the luteal phase after pituitary suppression with GnRH-a administration and ovarian stimulation with hMG, even though GnRH-a was discontinued on the day of hCG administration[83]. Others confirmed this observation by comparing the rate of ovarian quiescence, by the weekly fall in serum E_2 concentration, following stimulation with or without continuing GnRH-a after the administration of 10 000 IU of hCG. There was no difference between the two groups in terms of ovarian quiescence, and serum LH concentration remained low in all women, irrespective of the group[73]. According to these preliminary data, the majority of authors stopped GnRH-a after hCG administration.

Nevertheless, Endo *et al.*[84] assessed the efficacy of the continuous administration of GnRH-a for 1 week after the administration of 5000 IU of hCG and elective embryo cryopreservation to prevent early OHSS. In this prospective, randomized, controlled trial ($n = 138$), no high-risk patients treated with continued GnRH-a developed severe OHSS, compared with 10% in the control group with embryo cryopreservation alone. In addition to the luteolytic effect of continuous GnRH-a, the authors underline its possible local effect on the ovary in humans with a probable reduction of VEGF expression.

Summary

At present, there is insufficient evidence to support routine cryopreservation for the prevention of severe OHSS. It has not been established whether the elective freezing of all embryos completely eliminates the risk of OHSS. Early OHSS is not avoided, but late OHSS is avoided, or at least its duration and severity are reduced in high-risk patients. This is due to the absence of endogenous hCG, produced by the trophoblast. A recent study using GnRH-a administration during the luteal phase after elective cryopreservation decreased the incidence of early OHSS. In all but one report, the pregnancy rate after frozen–thawed embryo replacement was as high as when using fresh embryos.

ELECTROCAUTERY OR LASER VAPORIZATION OF ONE OR BOTH OVARIES

PCOS is the major risk factor for OHSS. The results of preventive methods for OHSS in these patients are unpredictable in terms of ovarian response and OHSS prevention. OHSS was observed despite using a low step-up regimen with gradual increase of the dose of gonadotropins. Moreover, the ovarian response may be unsatisfactory when decreased doses of gonadotropins are given after a previous experience of OHSS[8,10].

One of the possible treatments of PCOS is destruction of follicles at the surface of the ovary, by wedge resection or by multiple puncture using laparoscopic ovarian electrocauterization. The endocrine effects associated with this treatment include a reduction in serum LH and serum androgens, with corresponding ovulation improvement and conception. A reduction of multiple pregnancy, OHSS and probably miscarriage rates is also observed.

A number of authors have suggested treating patients suffering from PCOS by using these destructive techniques before starting to stimulate them for IVF[85–88]. This treatment can be performed on one or two ovaries with electrocautery or laser vaporization. The main undesirable side-effect of these methods is the development of postoperative adhesions.

Fukaya *et al.*[85] reported preliminary encouraging results after ovarian laser therapy in patients who suffered from PCOS and had developed OHSS in the past.

Table 3 Summary of main results concerning cryopreservation

Author	*Design*	*Control group (n)*	*Risk factors (n)*	*Pregnancy with thawed embryos*	*OHSS with cryopreservation (versus control)*	*Comment*
Amso[72]	Observational	—	25–45 follicles, abdominal pain (4)	100%/trsf	10% moderate	
Salat-Baroux[74]	Observational	—	$E_2 = 4722 + 1190$ pg/ml day after hCG (33)	27%/trsf	3% severe	
Wada[79]	Retrospective observational	Pregnant (49) and non-pregnant (154)	NA (38)	—	18% all grades only if $E_2 > 3500$ pg/ml (18 and 4%)	0% if $E_2 < 3500$ pg/ml with cryopreservation
Wada[75]	Retrospective observational	—	$E_2 > 3500$ pg/ml (78)	26%/trsf	27% all grades (8% severe)	
Wada[9]	Retrospective observational	Historical group without prevention (105)	$E_2 > 3500$ pg/ml (136)	21%/trsf	8.8%, only 6% severe (9.5%, 60% severe)	71.8% survival embryos
Pattinson[76]	Retrospective	General IVF without risk factors (564)	$E_2 \leq 4086$ pg/ml and > 50 follicles (69)	25.2%/trsf, 40%/patient	1.4% (1.8% severe)	84% survival embryos 14% canceling
Tiitinen[80]	Prospective	General IVF without risk factors (367)	$E_2 > 2724$ pg/ml and/or > 20 oocytes (33)	32.6%/trsf, 65.2%/patient	4.3% moderate (versus 0.5%)	22.7% implantation rate

continued

Table 3 *Continued*

Author	*Design*	*Control group (n)*	*Risk factors (n)*	*Pregnancy with thawed embryos*	*OHSS with cryopreservation (versus control)*	*Comment*
Awonuga[77]	Retrospective controlled	E_2 > 2724 pg/ml and/or > 15 oocytes (52)	E_2 > 2724 pg/ml and/or ≥ 15 oocytes (65)	17%/trsf	3% severe, 3% moderate (3.8% severe and moderate) (NS)	Significantly higher PR in controls (35%, $p < 0.05$)
Queenan[81]	Prospective non-controlled	—	E_2 ≥ 4500 pg/ml and > 15 oocytes (15)	58%/trsf, 67% delivery/ patient	13% severe 13% moderate	
Benavida[82]	Retrospective controlled	Coasting group (22)	E_2 ≥ 3000 pg/ml (26)	25.6%/trsf	7.6% (4.5%) (NS)	
Ferraretti[78]	Prospective randomized	E_2 > 1500 pg/ml and > 15 oocytes (67)	E_2 > 1500 pg/ml and > 15 oocytes (58)	35.4%/trsf, 48.3% per patient	0% (versus 6%)	

IVF, *in vitro* fertilization; E_2, estradiol; hCG, human chorionic gonadotropin; NA, not available; Trsf, embryo transfer; NS, not significant; PR, pregnancy rate

Only one prospective randomized study, involving 50 patients, affected by PCOS has been carried out[86]. PCOS patients who failed to become pregnant during a previous trial, or whose cycle had been canceled for high OHSS risk, were randomized between classical IVF treatment versus electrocautery of one ovary, 1 week before ovarian stimulation. The pregnancy and miscarriage rates were identical, but the rate of canceling for risk of OHSS was significantly lower in the cauterized group. There was no advantage in terms of miscarriage rate, which remained high in both groups.

Finally, a retrospective comparison was made of 15 women with clomiphene-resistant PCOS, treated by laparoscopic ovarian diathermy before IVF, and 16 PCOS patients who did not receive surgical pretreatment[88]. In this study there was only a trend toward a lower risk of miscarriage (28.6% vs. 66.7%) and OHSS (0% vs. 4.2%), and higher chances of pregnancy (29.4% vs. 10.5%) in the group which had been surgically pretreated, but these differences were not statistically significant.

Minimal ovarian destruction is necessary to sensitize PCOS to exogenous gonadotropins. However, in order to avoid OHSS, a considerable amount of healthy ovarian destruction is required, with the drawback that, under these conditions, the ovarian reserve may be hampered.

Summary

Since only preliminary data are available and in view of the possible side-effects (adhesions and loss of ovarian tissue) and its invasive character, this approach should be restricted to rebel cases of OHSS in patients suffering from PCOS, and applied only as a last resort.

REDUCTION OF THE NUMBER OF TRANSFERRED EMBRYOS

Late-onset OHSS may be induced or aggravated by the rising hCG produced by early pregnancy. As hCG secretion is higher in multiple pregnancies, it can be postulated that by reducing the number of conceptuses the incidence or severity of OHSS will decrease. In these conditions, a reduction of the number of transferred embryos could be an efficient preventive method for high-risk patients.

Koike *et al.*[89] observed, in a retrospective study, a higher number of days of hospital stay in relation to the number of conceptuses.

De Neubourg *et al.*[90] evaluated the incidence of single-embryo transfer (SET) and its subsequent decline in twin pregnancies. The authors evaluated the possible consequence of decreasing multiple pregnancy on OHSS incidence. Over a 5-year period, SET increased from 13 to 46%, which was associated with a decrease in multiple pregnancies from 33.6 to 11.7%. During this period, the incidence of OHSS did not decrease (0.5–2.4%). Moreover, the proportions of OHSS among singleton (3.32%) and twin (3.73%) conception cycles were similar. It seems clear from this study that the late form of OHSS is related more to the presence of hCG than to its level.

In a recent Belgian study[91], multiple pregnancies were equally high among early- and late-OHSS cases (40.0% and 45.5%, respectively), but only in the group of late-OHSS cases was significance compared with the non-OHSS population reached (45.5% vs. 29.1%). This late form, closely associated with multiple pregnancies, is more likely to be severe.

According to these three preliminary studies, it is more the severity than the incidence of OHSS that is dependent on the level of hCG, resulting from multiple pregnancy

CONCLUSIONS

In the prevention of any disease, it should be emphasized that the possibility of primary prevention depends on two main requirements: first, the etiology of the disease must be known, while causal and predisposing factors should be identified; and second, it must be feasible to avoid or manipulate such factors as part of a preventive strategy.

Secondary prevention requires knowledge of the pathophysiological mechanisms of the disease, availability of early detection methods, and means to intervene and correct the pathophysiological changes[46].

There is disagreement regarding the sensitivity and predictive values of the various patient characteristics which may be used to predict OHSS. The greater severity of late OHSS and its poor correlation with conventional ovarian response parameters is a major problem in clinical practice. None of the predictive data for late OHSS are ever available before oocyte retrieval.

Late OHSS is related to hCG levels and probably to the number of ovarian cells capable of producing the causal 'unidentified ovarian mediator' under the influence of hCG. It may be useful, therefore, to act at two levels: first, to attempt to limit the dose or concentration of hCG (level 1); and second, to find a way to induce luteolysis (level 2) without inducing a detrimental effect on endometrial and oocyte quality.

Intervening at level 1 can theoretically be achieved by decreasing the hCG dose for ovulation induction, by cryopreservation, by SET and by using progesterone instead of hCG supplementation in the luteal phase. Finally, intervening at level 2 may consist of enhancing luteolysis, as in EUFA, coasting and electrocautery of one or both ovaries. Albumin and HES constitute secondary prevention methods.

Finally, apart from canceling, none of these approaches is totally efficient, although most of the above-mentioned methods decrease the incidence in patients at high risk of OHSS.

The effect of combining methods which act at two different levels (1 and 2) should be assessed[92].

REFERENCES

1. Check JH, Goldberg BB, Kurtz A, et al. Serum estradiols versus pelvic sonography in monitoring HMG therapy. Int J Fertil 1985; 30: 61–3.

2. Delvigne A, Demoulin A, Smitz J, et al. The ovarian hyperstimulation syndrome in in-vitro fertilization: a Belgian multicentric study. I. Clinical and biological features. Hum Reprod 1993; 8: 1353–60.

3. Hancock KW, Stitch SR, Oakey RE, et al. Ovulation stimulation. Problems of prediction of response to gonadotrophins. Lancet 1970; 2: 482–5.

4. Schenker JG, Weinstein D. Ovarian hyperstimulation syndrome: a current survey. Fertil Steril 1978; 3: 255–68.

5. Balen AH, Braat DD, West C, et al. Cumulative conception and live birth rates after the treatment of anovulatory infertility: safety and efficacy of ovulation induction in 200 patients. Hum Reprod 1994; 9: 1563–70.

6. Jain T, Harlow BL, Hornstein MD. Insurance coverage and outcomes of in vitro fertilization. N Engl J Med 2002; 347: 661–6.

7. Forman RG, Frydman R, Egan D, et al. Severe ovarian hyperstimulation syndrome using agonists of gonadotropin-releasing hormone for in vitro fertilization: a European series and a proposal for prevention. Fertil Steril 1990; 53: 502–9.

8. Wada I, Matson PL, Troup SA, et al. Assisted conception using buserelin and human menopausal gonadotrophins in women with polycystic ovary syndrome. Br J Obstet Gynaecol 1993; 100: 365–9.

9. Wada I, Matson PL, Troup SA, et al. Does elective cryopreservation of all embryos from women at risk of ovarian hyperstimulation syndrome reduce the incidence of the condition? Br J Obstet Gynaecol 1993; 100: 265–9.

10. Amso NN, Shaw RW, Ahuja KK, et al. Prevention of ovarian hyperstimulation syndrome. Fertil Steril 1991; 55: 220–1.

11. Rabinovici J, Kushnir O, Shalev J, et al. Rescue of menotrophin cycles prone to develop ovarian

hyperstimulation. Br J Obstet Gynaecol 1987; 94: 1098–102.

12. Urman B, Pride SM, Yuen BH. Management of overstimulated gonadotrophin cycles with a controlled drift period. Hum Reprod 1992; 7: 213–17.

13. Sher G, Salem R, Feinman M, et al. Eliminating the risk of life-endangering complications following overstimulation with menotropin fertility agents: a report on women undergoing in vitro fertilization and embryo transfer. Obstet Gynecol 1993; 81: 1009–11.

14. Tozer AJ, Iles RK, Iammarrone E, et al. Characteristics of populations of granulosa cells from individual follicles in women undergoing 'coasting' during controlled ovarian stimulation (COS) for IVF. Hum Reprod 2004; 19: 2561–8.

15. Garcia-Velasco JA, Zuniga A, Pacheco A, et al. Coasting acts through downregulation of VEGF gene expression and protein secretion. Hum Reprod 2004; 19: 1530–8.

16. Delvigne A, Rozenberg S. Preventive attitude of physicians to avoid OHSS in IVF patients. Hum Reprod 2001; 16: 2491–5.

17. Delvigne A, Rozenberg S. A systematic review of coasting, a procedure to avoid ovarian hyperstimulation syndrome in in vitro fertilisation patients. Hum Reprod Update 2002; 8: 291–6.

18. Delvigne A, Rozenberg S. Epidemiology and prevention of ovarian hyperstimulation syndrome (OHSS): a review. Hum Reprod Update 2002; 8: 559–77.

19. Al-Shawaf T, Zosmer A, Hussain S, et al. Prevention of severe ovarian hyperstimulation syndrome in IVF with or without ICSI and embryo transfer: a modified 'coasting' strategy based on ultrasound for identification of high-risk patients. Hum Reprod 2001; 16: 24–30.

20. Aboulghar MA, Mansour RT, Serour GI, et al. Reduction of human menopausal gonadotropin dose before coasting prevents severe ovarian hyperstimulation syndrome with minimal cycle cancellation. J Assist Reprod Genet 2000; 17: 298–301.

21. Whelan JG 3rd, Vlahos NF. The ovarian hyperstimulation syndrome. Fertil Steril 2000; 73: 883–96.

22. Ulug U, Bahceci M, Erden HF, et al. The significance of coasting duration during ovarian stimulation for conception in assisted fertilization cycles. Hum Reprod 2002; 17: 310–13.

23. Isaza V, Garcia-Velasco JA, Aragonés M, et al. Oocyte and embryo quality after coasting: the experience from oocyte donation. Hum Reprod 2002; 17: 1777–82.

24. Delvigne A, Kostyla K, Murillo D, et al. Oocyte quality and IVF outcome after coasting to prevent ovarian hyperstimulation syndrome. Int J Fertil Womens Med 2003; 48: 25–31.

25. Egbase PE, Al-Sharhan M, Grudzinskas JG. 'Early coasting' in patients with polycystic ovarian syndrome is consistent with good clinical outcome. Hum Reprod 2002; 17: 1212–16.

26. Levinsohn-Tavor O, Friedler S, Schachter M, et al. Coasting – what is the best formula? Hum Reprod 2003; 18: 937–40.

27. Gonen Y, Powell WA, Casper RF. Effect of follicular aspiration on hormonal parameters in patients undergoing ovarian stimulation. Hum Reprod 1991; 6: 356–8.

28. Friedman CI, Schmidt GE, Chang FE, et al. Severe ovarian hyperstimulation following follicular aspiration. Am J Obstet Gynecol 1984; 150: 436–7.

29. Aboulghar MA, Mansour RT, Serour GI, et al. Follicular aspiration does not protect against the development of ovarian hyperstimulation syndrome. J Assist Reprod Genet 1992; 9: 238–43.

30. Vrtovec HM, Tomazevic T. Preventing severe ovarian hyperstimulation syndrome in an in vitro fertilization/embryo transfer program. Use of follicular aspiration after human chorionic gonadotropin administration. J Reprod Med 1995; 40: 37–40.

31. Egbase PE, Makhseed M, Al Sharhan M, et al. Timed unilateral ovarian follicular aspiration prior to administration of human chorionic gonadotrophin for the prevention of severe ovarian hyperstimulation syndrome in in-vitro fertilization: a prospective randomized study. Hum Reprod 1997; 12: 2603–6.

32. Egbase PE, Sharhan MA, Grudzinskas JG. Early unilateral follicular aspiration compared with coasting for the prevention of severe ovarian

hyperstimulation syndrome: a prospective randomized study. Hum Reprod 1999; 14: 1421–5.

33. Schröder K, Schöpper B, Al-Hasani S, et al. Unilateral follicular aspiration and in-vitro maturation before contralateral oocyte retrieval: a method to prevent ovarian hyperstimulation syndrome. Eur J Obstet Gynecol Reprod Biol 2003; 110: 186–9.

34. Gerris J, De Vits A, Joostens M, et al. Triggering of ovulation in human menopausal gonadotrophin-stimulated cycles: comparison between intravenously administered gonadotrophin-releasing hormone (100 and 500 micrograms), GnRH agonist (buserelin, 500 micrograms) and human chorionic gonadotrophin (10,000 IU). Hum Reprod 1995; 10: 56–62.

35. Abdalla HI, Ah-Moye M, Brinsden P, et al. The effect of the dose of human chorionic gonadotropin and the type of gonadotropin stimulation on oocyte recovery rates in an in vitro fertilization program. Fertil Steril 1987; 48: 958–63.

36. Schmidt DW, Maier DB, Nulsen JC, et al. Reducing the dose of human chorionic gonadotropin in high responders does not affect the outcomes of in vitro fertilization. Fertil Steril 2004; 82: 841–6.

37. Itskovitz-Eldor J, Levron J, Kol S. Use of gonadotropin-releasing hormone agonist to cause ovulation and prevent the ovarian hyperstimulation syndrome. Clin Obstet Gynecol 1993; 36: 701–10.

38. Shalev E, Giladi Y, Matilsky M, et al. Decreased incidence of severe ovarian hyperstimulation syndrome in high risk in-vitro fertilization patients receiving intravenous albumin: a prospective study. Hum Reprod 1995; 10: 1373–6.

39. Olivennes F, Fanchin R, Bouchard P, et al. Triggering of ovulation by a gonadotropin-releasing hormone (GnRH) agonist in patients pretreated with a GnRH antagonist. Fertil Steril 1996; 66: 151–3.

40. Kol S, Lewit N, Itskovitz-Eldor J. Ovarian hyperstimulation: effects of GnRH analogues. Ovarian hyperstimulation syndrome after using gonadotrophin-releasing hormone analogue as a trigger of ovulation: causes and implications. Hum Reprod 1996; 11: 1143–4.

41. Kol S, Itskovitz-Eldor J. Severe OHSS: yes, there is a strategy to prevent it! Hum Reprod 2000; 15: 2266–7.

42. Fauser BC, de Jong D, Olivennes F, et al. Endocrine profiles after triggering of final oocyte maturation with GnRH agonist after cotreatment with the GnRH antagonist ganirelix during ovarian hyperstimulation for in vitro fertilization. J Clin Endocrinol Metab 2002; 87: 709–15.

43. Imoedemhe D, Chan R, Pacpaco E. Preventing OHSS in at-risk patients: evidence from a long-term prospective study. Hum Reprod 1999; 14: 102–3.

44. Kol S. Luteolysis induced by a gonadotropin-releasing hormone agonist is the key to prevention of ovarian hyperstimulation syndrome. Fertil Steril 2004; 81: 1–5.

45. Tan SL, Balen A, el Hussein E, et al. The administration of glucocorticoids for the prevention of ovarian hyperstimulation syndrome in in vitro fertilization: a prospective randomized study. Fertil Steril 1992; 58: 378–83.

46. Lainas T, Petsas G, Stavropoulou G, et al. Administration of methylprednisolone to prevent severe ovarian hyperstimulation syndrome in patients undergoing in vitro fertilization. Fertil Steril 2002; 78: 529–33.

47. Orvieto R, Abir R, Kaplan B, et al. The role of intravenous albumin in the prevention of severe ovarian hyperstimulation syndrome. A pilot experimental study. Clin Exp Obstet Gynecol 1999; 26: 98–9.

48. Doldi N, Destefani A, Gessi A, et al. Human albumin enhances expression of vascular endothelial growth factor in cultured human luteinizing granulosa cells: importance in ovarian hyperstimulation syndrome. Hum Reprod 1999; 14: 1157–9.

49. Shaker A, Zosmer A, Dean N. Comparison of intravenous albumin and transfer of fresh embryos with cryopreservation of all embryos for subsequent transfer in prevention of ovarian hyperstimulation syndrome. Fertil Steril 1996; 65: 992–6.

50. Costabile L, Unfer V, Manna C, et al. Use of intramuscular progesterone versus intravenous albumin for the prevention of ovarian hyperstimulation syndrome. Gynecol Obstet Invest 2000; 50: 182–5.

51. Asch RH, Ivery G, Goldsman M, et al. The use of intravenous albumin in patients at high risk for severe ovarian hyperstimulation syndrome. Hum Reprod 1993; 8: 1015–20.

52. Shoham Z, Schacter M, Loumaye E, et al. The luteinizing hormone surge – the final stage in ovulation induction: modern aspects of ovulation triggering. Fertil Steril 1995; 64: 237–51.

53. Shahata M, Yang D, al-Natsha SD, et al. Intravenous albumin and severe ovarian hyperstimulation. Hum Reprod 1994; 9: 2186.

54. Ng E, Leader A, Claman P, et al. Intravenous albumin does not prevent the development of severe ovarian hyperstimulation syndrome in an in-vitro fertilization programme. Hum Reprod 1995; 10: 807–10.

55. Mukherjee T, Copperman AB, Sandler B, et al. Severe ovarian hyperstimulation despite prophylactic albumin at the time of oocyte retrieval for in vitro fertilization and embryo transfer. Fertil Steril 1995; 64: 641–3.

56. Orvieto R, Dekel A, Dicker D, et al. A severe case of ovarian hyperstimulation syndrome despite the prophylactic administration of intravenous albumin. Fertil Steril 1995; 64: 860–2.

57. Ben-Rafael Z, Orvieto R, Dekel A, et al. Intravenous albumin and the prevention of severe ovarian hyperstimulation syndrome. Hum Reprod 1995; 10: 2750–2.

58. Halme J, Toma SK, Talbert LM. A case of severe ovarian hyperstimulation in a healthy oocyte donor. Fertil Steril 1995; 64: 857–9.

59. Shalev E, Geslevich Y, Matilsky M, et al. Induction of pre-ovulatory gonadotrophin surge with gonadotrophin-releasing hormone agonist compared to pre-ovulatory injection of human chorionic gonadotrophins for ovulation induction in intrauterine insemination treatment cycles. Hum Reprod 1995; 10: 2244–7.

60. Isik AZ, Gokmen O, Zeyneloglu HB, et al. Intravenous albumin prevents moderate–severe ovarian hyperstimulation in in-vitro fertilization patients: a prospective, randomized and controlled study. Eur J Obstet Gynecol Reprod Biol 1996; 70: 179–83.

61. Orvieto R, Ben-Rafael Z. Prophylactic intravenous albumin for the prevention of severe ovarian hyperstimulation syndrome. Hum Reprod 1996; 11: 460–1.

62. Chen CD, Wu MY, Yang JH, et al. Intravenous albumin does not prevent the development of severe ovarian hyperstimulation syndrome. Fertil Steril 1997; 68: 287–91.

63. Ndukwe G, Thornton S, Fishel S, et al. Severe ovarian hyperstimulation syndrome: is it really preventable by prophylactic intravenous albumin? Fertil Steril 1997;68:851–4.

64. Koike T, Araki S, Ogawa S, et al. Does i.v. albumin prevent ovarian hyperstimulation syndrome? Hum Reprod 1999; 14: 1920.

65. Panay N, Iammarrone E, Zosmer A, et al. Does the prophylatic use of intravenous albumin prevent ovarian hyperstimulation syndrome? A randomized prospective sudy. In Edwards RG, Beard HK, Hansen R, eds. Abstracts of the 15th Annual Meeting of the European Society of Human Reproduction and Embryology. Oxford University Press, 1999: 105.

66. Gökmen O, Ugur M, Ekin M, et al. Intravenous albumin versus hydroxyethyl starch for the prevention of ovarian hyperstimulation in an in-vitro fertilization programme: a prospective randomized placebo controlled study. Eur J Obstet Gynecol Reprod Biol 2001; 96: 187–92.

67. Aboulghar M, Evers JH, Al-Inany H. Intravenous albumin for preventing severe ovarian hyperstimulation syndrome: a Cochrane review. Hum Reprod 2002; 17: 3027–32.

68. Bellver J, Munoz EA, Ballesteros A, et al. Intravenous albumin does not prevent moderate–severe ovarian hyperstimulation syndrome in high-risk IVF patients: a randomized controlled study. Hum Reprod 2003; 18: 2283–8.

69. Graf MA, Fischer R, Naether OG, et al. Reduced incidence of ovarian hyperstimulation syndrome by prophylactic infusion of hydroxyaethyl starch solution in an in-vitro fertilization programme. Hum Reprod 1997; 12: 2599–602.

70. König E, Bussen S, Sutterlin M, et al. Prophylactic intravenous hydroxyethyl starch solution prevents moderate–severe ovarian hyperstimulation in in-vitro fertilization patients: a prospective, randomized, double-blind and placebo-controlled study. Hum Reprod 1998; 13: 2421–4.

71. Penzias AS. Luteal phase support. Fertil Steril 2002; 77: 318–23.

72. Amso NN, Ahuja KK, Morris N, et al. The management of predicted ovarian hyperstimulation involving gonadotropin-releasing hormone analog with elective cryopreservation of all pre-embryos. Fertil Steril 1990; 53: 1087–90.

73. Wada I, Matson PL, Horne G, et al. Is continuation of a gonadotrophin-releasing hormone agonist (GnRHa) necessary for women at risk of developing the ovarian hyperstimulation syndrome? Hum Reprod 1992; 7: 1090–3.

74. Salat-Baroux J, Alvarez S, Antoine JM, et al. Treatment of hyperstimulation during in-vitro fertilization. Hum Reprod 1990; 5: 36–9.

75. Wada I, Matson PL, Troup SA, et al. Outcome of treatment subsequent to the elective cryopreservation of all embryos from women at risk of the ovarian hyperstimulation syndrome. Hum Reprod 1992; 7: 962–6.

76. Pattinson HA, Hignett M, Dunphy BC, et al. Outcome of thaw embryo transfer after cryopreservation of all embryos in patients at risk of ovarian hyperstimulation syndrome. Fertil Steril 1994; 62: 1192–6.

77. Awonuga AO, Pittrof RJ, Zaidi J, et al. Elective cryopreservation of all embryos in women at risk of developing ovarian hyperstimulation syndrome may not prevent the condition but reduces the live birth rate. J Assist Reprod Genet 1996; 13: 401–6.

78. Ferraretti AP, Gianaroli L, Magli C, et al. Elective cryopreservation of all pronucleate embryos in women at risk of ovarian hyperstimulation syndrome: efficiency and safety. Hum Reprod 1999; 14: 1457–60.

79. Wada I, Matson PL, Burslem RW, et al. Ovarian hyperstimulation syndrome in GnRH/hMG stimulated cycles for IVF or GIFT. J Obstet Gynecol 1991; 11: 88–9.

80. Tiitinen A, Husa LM, Tulppala M, et al. The effect of cryopreservation in prevention of ovarian hyperstimulation syndrome. Br J Obstet Gynaecol 1995; 102: 326–9.

81. Queenan JT Jr, Veeck LL, Toner JP, et al. Cryopreservation of all prezygotes in patients at risk of severe hyperstimulation does not eliminate the syndrome, but the chances of pregnancy are excellent with subsequent frozen–thaw transfers. Hum Reprod 1997; 12: 1573–6.

82. Benadiva CA, Davis O, Kligman I, et al. Withholding gonadotropin administration is an effective alternative for the prevention of ovarian hyperstimulation syndrome. Fertil Steril 1997; 67: 724–7.

83. Norman RJ, Warnes GM, Wang X, et al. Differential effects of gonadotrophin-releasing hormone agonists administered as desensitizing or flare protocols on hormonal function in the luteal phase of hyperstimulated cycles. Hum Reprod 1991; 6: 206–13.

84. Endo T, Honnma H, Hayashi T, et al. Continuation of GnRH agonist administration for 1 week, after hCG injection, prevents ovarian hyperstimulation syndrome following elective cryopreservation of all pronucleate embryos. Hum Reprod 2002; 17: 2548–51.

85. Fukaya T, Murakami T, Tamura M, et al. Laser vaporization of the ovarian surface in polycystic ovary disease results in reduced ovarian hyperstimulation and improved pregnancy rates. Am J Obstet Gynecol 1995; 173: 119–25.

86. Rimington MR, Walker SM, Shaw RW. The use of laparoscopic ovarian electrocautery in preventing cancellation of in-vitro fertilization treatment cycles due to risk of ovarian hyperstimulation syndrome in women with polycystic ovaries. Hum Reprod 1997; 12: 1443–7.

87. Egbase P, Al-Awadi S, Al-Sharhan M, et al. Unilateral ovarian diathermy prior to successful in vitro fertilisation: a strategy to prevent recurrence of ovarian hyperstimulation syndrome ? J Obstet Gynecol 1998; 18: 171–3.

88. Tozer AJ, Al-Shawaf T, Zosmer A, et al. Does laparoscopic ovarian diathermy affect the outcome of IVF–embryo transfer in women with polycystic ovarian syndrome? A retrospective comparative study. Hum Reprod 2001; 16: 91–5.

89. Koike T, Minakami H, Araki S, et al. Severity of ovarian hyperstimulation syndrome: its relation to number of conceptuses. Int J Fertil Womens Med 2004; 49: 36–42.

90. De Neubourg D, Mangelschots K, Van Royen E, et al. Singleton pregnancies are as affected by ovarian hyperstimulation syndrome as twin pregnancies. Fertil Steril 2004; 82: 1691–3.

91. Papanikolaou EG, Tournaye H, Verpoest W, et al. Early and late ovarian hyperstimulation syndrome: early pregnancy outcome and profile. Hum Reprod 2005; 20: 636–41.

92. Isik AZ, Vicdan K. Combined approach as an effective method in the prevention of severe ovarian hyperstimulation syndrome. Eur J Obstet Gynecol Reprod Biol 2001; 97: 208–12.

CHAPTER 22

The role of coasting in the prevention of threatening ovarian hyperstimulation syndrome: a European perspective

Marc Dhont

INTRODUCTION

Several strategies to prevent ovarian hyperstimulation syndrome (OHSS) have been tried, and their rationale and efficacy are dealt with in other chapters of this book. Coasting in *in vitro* fertilization (IVF) was introduced in 1993[1], and has since been applied by many infertility centers, although the ultimate proof of its efficacy remains to be provided by a prospective randomized trial. In this chapter, I consider a number of questions and try to give the currently available and generally accepted answers.

DEFINITION OF COASTING AND MECHANISM OF ACTION

The word coasting is a nautical term, and means slowing down the speed of a vessel when approaching the coast. In IVF, the word was introduced to describe the process of diminishing or stopping gonadotropin therapy for a variable number of days before administering human chorionic gonadotropin (hCG)[1]. It was suggested that this approach prevents severe OHSS by removing the follicle stimulating hormone (FSH) stimulation of granulosa cells, thereby inhibiting their proliferation and reducing the number of granulosa cells available for luteinization[2]. This would allow continued follicular growth and maturation while reducing the risk of OHSS. In addition, Tortoriello *et al.*[3] suggested that the falling FSH concentration induces increased apoptosis of granulosa cells, which results in a reduction of chemical mediators or precursors that augment fluid extravasation. It has also been postulated that follicles of varying size have a different threshold to gonadotropins, and smaller follicles appear to be more susceptible to gonadotropin deprivation than are larger follicles[4].

Enhanced production of vascular endothelial growth factor (VEGF) plays a central role in the pathogenesis of OHSS. The concentration of VEGF is increased in follicular fluid, ascites and plasma of patients with OHSS[5–7]. The expression and secretion of VEGF by human luteinized granulosa cells has been shown to be hCG-dependent[8,9]. It has also been demonstrated that there are differences in follicular fluid VEGF concentrations between coasted and non-coasted patients, which indicates that coasting may alter the capacity of the granulosa cells to produce VEGF and/or their response to hCG[10]. The same authors also demonstrated that coasting alters the functional capacity of granulosa cells cultured *in vitro*[11]. By coasting, VEGF expression seems to be down-regulated[12]. There are thus a number of plausible mechanisms which underpin the probability of coasting being effective in reducing the incidence of OHSS.

CRITERIA FOR COASTING

Although the occurrence and severity of OHSS cannot be reliably predicted, there are some predictive factors that can be taken into account for deciding when to consider coasting. Some patient characteristics are helpful in deciding particularly which patients to coast. There certainly is also a relationship between the number of growing follicles and/or the serum estradiol level and the risk of OHSS. In susceptible patients, however, OHSS can occur, after triggering ovulation with hCG, with fewer than ten mature follicles, while other patients with 30 mature follicles can sustain the same procedure with only minor discomfort. Cut-off levels for the number of follicles and/or the estradiol level, therefore, are arbitrary, and will differ according to various authors and the perceived risk of the individual patient. Criteria for coasting used by different authors are given in Table 1. Another factor that cannot be computed is the choice of the individual patient, and the well-reasoned risk that she is willing to sustain after having been informed about the size of the risk and equally well about the potential hazards of severe ovarian stimulation and the consequences of preventive procedures, from cancellation of the cycle to other measures that could reduce her chance for pregnancy.

Patient characteristics

Patients with typical polycystic ovaries are at increased risk for developing OHSS and, hence, ovarian stimulation should be adapted from the outset to the anticipated number of follicles that will develop upon full stimulation. Lean patients in particular are prone to OHSS, and coasting should be considered more readily in these patients.

Estradiol levels

Most authors have used a cut-off level for serum estradiol of between 2500 and 3000 pg/ml for coasting. There are, however, some limitations in the use of estradiol levels as a criterion for coasting. The estradiol level does not sufficiently take into account the number of smaller follicles, which also contribute to the development of OHSS. With pure FSH, estradiol levels tend to be lower than with human menopausal gonadotropin (hMG), and a useful cut-off level for serum estradiol in these cases has not yet been established. Finally, this parameter does not take into account the presence of numerous follicles in only one ovary. Although it seems logical that the total number of follicles is the most important factor in the risk assessment of OHSS, it cannot be excluded that the number of follicles in a single ovary independently contributes to this risk. It seems, therefore, that estradiol is not an absolute variable for deciding to coast, but it keeps its place for monitoring the duration of the coasting process.

Number of follicles

Although there is no linear relationship between the number of growing follicles and the risk of severity of hyperstimulation, common sense indicates that this is certainly the most reliable parameter to be taken into account, provided that all follicles ≥ 13 mm are included in the count. Because OHSS can occur in patients with a single ovary, and it is not yet clear whether the risk of OHSS is determined by the total number of follicles or by the number of follicles per ovary, I would therefore propose considering coasting when the total number of follicles in both ovaries exceeds 30, or when more than 20 growing follicles are present in a single ovary.

Table 1 Criteria for coasting

Authors	*Type of study*	*Number of patients*	*Initial E_2 concentration* (pg/ml)	*E_2 at hCG administration* (pg/ml)	*Duration of coasting* (days)	*Additional criteria for coasting*
Sher *et al.* (1995)[2]	Retrospective	51	> 3000	< 3000	6.1 (3–11)	> 29 follicles, 30% of follicles >15 mm
Benadiva *et al.* (1997)[15]	Retrospective	22	> 3000	< 3000	1.9 ± 0.9	
Tortoriello *et al.* (1998)[3]	Retrospective	22	> 3000	< 3000	2.6 ± 0.3	≥5 follicles > 16 mm and 2 follicles > 19 mm
Dhont *et al.* (1998)[16]	Retrospective case–control	120	> 2500	< 2500	1.9 ± 0.8	≥20 follicles
Lee *et al.* (1998)[17]	Retrospective	20	> 2724	Decreasing	2.8 ± 1.3	Many immature follicles but < 3 follicles > 18 mm
Egbase *et al.* (1999)[13]	Retrospective randomized	15	> 6000	< 3000	4.9 ± 1.6	
Waldenström *et al.* (1999)[18]	Retrospective	65	Variable	< 2724	4.3 (3–6)	> 25 large follicles, 3 follicles > 17 mm
Fluker *et al.* (1999)[4]	Retrospective	63	> 3000	25% decline	3.4 ± 0.1	
Al-Shawaf *et al.* (2001)[19]	Retrospective	50	> 3595	< 2724	3.4 ± 1.6	> 20 follicles, 25% of follicles > 15 mm
Ulug *et al.* (2002)[14]	Retrospective	207	> 4000	< 4000	2.9 ± 0.1	> 20 follicles, 30% of follicles > 15 mm

E_2, estradiol; hCG, human chorionic gonadotropin

TIMING OF COASTING

Coasting should not be initiated too early because follicular development could come to a complete standstill. When less than 30% of follicles have attained a mean diameter of 15 mm, an abrupt arrest in follicular development and a rapid decline in plasma estradiol usually compromises the oocyte quality. It has been shown that when the leading follicle reaches ≥ 15 mm, follicular growth continues after the withdrawal of gonadotropins[13]. On the other hand, if most follicles are > 15 mm in mean diameter when coasting is started, large cystic follicles are commonly encountered, and the quality of oocytes is also compromised[5]. It seems, therefore, that coasting should start when at least half the follicles have reached a mature size and have become independent of further gonadotropin stimulation for their final growth. The optimal threshold, both for estradiol and for follicular size, to start coasting remains to be determined. It is possible, but has not yet been firmly established, that the higher is the estradiol level at the beginning of coasting, the less effective is coasting in preventing OHSS irrespective of the length of the coasting period.

DURATION OF COASTING

Most authors agree that coasting should be maintained until the estradiol concentration drops below 3000 pg/ml (Table 1). After withholding gonadotropins, there is a further rise of serum estradiol for 1 or 2 days. Hence, the duration of coasting is dependent on the serum estradiol level at the time coasting starts; higher levels will require a longer coasting period. There is circumstantial evidence that the duration of coasting may impact on the success rate of IVF either by affecting oocyte and embryo quality or by altering endometrial receptivity. Ulug *et al.*[14] found that coasting for ≥ 4 days reduced pregnancy rates, although oocyte quality was not affected. Using the oocyte donation model, whereby endometrial receptivity is kept under control by the administration of estrogens followed by estrogens and progesterone in an artificial cycle, Isaza *et al.*[20] found that coasting for more than 4 days reduced pregnancy rates in the recipients, indicating that oocyte quality was affected by the duration of coasting. Alteration of endometrial receptivity can be an alternative or concomitant factor in the inverse relationship between the duration of coasting and pregnancy rate. The prolonged drop in estradiol level may compromise endometrial integrity and even induce estrogen-withdrawal bleeding. A rise of progesterone before the administration of hCG has been shown to occur more frequently in the coasted patient, which might affect the implantation window[21]. There is a consensus that coasting should not be extended beyond 4 days, but the optimal duration of coasting in terms of both prevention of OHSS and maintaining a normal pregnancy rate remains to be determined.

EFFICACY OF COASTING

There are no large-scale randomized controlled trials to establish firmly the effectiveness of coasting in preventing OHSS. There is only one randomized controlled trial in which coasting was compared with early unilateral follicular aspiration (EUFA) for the prevention of moderate and severe OHSS[13]. Thirty women undergoing superovulation for IVF/intracytoplasmic sperm injection (ICSI) treatment with gonadotropin-releasing hormone agonist (GnRH-a) down-regulation and gonadotropin stimulation were included in the study. The women were considered to be at risk of hyperstimulation when the estradiol concentration was > 6000 pg/ml and > 15 follicles in each ovary with at least two follicles > 18 mm in diameter were present. The number of oocytes retrieved was significantly lower in the coasting group (9.6) than in the EUFA group (15.4), but the clinical pregnancy rates were comparable. The incidence of moderate and severe OHSS (3/15 in the coasting group) was not different between the two groups ($n = 30$; odds ratio (OR) 0.76, 95% confidence interval (CI) 0.18–3.24).

We performed a case–control study in which we matched every case with 'non-coasted' IVF patients having comparable risk factors[16]. Outcomes were compared with those from 120 matched patients in whom serum estradiol levels and number of follicles at the time of hCG administration were comparable to those at the beginning of coasting (control group). The control group was selected from patients who had been stimulated for IVF before coasting had been introduced between 1989 and 1993 ($n = 120$). The main difference in the treatment protocol of the control group was that, in most of the patients, stimulation was performed using a long protocol (goserelin; Zeneca, Belgium), starting with 4 ampoules/day after complete pituitary desensitization was obtained. The case group consisted of 120 women undergoing ovarian stimulation for IVF who were considered to be at risk for ovarian hyperstimulation (serum estradiol levels > 2500 pg/ml or more than 20 follicles at the time of hCG administration). Gonadotropin administration was withheld when serum estradiol exceeded 2500 pg/ml, and hCG administration was delayed until estradiol levels dropped below 2500 pg/ml. The luteal phase was supported by progesterone intramuscularly (50 mg per day) in all cases and control patients. The incidence of moderate and severe OHSS, number of oocytes retrieved and pregnancy rate were compared in both groups. The incidence of moderate and severe OHSS was 5.8% in the coasting group versus 18.3% in the control group ($p < 0.005$; OR 0.27, 95% CI 0.11–0.67). The odds ratio of severe OHSS in the coasting group was 0.11 (95% CI 0.01–0.86). In fact, only one case with severe OHSS had to be hospitalized, in contrast with nine cases in the control group ($p < 0.01$), bringing the overall incidence of severe OHSS in our IVF program down to less than 0.1% since coasting was introduced. There was no significant difference in oocyte maturity (93.6% of retrieved oocytes in the coasting group were mature versus 93.2% in the control group), nor in fertilization rate. Although the number of oocytes was significantly lower in the coasting group (19.7 ± 0.6 vs. 22.1 ± 0.6), coasting did not affect the pregnancy rate (37.5% vs. 36.7%).

Second-hand evidence for the efficacy of coasting to prevent OHSS comes from retrospective observational studies (Table 2). In most of these studies, the incidence of severe OHSS after coasting was less than 2%. Differences in study design and the lack of standardized criteria for coasting and for the definition of severe OHSS are unfortunate limitations for estimating the real impact of coasting on the incidence of OHSS. Nevertheless, most studies agree that severe OHSS can be reduced to an incidence of lower than 2% in patients at risk. Two studies report much higher figures, but the criteria for starting coasting were less stringent, and only 15 and 20 patients were studied[13,17], respectively.

CONCLUSION

Coasting is one of the methods which is thought to be useful in preventing ovarian hyperstimulation syndrome. It involves withholding gonadotropin stimulation when estradiol levels exceed a certain threshold and waiting to give hCG until estradiol levels start dropping. There are a number of case–control and retrospective observational studies to support this strategy. However, there is a lack of prospective randomized trials to estimate the efficacy of coasting compared with placebo or other preventive measures.

Criteria for the initiation of coasting and its timing and duration are not yet uniformly established, but based on the literature, the following consensus can be proposed: coasting will be

Table 2 Comparison of outcome of coasting in terms of severe ovarian hyperstimulation syndrome and pregnancy rate

Authors	*Number of patients*	*Severe OHSS* (%)	*Fertilization rate* (%)	*Implantation rate* (%)	*Pregnancy rate/cycle* (%)
Sher *et al.* (1995)[2]	51	0	69	10	41
Benadiva *et al.* (1997)[15]	22	0	64	—	64
Tortoriello *et al.* (1998)[3]	22	0	61	19	57
Dhont *et al.* (1998)[16]	120	0.8	—	20	38
Lee *et al.* (1998)[17]	20	20	63	—	40*
Egbase *et al.* (1999)[13]	15	20	—	—	33
Waldenström *et al.* (1999)[18]	65	1.5	61	31	42
Fluker *et al.* (1999)[4]	63	0	71	14	37
Al-Shawaf *et al.* (2001)[19]	50	0.2	55	26	40
Ulug *et al.* (2002)[14]	207	1.9	71	19	51*

*Pregnancy rate expressed per embryo transfer

considered when > 20 follicles are developing; it should be initiated when the serum estradiol concentration exceeds 3500 pg/ml and when the largest follicle has reached a diameter of 18 mm. The administration of hCG should be delayed until the estradiol level drops below 3000 pg/ml, but the duration of coasting should be limited to ≤4 days because both the number of oocytes and the pregnancy rate drop considerably after a longer interval. By following these guidelines, the incidence of severe OHSS can be reduced to < 2% while the pregnancy rate will be unaffected.

Further studies are also needed to establish the most optimal timing and duration of coasting. Because with careful stimulation severe OHSS is rare, it seems unlikely that statistically solid proof of efficacy and data relating to timing and duration of stimulation will be forthcoming in the near future. For the time being, each IVF center should identify its own cut-off limit of serum estradiol and/or number of follicles and/or follicle size for the onset of coasting and for the timing of hCG administration.

REFERENCES

1. Sher G, Salem R, Feinman M, et al. Eliminating the risk of life-endangering complications following overstimulation with menotropin fertility agents: a report on women undergoing in vitro fertilization and embryo transfer. Obstet Gynecol 1993; 81: 1009–11.
2. Sher G, Zouves C, Feinman M, et al. 'Prolonged coasting': an effective method for preventing severe ovarian hyperstimulation syndrome in patients undergoing in-vitro fertilization. Hum Reprod 1995; 10: 3107–9.
3. Tortoriello DV, McGovern P, Colon JM, et al. 'Coasting' does not adversely affect cycle outcome in a subset of highly responsive IVF patients. Fertil Steril 1998; 69: 454–60.
4. Fluker MR, Hooper WM, Yuzpe A. Withholding gonadotropins ('coasting') to minimize the risk

of ovarian hyperstimulation during superovulation and in vitro fertilization–embryo transfer cycles. Fertil Steril 1999; 71: 294–301.

5. McClure N, Healy DL, Rogers PAW, et al. Vascular endothelial growth factor as capillary permeability agent in ovarian hyperstimulation syndrome. Lancet 1994; 344: 235–6.

6. Abramov Y, Barak V, Nisman B, et al. Vascular endothelial growth factor plasma levels correlate to the clinical picture in severe hyperstimulation syndrome. Fertil Steril 1997; 67: 261–5.

7. Agrawal R, Tan SL, Wild S, et al. Serum vascular endothelial growth factor concentrations in in vitro fertilization cycles predict the risk of ovarian hyperstimulation syndrome. Fertil Steril 1999; 71: 287–93.

8. Neulen J, Yan Z, Raczek S, et al. Human chorionic gonadotropin dependent expression of vascular endothelial growth factor/vascular permeability factor in human granulosa cells: importance in ovarian hyperstimulation syndrome. J Clin Endocrinol Metab 1995; 80: 1967–71.

9. Neulen J, Raczek S, Pogorzelski M, et al. Secretion of vascular endothelial growth factor/vascular permeability factor from human luteinized granulosa cells is human chorionic gonadotrophin dependent. Mol Hum Reprod 1998; 4: 203–6.

10. Tozer AJ, Iles RK, Iammarrone E, et al. The effects of 'coasting' on follicular fluid concentrations of vascular endothelial growth factor in women at risk of developing ovarian hyperstimulation syndrome. Hum Reprod 2004; 19: 522–8.

11. Tozer AJ, Iles RK, Iammarrone E, et al. Characteristics of populations of granulosa cells from individual follicles in women undergoing 'coasting' during controlled ovarian stimulation (COS) for IVF. Hum Reprod 2004; 19: 2561–8.

12. Garcia-Velasco JA, Zúñiga A, Pacheco A, et al. Coasting acts through downregulation of VEGF gene expression and protein secretion. Hum Reprod 2004; 19: 1530–8.

13. Egbase PE, Al Sharhan M, Grudzinskas JG. Early unilateral follicular aspiration compared with coasting for the prevention of severe ovarian hyperstimulation syndrome: a prospective randomized study. Hum Reprod 1999; 14: 1421–5.

14. Ulug U, Bahceci M, Erden HF, et al. The significance of coasting duration during ovarian stimulation for conception in assisted fertilization cycles. Hum Reprod 2002; 17: 310–13.

15. Benadiva CA, Owen D, Kligman I, et al. Withholding gonadotropin administration is an effective alternative for the prevention of ovarian stimulation syndrome. Fertil Steril 1997; 67: 724–7.

16. Dhont M, Van der Straeten F, De Sutter P. Prevention of severe ovarian hyperstimulation by coasting. Fertil Steril 1998; 70: 847–50.

17. Lee C, Tummon I, Martin J, et al. Does withholding gonadotrophin administration prevent severe ovarian hyperstimulation syndrome? Hum Reprod 1998; 13: 1157–8.

18. Waldenström U, Kahn J, Marsk L, et al. High pregnancy rates and successful prevention of severe hyperstimulation syndrome by 'prolonged coasting' of very hyperstimulated patients: a multicentre study. Hum Reprod 1999; 14: 294–7.

19. Al-Shawaf T, Zosmer A, Hussain S, et al. Prevention of severe ovarian hyperstimulation syndrome in IVF with or without ICSI and embryo transfer: a modified 'coasting' strategy based on ultrasound for identification of high-risk patients. Hum Reprod 2001; 16: 24–30.

20. Isaza V, Garcia-Velasco JA, Aragonés M, et al. Oocyte and embryo quality after coasting: the experience from oocyte donation. Hum Reprod 2002; 17: 1777–82.

21. Moreno L, Diaz I, Pacheco A, et al. Extended coasting duration exerts a negative impact on IVF cycle outcome due to premature luteinization. Reprod Biomed Online 2004; 9: 500–4.

CHAPTER 23

The role of coasting in the prevention of threatening ovarian hyperstimulation syndrome: an American perspective

Botros Rizk

INTRODUCTION

Coasting is the most popular method among physicians to prevent ovarian hyperstimulation syndrome (OHSS)[1]. This is absolutely true whether the patient is undergoing *in vitro* fertilization (IVF) in the United States or in Europe. Withholding gonadotropins and delaying the administration of human chorionic gonadotropin (hCG) have been employed in ovulation induction since the late 1980s and early 1990s[2–5]. Shortly afterwards, coasting was used to prevent severe OHSS in IVF cycles[6]. More than 15 studies (Tables 1–3) have been published, and several reviews have critically evaluated the effect of coasting on OHSS[1,7–9]. In this chapter, the advantages and the mechanism of action of coasting are discussed in detail. The impact of the points of initiation and termination of coasting as well as the duration are analyzed for the various publications based on our previous reviews and critical analyses[10,11].

PHILOSOPHY OF COASTING

Serum estradiol levels at the time of ovulation triggering are considered to be a clinical predictor of the risk of developing OHSS[12]. It has therefore been proposed to postpone hCG administration to allow the serum estradiol levels to drop below a certain threshold. This has been coined 'coasting' or 'controlled drift period'.

ADVANTAGES OF COASTING

The advantages of coasting are obvious for three reasons[10,11]. The first advantage of coasting is that the cycle is rescued and not canceled. The second advantage is that the embryos that are generated during the treatment cycle will be transferred, and hence there is no need for cryopreservation. The third advantage is that there is no need for gonadotropins or other medications nor for any supplementary procedures.

HOW DOES COASTING WORK?

The association between OHSS and high estradiol levels is very well established[12]. This certainly does not mean that the high estradiol levels *per se* result in the manifestations of increased permeability associated with OHSS[8,9,13].

Table 1 Population characteristics of the study, design and selection criteria used for coasting. Reproduced with permission from reference 7

*Authors** (n)	*Mean age* (years) ± *SD (range)*	*Selection criteria E_2* (pg/ml), *additional criteria*	*Design/control group(s)*
Sher *et al.*[25], 1995 (51)	37.3 (28–42)	E_2 > 3000, follicle number > 29 and 30% follicles ≥ 15 mm	Descriptive/NA
Benadiva *et al.*[27], 1997 (22)	34.5 ± 3.6	E_2 ≥ 3000	Retrospective/cryopreserved patients
Tortoriello *et al.*[29], 1998 (44)	32.6 ± 0.7	E_2 > 3000 and five or more follicles ≥ 16 mm and two follicles ≥ 19 mm	Retrospective/subgroup of coasted versus two control groups
Dhont *et al.*[13], 1998 (120)	NA	E_2 > 2500 and follicle number ≥ 20	Retrospective/historical cohort
Lee *et al.*[28], 1998 (20)	NA	E_2 > 2777 and many immature follicles > 18 mm	
Fluker *et al.*[5], 1999 (63)	32.2 ± NA	E_2 rose rapidly and generally > 3000	Descriptive/NA
Waldenström *et al.*[15], 1999 (65)	31.5 (23–39)	'Very high E_2' and > 25 'large follicles' of which the three largest ≥ 17 mm	Descriptive/NA
Egbase *et al.*[43], 1999 (15)	33.5 ± 2.8	E_2 > 6000 and > 15 follicles/ovary and two or more > 18	Prospective randomized early follicular aspiration
Dechaud *et al.*[46], 2000 (14)	NA	E_2 ≥ 5000 and/or > 20 follicles of which three or more follicles ≥ 18 mm without abdominal pain	Descriptive/NA
Ohata *et al.*[32], 2000 (5)	32 (25–37)	≥ 30% follicles ≥ 16 mm and severe OHSS in previous cycle	Descriptive/NA
Aboulghar *et al.*[31], 2000 (24)	29.9 ± 4.6	E_2 > 3000 and > 20 follicles with a dominant follicle ≥ 16 mm	Retrospective/historical group
Al-Shawaf *et al.*[14], 2001 (50)	32.5 ± 4.5	> 20 follicles and 25% ≥ 15 mm, E_2 ≥ 3596	Prospective/observational normal cycle

*Reference numbers refer to this article; NA, not available; E_2, estradiol

Coasting may diminish the *functional granulosa cell cohort*, resulting in a gradual decline in circulating estradiol levels, but more important, reduction of the chemical mediators that augment capillary permeability and fluid retention. Al-Shawaf *et al.* in 2001[14] postulated that coasting may reduce the incidence of severe OHSS in several ways. Follicle stimulating hormone (FSH) is known to induce luteinizing hormone (LH) receptors on granulosa cells; withholding gonadotropin will result in a decrease in FSH concentration and down-regulation of the LH receptors[14,15]. Through this mechanism, the number of granulosa cells available for luteinization will become less and the vasoactive substances responsible for the manifestations of OHSS will become less concentrated. Follicles of varying sizes may have different thresholds to gonadotropins[10]. Smaller follicles have a higher threshold than do larger follicles[5]. Withholding gonadotropins may therefore cause apoptosis of the granulosa cells and atresia of a large number of small follicles. Longer periods of coasting will cause a further reduction in FSH concentration followed by atresia of medium-sized follicles. When the FSH concentration falls further, it is possible that mature follicles > 15 mm will also undergo atresia, resulting in large follicular cysts with poor-quality and lower number of oocytes[14].

During coasting, estradiol levels initially increase because dominant follicles may continue their growth (Figure 1), despite the lack of hormonal stimulus, whereas intermediate follicles may undergo atresia[10]. Presumably, this is one mechanism of the efficacy of coasting in preventing OHSS.

The characteristics of granulosa cells in the follicles of women undergoing coasting in controlled ovarian stimulation for IVF have recently been described[16]. The effect of withholding gonadotropins during controlled ovarian stimulation in women at risk of developing OHSS was recently evaluated[17]. Individual follicles of variable sizes were assessed in relation to the granulosa cell number, oocytes retrieved, fertilization and embryo quality. The authors acknowledged that the ideal control group of women would be those identified to be at risk of developing OHSS, but not coasted. However, this was not ethically possible, since coasting has been successfully used to prevent severe OHSS in their unit for several years[14]. The control group was selected from optimally responsive women, excluding all poor and hyper-responders. The authors observed wide variations of follicular fluid levels of vascular endothelial growth factor (VEGF) in follicles of the same size, both in different patients and in the same patient, which reflects the unique and individual composition of each follicular environment. Despite these wide variations, VEGF levels in follicular fluid in the coasted group were constantly lower than the VEGF follicular fluid levels in the control group.

VEGF concentration in follicular fluid may depend on the quality and number of granulosa cells[18,19]. Tozer *et al.*[17] observed a negative correlation between follicular fluid VEGF and granulosa cell number, which was independent of follicle size. Greater granulosa cell numbers have been associated with more competent follicles[20], and lower follicular fluid VEGF levels with more oocytes[21] and better embryo quality[22]. Tozer *et al.*[17] suggested that this correlation, which was more significant in the coasted group, may be due to the differential effect of gonadotropin withdrawal on individual follicles in favor of those follicles with a greater number of granulosa cells/more competent follicles. The study did not confirm or refute VEGF as the cornerstone of OHSS pathophysiology, but established that VEGF follicular fluid concentrations in highly responsive women who had undergone coasting were significantly lower than in the control group of women studied.

Garcia-Velasco *et al.*, in 2004[23], suggested that coasting acts through down-regulation of VEGF gene expression and protein secretion. The fact that medium and small follicles are

Table 2 *In vitro* fertilization (IVF) data for the coasted cycle: estradiol (E_2) data are in pg/ml, means (ranges) or ± SD are given. Reproduced with permission from reference 7

Study	*E_2 day of coasting*	*E_2 day hCG received*	ΔE_2	*Coasting duration* (days)	*Oocytes* (*n*)	*Fertilization rate* (%)	*Pregnancy rate* (%)	*Patients with ascites* (*n*)	*Patients with hemo-concentration* (*n*)
Sher *et al.*, 1995	NA	2163 (560–2920)	5487	6.1 (3–11)	21	69	41†	12	0
Benadiva *et al.*, 1997	3802 ± 731	2206 ± 932	1597	1.9 ± 0.9	15 ± 6.5	62.2	63.6†	NA	NA
Tortoriello *et al.*, 1998	4015 ± 112	2407 ± 130	2475	2.6 ± 0.3	15.8 ± 1.2	59.8	44.45†	6 (5 clinically and 1 at ultrasound)	3
Dhont *et al.*, 1998	3834 ± 872	2348 ± 472.2	1486	1.94 ± 0.8	19.7 ± 0.6	NA	37.5*	NA	1
Lee *et al.*, 1999	NA	NA	NA	2.8 ± 1.3	NA	63	40‡	4 (2 paracentesis)	NA
Fluker *et al.*, 1999	NA	2832 ± 129	2245	5.3 ± 0.2	10.8 ± 0.5	71	36.5*	1	1
Waldenström *et al.*, 1999	> 6483 (3541–7764) 4471 (2821–7353)	1569 (472–2507)	4576	4.3 (3–6)	10 (3–21)	61	42*	< 300–800 ml: 300–800 ml: > 800 ml:	3/61 3/61 2/61
Egbase *et al.*, 1999	10 055 ± 965	1410 ± 246	NA	4.9 ± 1.6	9.6 ± 3.2	58.4 ± 2.1	33.3*	3	NA

continued

Table 2 *Continued*

Study	*E_2 day of coasting*	*E_2 day hCG received*	ΔE_2	*Coasting duration* (days)	*Oocytes* (*n*)	*Fertilization rate* (%)	*Pregnancy rate* (%)	*Patients with ascites* (*n*)	*Patients with hemo-concentration* (*n*)
Dechaud *et al.*, 2000	5761	3596	NA	1.6 (1–3)	15	36.7	$30^{\dagger}$	NA	0/10
Ohata *et al.*, 2000	NA	1242.6 (425–1800)	NA	4 (3–6)	9.2 (6–15)	NA	20*	5	0
Aboulghar *et al.*, 2000	7150 ± 1050	4640 ± 1100	NA	2.92 ± 0.92	16 ± 3.5	59	$35^{\dagger}$	4	0
Al-Shawaf *et al.*, 2001	NA	NA	NA	3.4 ± 1.6	11.0 ± 5.5 (0–22)	55.1	40*	1/50	NA

*Pregnancy rate/cycle; †pregnancy rate/retrieval; ‡pregnancy rate/embryo transfer; NA, not available; hCG, human chorionic gonadotropin

Table 3 Clinical description of registered OHSS cases. Reproduced with permission from reference 7

Authors (*n*)	*Patients with ascites* (*n*)	*Hemoconcentration* (*n*)	*Comments, OHSS classification*
Sher *et al.*, 1995 (51)	12	0	
Benadiva *et al.*, 1997 (22)	NA	NA	1 moderate OHSS/classification non-precise
Tortoriello *et al.*,1998 (44)	6 (5 clinically and 1 at ultrasound)	3	
Dhont *et al.*, 1998 (120)	NA	1	5.8% of moderate (involves ascites) and severe OHSS
Lee *et al.*, 1998 (20)	4 (2 paracentesis)	NA	4 severe OHSS (distress with ovarian enlargement and ascites)
Fluker *et al.*, 1999 (63)	1	1	Cumulated results of 2 groups (classical and modified coasting $n = 93$); 9/93 had nausea and vomiting; 2 had ascites
Waldenström *et al.*, 1999 (65)	< 300 ml: 6/61 300–800 ml: 3/61 > 800 ml: 2/61	2/61	1 paracentesis
Egbase *et al.*, 1999 (15)	3	NA	3 additional cases of moderate OHSS when considering the classification of Schenker
Dechaud *et al.*, 2000 (14)	NA	0/10	Refers only to severe forms of OHSS
Ohata *et al.*, 2000 (5)	5	0	Ascites at ultrasound
Aboulghar *et al.*, 2000 (24)	4	0	Ascites at ultrasound (moderate according to the classification of Goland)
Al-Shawaf *et al.*, 2001 (50)	1*/50	NA	2 moderate OHSS according to the classification of Navot
Total	46/283 (16.3%)	7/378 (2.8%)	

*This patient was excluded concerning a protocol violation; NA, not available

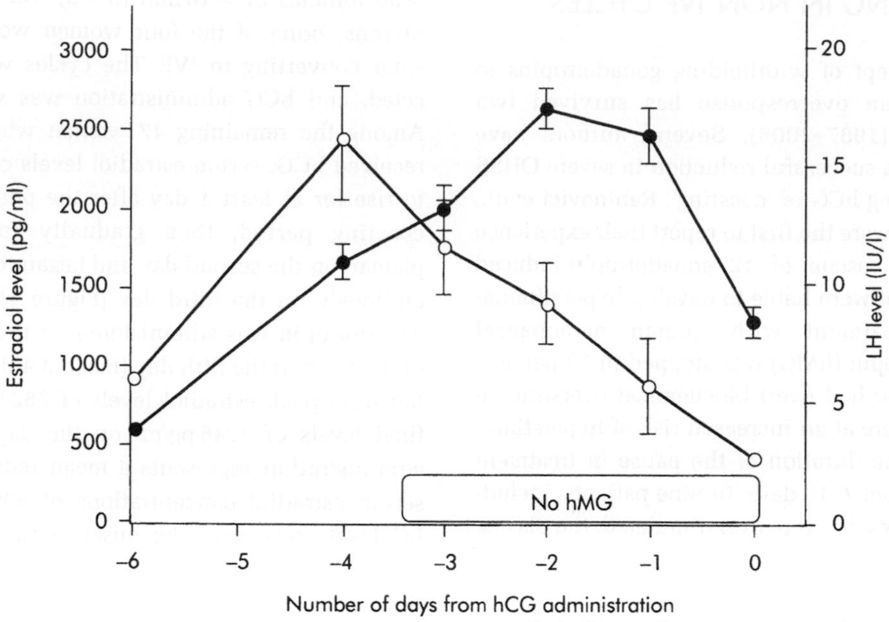

Figure 1 Mean ± SE estradiol and luteinizing hormone (LH) concentrations before and during the coasting period in superovulation cycles. Mean LH levels rose spontaneously just before the coasting period, coinciding with the rapid rise in estradiol concentrations. The line with open circles represents LH concentrations, whereas the line with solid circles represents estradiol concentrations. hMG, human menopausal gonadotropin; hCG, human chorionic gonadotropin. Reproduced with permission from reference 5

more sensitive to undergoing atretic changes is of crucial relevance in both steroid and vasoactive mediator secretion. They also observed that a significantly higher percentage of granulosa lutein cells become apoptotic after coasting. This difference is even greater for immature follicles.

PHYSICIAN ATTITUDES TOWARDS COASTING

Physicians' practice in infertility has been more of an art and is now developing into science. Physicians' attitudes are still more on the artistic side than the scientific side. Delvigne and Rozenberg[1] assessed whether physicians would modify the preventive attitude in relation to clinical factors and the estradiol response. They constructed case scenarios with three levels of risk factors for OHSS. At random, three of the 12 artificially constructed case scenarios were sent to 573 physicians who are members of the European Society for Human Reproduction and Embryology (ESHRE). Among the selected preventive measures, coasting was by far the most popular choice (60%), followed by the use of intravenous albumin or hydroxyethyl starch solution (36%), and cryopreservation of all embryos (33%).

COASTING IN NON-IVF CYCLES

The concept of withholding gonadotropins to prevent an overresponse has survived two decades (1987–2005). Several authors have reported a successful reduction in severe OHSS by delaying hCG or 'coasting'. Rabinovici *et al.*, in 1987[2], were the first to report their experience with the rescue of 12 gonadotropin-induced cycles that were liable to develop hyperstimulation. Treatment with human menopausal gonadotropin (hMG) was stopped in 12 patients who either had overt biochemical overstimulation or were at an increased risk of hyperstimulation. The duration of the pause in treatment ranged from 2–10 days. In nine patients, including the six who were overstimulated, the plasma estradiol levels declined, despite the continuing growth of most follicles. None of these patients conceived following hCG. Pregnancies occurred in three patients whose estradiol levels continued to rise until the day of hCG. They therefore concluded that, although rescue of the overstimulated cycles is sometimes possible, the resulting conceptions seem to be associated with a continuing rise of estradiol during the period of treatment pause.

Urman *et al.*[3] studied 40 cycles in 32 patients with polycystic ovarian syndrome (PCOS). The authors withheld gonadotropins and continued to monitor by daily assay for estradiol and frequent ultrasound examination. They used the term 'controlled drift period' to explain coasting. The mean duration of coasting was 2.8 days. The clinical pregnancy rate per cycle was 25% (10/40). OHSS occurred in 2.5% (1/40). The authors did not share the same conclusion about the relationship between pregnancy and the rise of estradiol as suggested by Rabinovici *et al.*[2].

Fluker *et al.*[5] also used coasting in 51 women undergoing superovulation who had estradiol levels of >3000 pg/ml. In four of the 51 women, excessive follicular diameter was observed by the presence of 8–10 follicles ≥ 18 mm ($n = 2$) or > 30 follicles of > 10 mm ($n = 2$). For religious reasons, none of the four women would consider converting to IVF. The cycles were canceled, and hCG administration was withheld. Among the remaining 47 women who indeed received hCG, serum estradiol levels continued to rise for at least 1 day after the onset of the coasting period, then gradually reached a plateau on the second day and began to fall precipitously on the third day (Figure 1). Human gonadotropin was administered on the evening of the third to the fifth day (mean 3.4 days). The fall from peak estradiol levels of 2824 pg/ml to final levels of 1246 pg/ml on the day of hCG administration represents a mean reduction in serum estradiol concentrations of 56%. Mean LH levels rose near the onset of the coasting period and decreased spontaneously while follicular growth continued. Moderate OHSS occurred in three (6%) of the 47 women to whom hCG was administered. A small amount of ascites was noted sonographically, and ovaries were enlarged to 6–10 cm. This was not accompanied by significant abnormalities in renal function or hematological parameters. Spontaneous resolution occurred with bedrest at home. Eleven pregnancies occurred among the 47 women (23.4%), including eight singletons, one twin, one triplet and one ectopic pregnancy.

COASTING IN GONADOTROPIN-RELEASING HORMONE AGONIST IVF CYCLES

Between 1993 and 2005, more than 15 studies were published on coasting[10]. The long gonadotropin-releasing hormone (GnRH) agonist protocol was used in almost all cycles, and the short protocol was used in only one study[13]. This is not surprising, because GnRH agonist (GnRH-a) protocols were the most widely used for IVF stimulation during that period, and they are also associated with the highest probability of OHSS development[4,24].

Sher *et al.*[6] suggested that prolonged coasting in GnRH-a/hMG/FSH cycles could prevent life-endangering complications of OHSS. They withheld gonadotropins in 17 patients whose serum estradiol exceeded 6000 pg/ml, and continued daily GnRH-a until estradiol levels had fallen below 3000 pg/ml. hCG (10 000 IU) was administered to trigger ovulation. The estradiol levels continued to rise rapidly in the 48 h following initiation of the coasting period, then plateaued and began to fall 96–168 h after gonadotropins were stopped. The coasting period lasted between 4 and 9 days, and the day of hCG administration fell on cycle days 12–16. Six of the 17 cycles (35%) produced viable pregnancies. All 17 patients developed signs of grade 2 or 3 OHSS, but none developed severe OHSS. In 1995, the same authors treated 51 women at risk of developing OHSS by coasting, and also waited until the estradiol level dropped to below 3000 pg/ml[25]. The clinical pregnancy rate was 41% per oocyte retrieval (21/51). None of the patients developed severe OHSS; however, the mean number of embryos transferred was 5.4, which was extremely high.

Ben-Nun *et al.*, in 1993[26], conducted a pilot study of 66 patients at risk of developing OHSS. These patients were coasted, and hCG was given when the estradiol level reached 2500 pg/ml. Four of the 66 patients developed OHSS.

Benadiva *et al.*, in 1997[27], compared coasting with cryopreservation. Gonadotropins were withheld in 22 patients at risk of OHSS. hCG was administered when the estradiol levels dropped to ≤ 3000 pg/ml. The control group consisted of 26 patients in whom no fresh embryo transfer was performed, and all the embryos were cryopreserved and transferred during a subsequent unstimulated cycle. Fertilization and delivery rates were not significantly different between the two groups, and Benadiva *et al.* concluded that coasting could produce high pregnancy rates without the need for multiple frozen/thawed cycles.

Dhont *et al.*[13] published one of the largest retrospective studies of 120 women undergoing IVF between 1994 and 1996 at risk of OHSS. This large study is discussed in detail by the above author in Chapter 22 of this book. Briefly, patients were coasted when the estradiol levels exceeded 2500 pg/ml, and hCG was withheld, and then administered when the estradiol levels dropped below 2500 pg/ml. The authors compared the outcome with those of 120 matched OHSS high-risk patients who did not undergo coasting. Coasting significantly decreased the incidence of moderate and severe OHSS with an odds ratio of 0.11 and confidence interval (CI) 0.01–0.89.

Lee *et al.*, in 1998[28], carried out a pilot study of coasting in 20 patients at risk of OHSS. The mean duration of coasting was 3 days. hCG was administered on the day that the serum estradiol levels began to fall, and four of the 20 patients developed severe OHSS despite coasting. The authors observed more severe OHSS cases (20%) within the group of coasted women than in the general reference population (1%). The general population presented no risk factors for OHSS. They concluded that hCG administration was too early to prevent OHSS.

Tortoriello *et al.* performed a very interesting study[29]. The authors investigated three groups of patients. The first group consisted of highly responsive coasted patients. The second group consisted of equally responsive patients who did not undergo coasting. The third group was a control group consisting of age-matched normally responsive patients. The rates of moderate and severe OHSS did not differ statistically among the three groups. No patient in group three developed OHSS. Moderate OHSS was diagnosed in one patient from group one on the basis of sonographically demonstrable minimal ascites. One patient in group two obtained a singleton pregnancy and developed critical OHSS with severe hemoconcentration, oliguria and a large pleural effusion that required 7 days of hospitalization.

Two subsets of coasted patients were also compared, to assess the effect of estradiol levels at the time they met the criteria for hCG (Table 4). Subset one was identical to group one, consisting of those 22 coasted patients who achieved an estradiol level between 3000 and 3999 pg/ml at the time they met the criteria. Subset two consisted of the remaining 22 coasted patients excluded from the comparison analysis who achieved estradiol levels of > 4000 pg/ml at the time they met the criteria. The two subsets did not differ regarding age, FSH level, prevalence of polycystic ovaries, number of oocytes retrieved or oocyte maturity, fertilization and cleavage. These patients on average coasted approximately 1 day longer than the less responsive subset ($p = 0.0463$). The authors observed a significantly higher implantation rate, and the trends suggested a higher clinical and multiple pregnancy rate in subset one. There were no significant differences in severe or moderate OHSS between the two subsets. However, all three patients who developed severe OHSS were in subset two, and two of them were hospitalized for 2 days[29].

The estradiol and progesterone levels in all 44 coasted patients were significantly reduced by the end of coasting periods lasting longer than 2 days. Linear regression analysis demonstrated a statistically significant positive relationship between the duration of coasting and peak estradiol level achieved ($p < 0.0001$), as well as a significant negative relationship between coasting duration and the total number of mature oocytes retrieved ($p = 0.036$). Logistic regression analysis of coasting interval duration also suggested an inverse relationship to the clinical pregnancy rate ($p = 0.09$).

Table 4 Outcome parameters for 'coaster' subsets depending on estradiol (E_2) levels and maturity of follicles at time of initiation of coasting. Reproduced with permission from reference 29

	Coasted group		
Variable	*E_2 level of 3000–3999 pg/ml (n = 22)*	*E_2 level of ≥ 4000 pg/ml (n = 22)*	*p Value*
Mean (± SEM) number of oocytes retrieved	15.9 ± 1.2	15.6 ± 1.2	NS
Maturity rate (%)	80.4	78.9	NS
Fertilization rate (%)	60.9	58.8	NS
Cleavage rate (%)	85.2	93.1	NS
Mean (± SEM) number of embryos transferred	4.6 ± 0.3	5.2 ± 0.3	NS
Mean (± SEM) number of embryos frozen	3.1 ± 0.8	2.8 ± 0.8	NS
Clinical pregnancy rate (%)	57.1	31.8	NS
Implantation rate (%)	19.0	6.7	0.04*
Multiple pregnancy rate (%)	41.6	28.6	NS
Severe OHSS rate (%)	0	13.6	NS

*Significance determined by Kruskal–Wallis test; NS, not significant

Tortoriello *et al.*[30] also observed severe OHSS, despite coasting, as gonadotropins were withheld when serum estradiol levels were 14 700 pmol/l. An important finding was that there was a higher than expected incidence of severe OHSS (33%) when coasting was started with serum estradiol levels > 29 000 pmol/l, and a large number of follicles with diameter larger than 18 mm.

Waldenström *et al.* performed a multicenter trial of coasting in 65 IVF cycles considered to be severely hyperstimulated. hCG was given when the estradiol levels fell below 10 000 pmol/l. The mean duration of coasting was 4.3 days, and four cycles were canceled. The pregnancy rate was 42% and the implantation rate was 31%, and only one patient developed severe OHSS[15].

Fluker *et al.*[5] studied two groups of IVF patients undergoing coasting, with mature and immature follicles. In the first group ($n = 63$), the estradiol concentration rose rapidly and exceeded 3000 pg/ml. Exogenous gonadotropins were withheld to allow estradiol concentrations to decrease by at least 25% before hCG administration. Each subject met the follicular criteria for hCG administration and oocyte retrieval, ≥ 3 follicles of ≥ 18 mm before or during the coasting period. Oocyte retrieval was performed 34 h later. The luteal phase was supported with micronized progesterone at a dosage of 200 mg twice daily. In the second group ($n = 30$), estradiol concentrations rose rapidly in the presence of numerous intermediate-size follicles. In anticipation of overstimulation, the hMG dosage was reduced. This was followed by an abrupt and inadvertent decline in estradiol concentrations before the attainment of appropriate follicular maturity. Gonadotropin treatment was then reinstituted to restimulate follicular growth. Then 10 000 IU of hCG was administered once three or more follicles ≥ 18 mm were achieved. Oocyte retrieval was performed as per the routine protocol. The mean age, etiology and duration of infertility were similar between the two groups. The average duration of rise was longer in the first group, 3.3 days, than in the second group, 1.37 days (Figure 2), in keeping with the larger follicles and more established steroid oogenesis[5]. Clinical pregnancies occurred in 23 of 63 cycles (36.5%) and in 12 of 30 cycles (40%), and the implantation rate per embryo was 14.3% and 17.8%, respectively. Eleven women (12%) had evidence of moderate OHSS, which was managed conservatively at home. One woman (1.1%) from the second group was hospitalized with severe OHSS that required treatment with paracentesis and intravenous albumin. The authors noted that their implantation rates compared favorably with those of Sher *et al.*[6], 15.4% vs. 9.5%, respectively, as did the clinical pregnancy rates, 37.5% vs. 41%, respectively, despite the difference in the number of embryos transferred, 2.9 vs. 5.4, respectively. The authors suggested that IVF cycles do not have to be markedly overstimulated to have enough reserve to withstand the coasting period. Rather, a limited period of coasting before the administration of hCG may improve the margin of safety and still be well tolerated, even in cycles in which the response is only slightly increased. The approach in IVF cycles in the study by Fluker *et al.*[5], was different from that in those studied by Sher *et al.*[6,25]. An aggressive stimulation was used in the studies by Sher *et al.*: the estradiol levels were > 6000 pg/ml, or patients had > 30 follicles and received hCG after their estradiol levels decreased to < 3000 pg/ml. In contrast, the more conservative approach to stimulation in the study by Fluker *et al.* resulted in lower peak estradiol levels and a less precipitous decline in estradiol concentration. As a result, only 18 of 93 patients undergoing IVF in their study had estradiol levels of > 6000 pg/ml and 28 received hCG, even though their estradiol levels remained > 3000 pg/ml. Fluker *et al.* highlighted that the only woman in whom severe OHSS developed in their study had an estradiol level of 2762 pg/ml, which is below the limit sug-

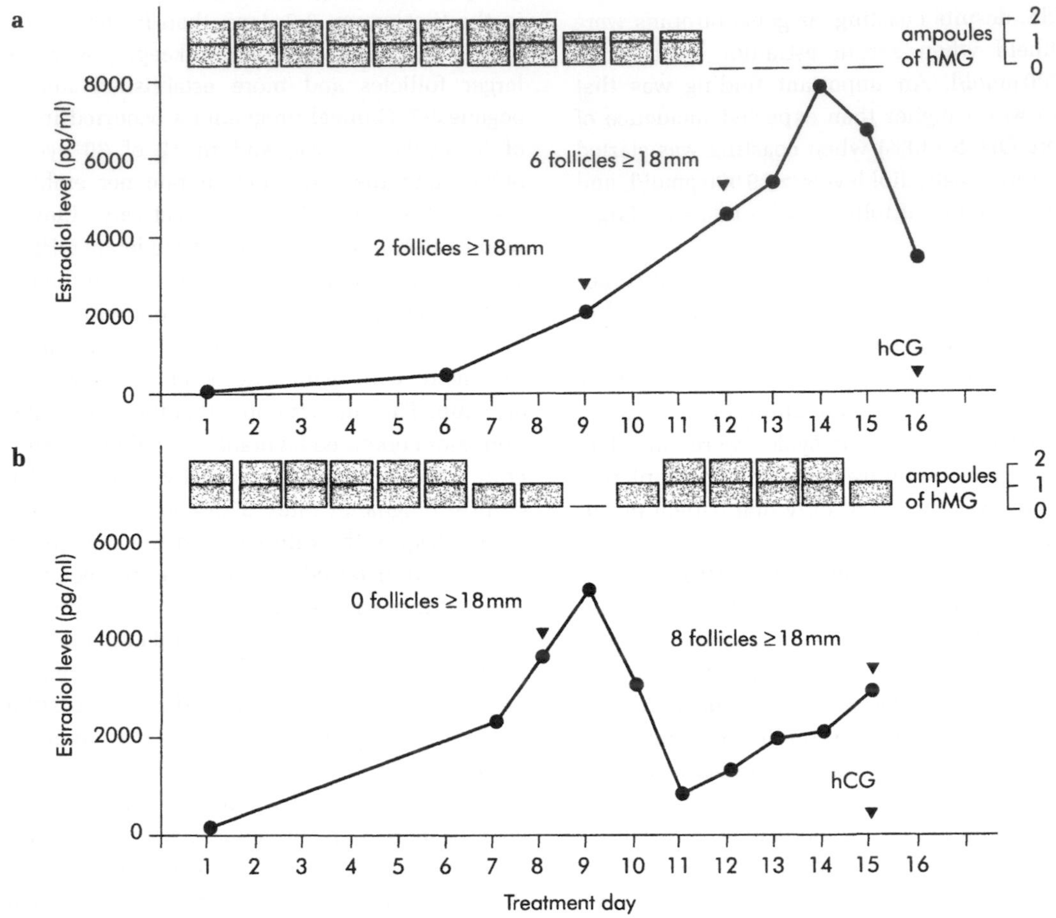

Figure 2 Characteristics of representative *in vitro* fertilization–embryo transfer (IVF–ET) cycles in which coasting was used to restrain rapidly rising estradiol levels in two patient subgroups: (a) after the attainment of follicular maturity (group 2A) and (b) before reaching follicular maturity (group 2B). Conception occurred in both cycles. hMG, human menopausal gonadotropin; hCG, human chorionic gonadotropin. Reproduced with permission from reference 5

gested by most investigators as a safe point to give hCG and have success with coasting.

Aboulghar *et al.* performed a prospective randomized study to evaluate the incidence of OHSS in 49 high-risk patients, using a reduced hMG dose in one arm and continuation of the same dose in the other arm before coasting. There were no cases of severe OHSS in either group after coasting; however, the duration of coasting was significantly reduced when the dose of hMG was reduced. The authors used a historical control group as reference for the two subsets of coasted patients. The incidence of severe OHSS in the historical group with high estradiol levels (mean 7200 pg/ml) was 25% (eight cases out of 32), as compared with 17% (four cases out of 24) in the coasted group[31].

Ohata *et al.*[32] performed coasting in five patients with PCOS who had developed severe OHSS in a previous cycle. Coasting was effective in preventing OHSS in these patients.

Grochowski *et al.*[33] performed a coasting study in 112 hyperstimulated IVF patients when the estradiol level was over 3000 pg/ml and the leading follicle's diameter was ≥ 18 mm. Fertilization failed in six patients. All the embryos were frozen in another ten patients. The pregnancy rate was 30.4% and the implantation rate was 18.1%. Moderate OHSS occurred in six patients and severe OHSS occurred in another two patients.

Al-Shawaf *et al.*[14] performed a modified coasting protocol in patients at risk of severe OHSS based on ultrasound monitoring. Serum estradiol levels were measured only in patients with > 20 follicles on ultrasound. Moderate OHSS occurred in three patients (0.7%) and severe OHSS in one patient (0.2%). Pregnancy rates were 39.6% and 40% in cycles where the gonadotropin dose was reduced or withheld, respectively.

Al-Shawaf *et al.*, in 2002[34], determined that measuring serum FSH in addition to estradiol levels during coasting could assist in predicting the point at which the serum estradiol level had declined to a sufficiently safe point for hCG administration.

The time of initiation of coasting has always been considered to be a crucial point. Tortoriello *et al.*[30] suggested that if coasting was initiated at very high estradiol levels, severe OHSS may occur in one out of three patients. Egbase *et al.*[35] therefore performed a pilot study to determine the impact of withholding gonadotropins at an earlier stage in patients at risk of developing OHSS. The authors concluded that early withholding of gonadotropins is also associated with a good outcome.

Ulug *et al.*[36] carried out a retrospective study to define the optimal interval of coasting in patients at high risk of developing OHSS. In their study, patients were characterized according to the number of days between the cessation of gonadotropins and hCG administration. Patients in whom coasting lasted ≥ 4 days had significantly reduced implantation, compared with patients with a shorter coasting interval.

COASTING IN GONADOTROPIN-RELEASING HORMONE ANTAGONIST IVF CYCLES

Delvigne *et al.*[37] reported two cases in which coasting was used in a stimulation regimen that included a GnRH antagonist and gonadotropins. The first case had an estradiol level of 7851 pg/ml on day 16 of the cycle, and the second patient, a level of 6701 pg/ml on day 13 of her cycle. The first patient increased her level of estradiol on the first day after coasting and then had a rapid and clinically significant 83% decrease in the level of estradiol. The second patient experienced a more progressive decrease of estradiol, but her estradiol level did not increase after hMG administration was stopped. Neither patient developed OHSS. The authors suggested that coasting could be used when stimulation involves hMG and a GnRH antagonist.

WHEN TO INITIATE COASTING?

Levinsohn-Tavor *et al.*[38] appraised the three factors that should be considered for the initiation of coasting:

(1) Plasma estradiol concentration, which reflects the total functional granulosa cell population;

(2) The number of ovarian follicles, which predicts the potential for further granulosa cell population and estradiol rise;

(3) The diameter of the leading follicles.

Most publications addressing coasting reflect that an estradiol concentration of 2500–3000 pg/ml was the value most commonly chosen by clinicians[5,6,13,14,27–29]. The relatively low threshold for coasting has been shown to reduce the incidence of OHSS effectively without compromising the cycle outcome[38]. High cut-off levels of around 6000 pg/ml are associated with a higher incidence of OHSS and the need for longer periods of coasting[15].

Since the first study by Rabinovici *et al.*[2], it has been demonstrated that even after withholding gonadotropins there is an additional subsequent rise in serum estradiol for 1 or more days[5,6,35] (Figures 1 and 2). When coasting was initiated at a plasma estradiol value of over 3000 pg/ml, the plasma estradiol increased to over 6000 pg/ml during the coasting period.

WHEN TO ADMINISTER hCG AND WHEN TO END COASTING?

Administration of hCG when the estradiol level drops below 2500–3000 pg/ml has been termed to be effective in lowering the risk of OHSS[5,13,14,27,29]. Dhont *et al.*[13] compared a coasting group with a matched control group. Both had a similar maximum estradiol level (3830 pg/ml) and number of follicles ($n = 24$). On the day of hCG administration, estradiol levels were 2348 pg/ml in the coasted group compared with 3833 pg/ml in the control group. Only one patient in the coasted group developed severe OHSS, compared with nine patients in the control group.

Levinsohn-Tavor *et al.*[38] advised that when an appropriate threshold for administering hCG is attained, the serum estradiol should be followed and not allowed to fall too low below this level. We fully agree with this excellent clinical remark. However, the greatest difficulty that we have encountered is the significant drop in estradiol level that could occur in 1 day. Rizk *et al.* encountered two patients whose estradiol level was above 4000 pg/ml during coasting and dropped to below 1000 pg/ml over a 24-h period, with a detrimental effect on the quality of oocytes and pregnancy outcome[11]. Waldenström *et al.* reported two cases in which they delayed hCG for an additional 2 days after the serum estradiol level had dropped below the threshold level of 2724 pg/ml, which led to bleeding and cycle cancellation. In three other cases, serum estradiol was allowed to fall below the threshold value, resulting in the retrieval of 1–3 oocytes of poor quality[15].

DURATION OF COASTING

The number of recorded days of coasting has varied between 1 and 11 (Table 2). The effect of duration of coasting has remained controversial. While some studies suggested that gonadotropins could be withheld for 10 or more days without compromise of the outcome, others have experienced a decrease in pregnancy rate when the duration has exceeded 4 days[11,29,36,39]. Ulug *et al.* found that coasting for 4 or more days reduces the implantation and pregnancy rates, while oocyte quality does not appear to be affected[36].

Moreno *et al.*, in 2004[40], performed a retrospective study of 132 patients who demonstrated a high response to ovarian stimulation with estradiol > 4500 pg/ml and/or more than 20 follicles > 17 mm and were coasted due to the high risk of developing OHSS. The authors investigated the impact of duration of coasting on IVF cycle outcome. In addition, serum progesterone and LH were measured, to investigate whether premature luteinization was present in the cycles and whether it might be related to coasting duration. A significant difference in implantation rate was observed when coasting was required for more than 4 days, together with a trend toward a high cancellation rate. Premature luteinization was significantly elevated in women undergoing coasting compared with control women, 34% vs. 15.6% ($p < 0.05$). In the majority of patients who showed premature luteinization, coasting lasted 3 days. The authors concluded that prolonged coasting may affect the endometrium in relation to the implantation window. These findings may explain why some patients undergoing extended coasting demonstrate a lower implantation rate compared with controls.

HOW SUCCESSFUL IS COASTING IN ELIMINATING OHSS?

There is no question that coasting has made a tremendous impact on the clinical management of OHSS. Delvigne and Rozenberg, after analyzing 12 studies including almost 500 coasted patients, reported a 2.5% incidence of severe OHSS, and that ascites developed in 16% of cases[41]. One of the factors of prime importance is the difference in classification of OHSS: whereas some cases will be referred to in some publications as moderate, others consider them as severe[42].

Most investigators have included coasting at least as part of their approach to prevent OHSS. From an evidence-based medicine point of view, there are few data in terms of prospective randomized trials. The reason for that is obvious: it would be difficult to have a randomization in which one of the arms would not be coasted and subjected to the risk of severe OHSS. Therefore, many investigators have included a control group of another modality of OHSS prevention, or a group of normo-responders[11,13,27,43].

COCHRANE REVIEW

D'Angelo and Amso[44] performed a Cochrane review of coasting for the prevention of OHSS. They identified 13 studies, but only one trial met the inclusion criteria. Therefore, it was concluded that there was insufficient evidence available to determine whether coasting was an effective strategy in preventing the occurrence of OHSS. In the only one prospective study, 15 patients were included in each study arm comparing coasting with unilateral follicular aspiration, a technique that is seldom used. The Cochrane review stressed the absence of high-quality studies that limited to a great extent the conclusions that could be drawn.

IS THERE A PROBLEM WITH COASTING?

The greatest concern about adopting a policy of coasting or withholding gonadotropins is a decrease in the quality or number of oocytes and a subsequent drop in the pregnancy rate[11]. One of the studies that could be used for background information is the investigation by Aboulghar *et al.*[45], evaluating the quality of oocytes in patients with severe OHSS. They reported that the inferior quality and maturity of oocytes in OHSS reduced the fertilization rate, but did not affect the quality or the number of embryos transferred, or the pregnancy rate. The effect on oocyte quality was attributed to the prevalence of polycystic ovaries in this group of patients. Whether one agrees or not about the impact of coasting on the quality of oocytes or embryos, this study serves to make the point that in patients with OHSS there might be a negative impact on the quality of oocytes, even without coasting.

The impact of coasting on oocyte quality has been discussed in coasted patients compared with a control group[10]. The literature is divided between those who believe that coasting has some negative impact on oocyte quality and those who believe that coasting has no impact on the quality of oocytes[11,39,46]. The criteria used for the initiation and determination of coasting that have been published in the literature are very heterogeneous. This probably explains some of the differences between reports. Ulug *et al.* found that coasting for 4 days or more reduces the implantation and pregnancy rate, while oocyte quality does not appear to be affected[36]. Isaza *et al.* compared cycle outcome in recipients of oocytes from donors who underwent coasting and donors who did not[39]. The outcome of oocyte donation from donors undergoing coasting was not impaired, with similar implantation and pregnancy rates. If the duration of coasting was > 4 days, a significant decrease in implantation and pregnancy rates was found. Delvigne *et al.* performed a retrospective cohort study of 157 patients compared with a control group of 208 IVF cycles, who had reached serum estradiol levels of at least 4000 pg/ml without being coasted[46]. In the group of coasted cycles, the question of whether indirect parameters related to coasting had an effect on IVF outcome was also analyzed. The authors observed that patients who had undergone coasting had higher maximum estradiol levels and greater numbers of large follicles ($p < 0.001$) and lower oocyte recovery rates ($p < 0.001$) than those of the control group. The IVF outcomes were similar between the two groups. The authors also observed that within the group of patients who had undergone coasting, no significant relationship was observed between the number of coasting days, estradiol levels on the day of hCG or fallen estradiol level and the outcome, whether measured in terms of oocyte quality, pregnancy rate or OHSS occurrence.

Rizk *et al.* similarly observed a decline in the implantation and pregnancy rates in those who underwent coasting[11]. The decrease in implantation and pregnancy rates was not statistically significant. However, in the subset of patients who received a lower dose of hCG (5000 IU vs. 10 000 IU), the difference was statistically significant ($p < 0.05$). In the reported publications, ovulation was induced in three studies by administering 5000 units of hCG[15,32,47], but more often with 10 000 units[5,6,13,14,29,43,45]. Therefore, the impact of combining coasting with reducing the dose of hCG has to be taken into consideration. The combination in our experience has led to a lower number of oocytes and lower quality of embryos.

CONCLUSIONS

Coasting is the most popular method for preventing OHSS. Prospective randomized studies regarding its efficacy are limited because it is unacceptable to have a control group subjected to the risk of severe hyperstimulation syndrome. A large multicenter trial with selected control group(s) could result in a definitive answer. The major advantage of such a clinical trial would be to have the same initiation point, a consensus of duration and the same finish line. To design such a trial, we should predetermine whether coasting would be initiated at a certain level of estradiol regardless of the size or maturity of the follicles, or should we include only patients with a specific estradiol level *and* follicular size? The optimal duration of coasting should also be analyzed. Finally, the point at which to end coasting and at which to administer hCG could also be a determining factor. It is necessary to highlight that the starting dose of gonadotropins used to vary between the two continents compared in the Appendix, but now the difference is less, ranging from 75 to 150 IU in the United States compared with Europe. This must be accounted for if such a trial is conducted with centers in the two continents. It would be interesting to perform a study separately in each continent among the authors of this book and perhaps with some variation of the defining landmarks, as the approach could address the same problems from a different angle[11,13,41].

REFERENCES

1. Delvigne A, Rozenberg S. Preventive attitude of physicians to avoid ovarian hyperstimulation syndrome in IVF patients. Hum Reprod 2001; 16: 2491–5.
2. Rabinovici J, Kushnir O, Shalev J, et al. Rescue of menotropin cycles prone to develop ovarian hyperstimulation. Br J Obstet Gynaecol 1987; 94: 1098–102.
3. Urman B, Pride SM, Ho Yuen B. Management of over-stimulated gonadotrophin cycles with a controlled drift period. Hum Reprod 1992; 7: 213–17.
4. Rizk B. Ovarian hyperstimulation syndrome. In Brinsden PR, Rainsbury PA, eds. A Textbook of In Vitro Fertilization and Assisted Reproduction. Carnforth, UK: Parthenon Publishing, 1992: 369–83.
5. Fluker MR, Hooper WM, Yuzpe AA. Withholding gonadotropins ('coasting') to minimize the risk of ovarian hyperstimulation during superovulation and in-vitro fertilization–embryo transfer cycles. Fertil Steril 1999; 71: 294 301.
6. Sher G, Salem R, Feinman M, et al. Eliminating the risks of life-endangering complications following over-stimulation with menotropin fertility agents: a report on women undergoing in-vitro fertilization and embryo transfer. Obstet Gynecol 1993; 81: 1009–11.
7. Delvigne A, Rozenberg S. A qualitative systematic review of coasting, a procedure to avoid ovarian hyperstimulation syndrome in IVF patients. Hum Reprod Update 2002; 8: 291–6.
8. Aboulghar MA, Mansour RT. Ovarian hyperstimulation syndrome: classifications and critical analysis of preventive measures. Hum Reprod Update 2003; 9: 275–89.
9. Rizk B, Aboulghar MA. Classification, pathophysiology and management of ovarian hyperstimulation syndrome. In Brinsden P, ed. A Textbook of In Vitro Fertilization and Assisted Reproduction. London: Taylor & Francis, 2005: 217–58.
10. Rizk B. Prevention of OHSS. In Rizk B, ed. Epidemiology, Pathophysiology, Prevention and Management of Ovarian Hyperstimulation Syndrome. Cambridge: Cambridge University Press, 2005: 264–94.
11. Rizk B, Grace J, Mulekhar M. Coasting is effective for abolishing the risk of OHSS but possibly decreases the quality of oocytes and pregnancy rates. Is that the price we pay? Fertil Steril 2006; in press.
12. Rizk B, Aboulghar M. Modern management of ovarian hyperstimulation syndrome. Hum Reprod 1991; 6: 1082–7.
13. Dhont M, Van der straiten F, De Sutter P. Prevention of severe ovarian hyperstimulation by coasting. Fertil Steril 1998; 70: 847–50.
14. Al-Shawaf T, Zosmer A, Hussain S, et al. Prevention of severe ovarian hyperstimulation syndrome in IVF with or without ICSI and embryo transfer: a modified 'coasting' strategy based on ultrasound for identification of high-risk patients. Hum Reprod 2001; 16: 24–30.
15. Waldenström U, Kahn J, Marsk L, et al. High pregnancy rates and successful prevention of severe ovarian hyperstimulation syndrome by 'prolonged coasting' of very hyperstimulated patients: a multi-centre study. Hum Reprod 1999; 14: 294–7.
16. Tozer AJ, Iles RK, Iammarrone E, et al. Characteristics of populations of granulosa cells from individual follicles in women undergoing 'coasting' during controlled ovarian stimulation (COS) for IVF. Hum Reprod 2004; 19: 2561–8.
17. Tozer AJ, Iles RK, Iammarrone E, et al. The effects of 'coasting' on follicular fluid concentrations of vascular endothelial growth factor in women at risk of developing ovarian hyperstimulation syndrome. Hum Reprod 2004; 19: 522–8.
18. Van Blerkom J, Antczak M, Schrader R. The developmental potential of the human oocyte is related to the dissolved oxygen content of follicular fluid: association with vascular endothelial growth factor levels and perifollicular blood

flow characteristics. Hum Reprod 1997; 12: 1047–55.

19. Rizk B, Aboulghar M, Smitz J, et al. The role of vascular endothelial growth factor and interleukins in the pathogenesis of severe ovarian hyperstimulation syndrome. Hum Reprod Update 1997; 3: 255–66.

20. McNatty KP, Makris A, DeGrazia C, et al. The production of progesterone, androgens and estrogens by granulosa cells, thecal tissue, and stromal tissue from human ovaries in vitro. J Clin Endocrinol Metab 1979; 49: 687–99.

21. Friedman CI, Seifer DB, Kennard EA, et al. Elevated level of follicular fluid vascular endothelial growth factor is a marker of diminished pregnancy potential. Fertil Steril 1998; 64: 268–72.

22. Barroso G, Barrionuevo M, Rao P, et al. Vascular endothelial growth factor, nitric oxide, and leptin follicular fluid levels correlate negatively with embryo quality in IVF patients. Fertil Steril 1999; 72: 1024–6.

23. Garcia-Velasco JA, Zuniga A, Pacheco A. Coasting acts through downregulation of VEGF gene expression and protein secretion. Hum Reprod 2004; 19: 1530–8.

24. Rizk B, Smitz J. Ovarian hyperstimulation syndrome after superovulation using GnRH agonists for IVF and related procedures. Hum Reprod 1992; 7: 320–7.

25. Sher G, Zouves C, Feinman M, et al. Prolonged coasting: an effective method. Hum Reprod 1995; 10: 3107–9.

26. Ben-Nun I, Shulman A, Ghetler Y, et al. The significance of 17β-estradiol levels in highly responding women during ovulation induction in IVF treatment: its impact and prognostic value with respect to oocyte maturation and treatment outcome. J Assist Reprod Genet 1993; 10: 213–15.

27. Benadiva CA, Davis O, Kligman I, et al. Withholding gonadotropin administration is an effective alternative for the prevention of ovarian hyperstimulation syndrome. Fertil Steril 1997; 67: 724–7.

28. Lee C, Tummon I, Martin J, et al. Does withholding gonadotrophin administration prevent severe ovarian hyperstimulation syndrome? Hum Reprod 1998; 13: 1157–8.

29. Tortoriello DV, McGovern PG, Colon JM, et al. 'Coasting' does not adversely affect cycle outcome in a subset of highly responsive in-vitro fertilization patients. Fertil Steril 1998; 69: 454–60.

30. Tortoriello DV, McGovern PG, Colon JM, et al. Critical ovarian hyperstimulation syndrome in a coasted in-vitro fertilization patient. Hum Reprod 1998; 13: 3005–8.

31. Aboulghar MA, Mansour RT, Serour GI, et al. Reduction of human menopausal gonadotropin dose before coasting prevents severe ovarian hyperstimulation syndrome with minimal cycle cancellation. J Assist Reprod Genet 2000; 17: 298–301.

32. Ohata Y, Harada T, Ito M, et al. Coasting may reduce the severity of the ovarian hyperstimulation syndrome in patients with polycystic ovary syndrome. Gynecol Obstet Invest 2000; 50: 186–8.

33. Grochowski D, Wolczynski S, Kuczynski W, et al. Correctly timed coasting reduces the risk of ovarian hyperstimulation syndrome and gives good cycle outcome in an in vitro fertilization program. Gynecol Endocrinol 2001; 15: 234–8.

34. Al-Shawaf T, Zosmer A, Tozer A, et al. Value of measuring serum FSH in addition to serum estradiol in a coasting programme to prevent severe OHSS. Hum Reprod 2002; 17: 1217–21.

35. Egbase PE, Al-Sharhan M, Grudzinskas JG. Early 'coasting' in patients with polycystic ovarian syndrome is consistent with good clinical outcome. Hum Reprod 2002; 17: 1212–16.

36. Ulug U, Bahceci M, Erden HF, et al. The significance of coasting duration during ovarian stimulation for conception in assisted fertilization cycles. Hum Reprod 2002; 17: 310–13.

37. Delvigne A, Carlier C, Rozenberg S. Is coasting effective for preventing ovarian hyperstimulation syndrome in patients receiving a gonadotropin-releasing hormone antagonist during an in vitro fertilization cycle? Fertil Steril 2001; 76: 844–6.

38. Levinsohn-Tavor S, Friedler M, Schachter A, et al. Coasting – what is the best formula? Hum Reprod 2003; 18: 937–40.

39. Isaza V, Garcia-Velasco JA, Aragones M, et al. Oocyte and embryo quality after coasting: the experience from oocyte donation. Hum Reprod 2002; 17: 1737–58.

40. Moreno L, Diaz I, Pacheco A, et al. Extended coasting duration exerts a negative impact on IVF cycle outcome due to premature luteinization. Reprod Biomed Online. 2004; 9: 500–4.

41. Delvigne A, Rozenberg S. Epidemiology and prevention of ovarian hyperstimulation syndrome (OHSS): a review. Hum Reprod Update 2002; 8: 559–77.

42. Rizk B. Classification of OHSS. In Rizk B, ed. Epidemiology, Pathophysiology, Prevention and Management of Ovarian Hyperstimulation Syndrome. Cambridge: Cambridge University Press, 2005: 6–26.

43. Egbase PE, Sharhan MA, Grudzinskas JG. Early unilateral follicular aspiration compared with coasting for the prevention of severe ovarian hyperstimulation syndrome: a prospective randomized study. Hum Reprod 1999; 14: 2922–3.

44. D'Angelo A, Amso N. 'Coasting' (withholding gonadotrophins) for preventing ovarian hyperstimulation syndrome. Cochrane Database Syst Rev 2002; (3): CD002811.

45. Aboulghar MA, Mansour RT, Serour GI, et al. Oocyte quality in patients with severe ovarian hyperstimulation syndrome. Fertil Steril 1997; 68: 1017–21.

46. Dechaud H, Anahory T, Aligier N, et al. Coasting: a response to excessive ovarian stimulation. Gynecol Obstet Fertil 2000; 28: 115–19.

47. Delvigne A, Manigart Y, Kostyla K, et al. Oocyte quality after coasting for ovarian hyperstimulation syndrome prevention. Hum Reprod 2002; 17: 153.

APPENDIX

Comparative table of differences in approach to OHSS between the USA and Europe

	*USA**	*Europe**
Starting dose of gonadotropins in the normal patient	225 IU for most patients, 150 IU or less for PCOS patients	225 IU hMG or 200 IU recFSH, 150 IU (100 IU) in patients at risk
Triggering dose of hCG usually used	10 000 IU, 5000 IU for patients at risk	10 000 IU, 5000 IU in patients at risk
Start coasting when E_2 exceeds ??? pg/ml (or pmol/ml)	3000 pg/ml	3500 pg/ml
Start coasting when number of follicles per ovary exceeds ???	30 follicles	Total 30 follicles in both ovaries or > 20 follicles in a single ovary
Start coasting when > 50% of follicles exceed ??? mm	14 mm	18 mm
Start coasting at any of the following combinations of serum E_2/sonography or other criteria	3000 pg/ml and 30 follicles	The threshold criteria for coasting can be lowered in very lean patients or patients with a previous history of OHSS
Maximum duration of coasting	No maximum, but some believe worse results for patients coasted longer than 4 days	4 days
Lower threshold at which hCG will be given	Wait until hCG drops below 3000 pg/ml	From 3000 pg/ml onwards
Other differences regarding coasting between USA and Europe	Most commonly used technique	
Out-patient management until severe OHSS grade A (Rizk and Aboulghar, 2005)	Most patients are managed as out-patient with aspiration and rehydration unless there is respiratory difficulty, kidney problems or biochemical problems	Ascites, severe discomfort and hematocrit of > 45

*USA data provided by Botros Rizk, European data provided by Marc Dhont; hCG, human chorionic gonadotropin; E_2, estradiol; PCOS, polycystic ovarian syndrome; hMG, human menopausal gonadotropin; recFSH, recombinant follicle stimulating hormone

CHAPTER 24

Health-economic reflections on ovarian hyperstimulation syndrome and the importance of registries

Petra De Sutter and Jan Gerris

HEALTH-ECONOMIC ASPECTS OF OVARIAN HYPERSTIMULATION SYNDROME

General considerations

Not much has been published on the costs induced by the occurrence of the ovarian hyperstimulation syndrome (OHSS) as part of a treatment with *in vitro* fertilization/intracytoplasmic sperm injection (IVF/ICSI) or as part of non-IVF treatments. In several of the more important papers on the cost-effectiveness of infertility treatment, no specific mention of the relative cost of OHSS is made[1–6]. In a paper by Philips *et al.*[7], IVF costs were analyzed in general and compared with other treatment options, and these authors estimated OHSS to yield an extra cost of 236.69 GBP (around €355) per unit, and the incidence of OHSS in their model was estimated to be 4%. In their calculations, OHSS contributed 0.5% to the total cost of IVF. The costs they used, however, were not real costs, but were derived from a separate cost model.

To calculate the costs associated with OHSS, one has to take into account several preliminary and interconnected considerations.

The management of the more serious forms of OHSS differs from one place to another. To try to save costs, in some countries or centers patients may be hospitalized only when severe symptoms and signs occur, whereas in others they may be hospitalized more readily, to avoid further deterioration of the patient. The standard operating procedures may be influenced by previous personal bad experience with OHSS patients. Criteria for hospitalization are not very strict, although there is some agreement, as shown by the publication of both American and European[8–10] guidelines. Frequently, specific national guidelines for the diagnosis and management of OHSS are in existence as well. Differences between American and European approaches are to be expected with respect to a technique such as coasting, but also with respect to indications for hospitalization. A hematocrit level of more than 45% is an absolute indication for hospitalization. If the hematocrit is between 42 and 45%, it is the clinical situation of the patient which determines whether hospital admission is required in order to monitor the patient closely or relieve symptoms. Also, costs in absolute terms may be very different from one hospital to another. Finally, both direct costs and indirect costs have to be taken into consideration.

A specific consideration is that if a human life is lost because of uncontrollable events linked to severe OHSS, this will be considered as an unacceptable outcome.

Apart from costs incurred by hospitalization in the case of severe OHSS, which can to a certain extent be calculated on the basis of real costs, there are extra costs which are the consequence of mild and moderate forms of OHSS not necessitating hospitalization. These include repeat visits to the center, repeat sonograms and blood examinations, the administration of symptomatic drugs and indirect costs due to incapacity to work.

In an attempt to construct a detailed cost analysis of ovarian hyperstimulation in its many and varied forms, including the tip of the iceberg called OHSS, all of these have to be taken into consideration.

Data analysis

To obtain an idea of the direct costs incurred by hospitalization of an average OHSS patient, we analyzed hospital bills of 77 patients who were hospitalized from 2001 until 2004 after IVF/ICSI in two Flemish centers (25 in the Middelheim Hospital (AZM) Antwerp and 52 in the University Hospital (UZ) Ghent). These 77 cases of OHSS occurred as complications in a total of 6238 IVF/ICSI treatments in the same period (1585 in AZM Antwerp and 4653 in UZ Ghent), leading to an observed incidence of 77/6238 = 1.23%, which corresponds to published incidence data as well as to the national average for Belgium (142/9494 = 1.49% for 2002). It should be noted, however, that some patients treated in either hospital and having developed OHSS, may have been subsequently hospitalized elsewhere and therefore were not included in the present analysis. This is definitely the case for patients coming from The Netherlands, who are often treated by microsurgical epididymal sperm aspiration/testicular sperm extraction (MESA/TESE) plus ICSI in Belgium because of differences in regulations between the two countries, but who are subsequently treated in their country of origin.

The mean age of the patients was 30.7 ± 4.3 years, which is significantly younger than the mean age of the total population of patients treated with IVF/ICSI in both centers (32.82 ± 4.50 in Antwerp and 34.1 ± 4.85 in Ghent).

Clinical data of the patients hospitalized for OHSS were not analyzed in detail for the purpose of this study. The number of oocytes obtained in the patient group at the time of egg retrieval was 18.4 ± 10.6 (median 15.5, range 4–53), which is, as expected, significantly higher than the mean number of oocytes in the whole population treated in both programs (median 10 for both hospitals) (Figure 1).

Hospitalization lasted between 1 and 20 days with a median of 4 days. Costs were divided into hospitalization cost (room cost), costs for drugs (the main cost driver being intravenous albumin), costs for medical fees and technical procedures (mainly sonography and ascites puncture) and miscellaneous other costs, and were found to vary between a minimum of €407 and a maximum of €7633 with a mean of €1539 ± 1247 (median €1012) (Figure 2). Table 1 shows that of this total cost of €1539, the room cost was €1004 (65%), the cost for drugs was €138 (9%), physician's costs were €350 (23%) and other costs €48 (3%). Because all patients included in this study benefited from reimbursement by the Belgian social security system, they had to pay on average €320 (21% of the total costs), whereas €1219 (79%) was paid by social security.

A multivariate analysis could not identify any correlation between patient-related parameters and either length of stay or cost parameters. This means that the duration and cost of the management of OHSS are as unpredictable as its occurrence in the first place. Prevention, therefore, once more, is the only sensible solution to the problem of OHSS.

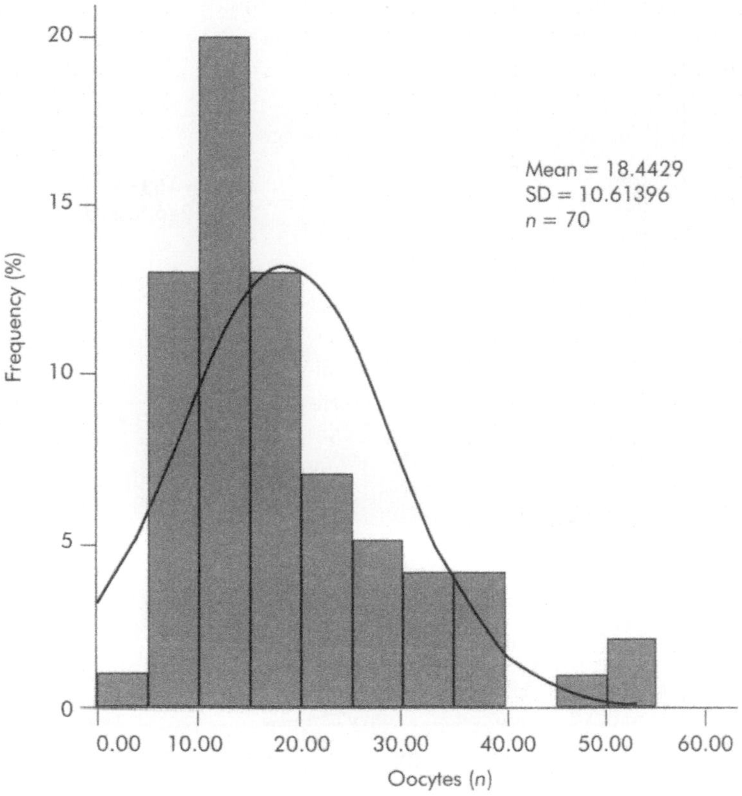

Figure 1 Frequency distribution of number of oocytes in patients hospitalized with OHSS

Exactly half of the patients hospitalized were pregnant and the other half were not. Neither the multivariate analysis nor a direct comparison of the groups of pregnant versus non-pregnant women hospitalized because of severe OHSS showed any difference in cost between groups (€1299 ± (SD) 941 versus €1445 ± (SD) 989 for non-pregnant versus pregnant patients, respectively).

Discussion

In Belgium, the total cost of one IVF/ICSI cycle, including gonadotropins, averages about €4000. When considering only treatments conducted in both centers as contributing to this analysis, this means that for a total expense of 6238 (total number of cycles) × €4000 = €24 952 000 needed for primary treatment over the period of time considered, an additional total expense of 77 (hospitalized OHSS cases) × €1539 = €118 503 is incurred for direct costs due to OHSS hospitalization. This does not include indirect costs due to working incapacity, and additional direct and indirect costs for OHSS patients who manage to escape hospitalization but nevertheless need extra consultation, sonography, blood tests and mostly analgesic drugs. These costs were not analyzed in this study, but may be estimated to be at least the same amount as the direct costs. This means that the total costs for OHSS

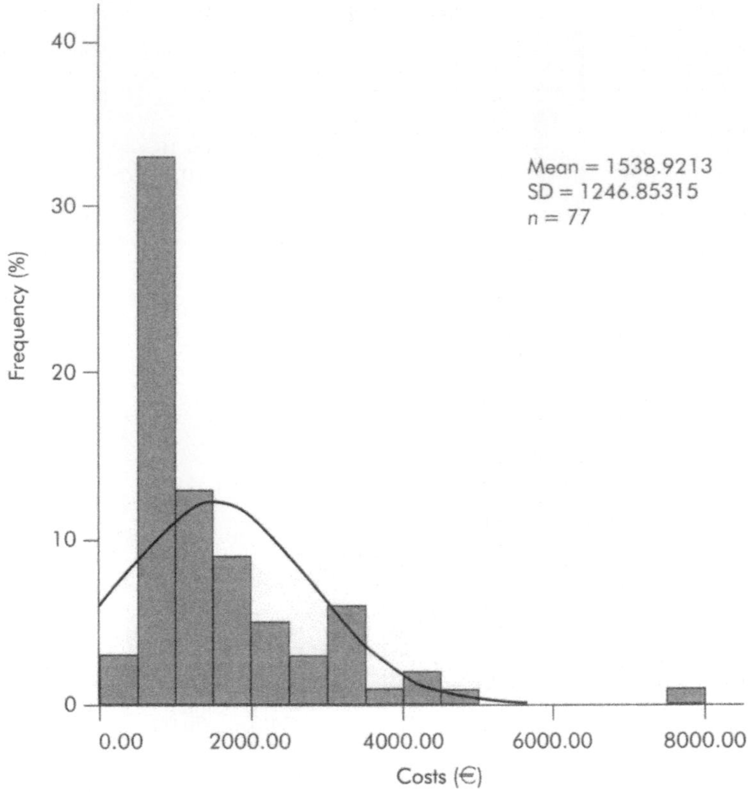

Figure 2 Frequency distribution of costs for hospitalized patients with OHSS

(about €237 000 with 1.23% severe cases) constitute approximately 1% of the primary treatment costs (€237 000 from €24 952 000).

More than half of these patients obtained an ongoing pregnancy, and it is therefore not possible to say that all these cases could have been prevented by not administering human chorionic gonadotropin (hCG) as an ovulation trigger. However, about two-thirds of patients clearly had the early form of the syndrome with a short hospitalization period, whereas one-third had a pregnancy enhanced form. Therefore, it makes sense to consider what the effect would have been if another ovulation trigger, e.g. recombinant luteinizing hormone (LH), had been used. It may be assumed that two-thirds of all OHSS cases could have been prevented in doing so, resulting in a saving of at least two-thirds of €237 000, i.e. approximately €158 000.

In terms of prevention, the administration of recombinant (rec)LH could theoretically reduce the incidence of OHSS if compared with the use of hCG to induce ovulation. We tried to calculate what the savings would be if recLH were to be used in all patients treated with IVF, or in a risk group. In Belgium, 1 ampoule of 5000 IU of hCG (required to induce ovulation in a patient at risk of OHSS) costs €4.65. If we hypothesize that (at least) two-thirds of all cases of OHSS could be prevented by administering recLH instead of hCG, the dose required might cost €158 000/6238 = approx. €25 as an equivalent.

Table 1 Costs of hospitalization (in €) of OHSS patients

	Mean	*Median*	*Standard deviation*	*Minimum*	*Maximum*
Hospital stay	1003.7	471.1	1094.8	200.5	6469.4
Pharmacy	137.8	62.8	233.0	2.2	1318.7
Physician	349.6	301.8	162.4	168.8	958.8
Other	47.9	13.5	202.4	0.0	1713.9
Total	1538.9	1012.1	1246.9	407.4	7633.0

In other words, even at a price five times as high as that of the currently used hCG, recLH would be cost-effective in preventing OHSS. Unfortunately, this product is not available at this price in the required dose, and until now the manufacturer has not (yet) decided to market this product further for this indication. However, whether this theoretical calculation holds is uncertain, because from the few data available to date, there seems not to be a lower incidence of OHSS after using recLH, although this has yet to be confirmed[11].

Besides the use of recLH, there could be other measures to prevent OHSS, such as the administration of methylprednisolone[12,13], coasting[14], unilateral ovarian aspiration[15] or avoiding transfer, and freezing all embryos[16]. The cost-effectiveness of these other measures to prevent OHSS must be computed to establish the most appropriate way to prevent OHSS from a health-economic perspective.

It is probable that even more is to be gained if one considers the predictive factors for the early form of OHSS as well as the reduction in morbidity in cases treated on an out-patient basis.

THE IMPORTANCE OF REGISTRIES

An issue that is linked to the problem of cost is the problem of correct registration of complications. The two most important complications of IVF/ICSI are multiple pregnancies and the ovarian hyperstimulation syndrome. Registration of the former has been part of national and supranational IVF/ICSI registries for a number of years now. Although at present not the case, it seems likely that at some time in the future there will be a reliable registration of the percentage of singletons and twins. The relative occurrence of singletons and twins may even be part of the way of reporting quality, using the acronym CUSIDERA (cumulative singleton delivery rate) as a measure of efficiency and CUTWIDERA (cumulative twin delivery rate) as a measure of safety[17].

For OHSS, the situation is more complex. There is a problem of definition to start with. What are mild, moderate and severe OHSS? May mild OHSS become severe OHSS? What do we want to register: only cases with hospitalization because they tend to be costly, or all cases with a minimal clinical impact because they tend to give an idea of how aggressively stimulations are conducted? Or, perhaps, do we want to register just lethal cases with the more than certain risk of severe underreporting?

Nevertheless, registration of OHSS makes sense for several reasons.

OHSS can lead to a potentially lethal outcome, and the symptomatology of its complications (mainly of a thromboembolic nature) may be masked by the other signs and symptoms of the syndrome. It can be hoped that the immediate reasons for any death due to OHSS can be properly understood so that future similar cases might eventually be saved. We should not be scared by the perfidious sensationalism of the modern-day press, but strive towards anonymous registration.

This is not an easy task. If a major complication occurs, the patient will be transferred to an intensive-care unit and treatment will be taken over by other health professionals. If there is no good registration and/or reporting of the major complications or even mortality of OHSS, and if a major complication or mortality occurs, the patient will be mentioned in the registries under the final diagnosis (often thrombosis and/or embolism), but the link with the OHSS cause could be lost. In our opinion, it is therefore mandatory that IVF registries track down all cases of severe OHSS and record their complications and outcome. Only in this way will the real size of the OHSS problem be known and the necessity of its prevention be obvious to everyone treating patients for infertility through assisted reproductive technologies (ART).

ACKNOWLEDGMENT

We thank Prof. dr. Lieven Annemans, Department of Health Economics, University Hospital Ghent, for his valuable help in performing the cost calculations.

REFERENCES

1. Collins J, Feeny D, Gunby J. The costs of infertility diagnosis and treatment in Canada in 1995. Hum Reprod 1997; 12: 951–8.
2. Van Voorhis BJ, Sparks AE, Allen BD, et al. Cost-effectiveness of infertility treatments: a cohort study. Fertil Steril 1997; 67: 830–6.
3. Wølner-Hanssen P, Rydhstroem H. Cost-effectiveness analysis of in-vitro fertilisation: estimated costs per successful pregnancy after transfer of one or two embryos. Hum Reprod 1998; 13: 88–94.
4. De Sutter P, Gerris J, Dhont M. A health-economic decision-analytic model comparing double with single embryo transfer in IVF/ICSI. Hum Reprod 2002; 17: 2891–6.
5. Garceau L, Henderson J, Davis LJ, et al. Economic implications of assisted reproductive techniques: a systematic review. Hum Reprod 2002; 17: 3090–109.
6. Mansour R, Aboulghar M, Serour GI, et al. The use of clomiphene citrate/human menopausal gonadotrophins in conjunction with GnRH antagonist in an IVF/ICSI program is not a cost effective protocol. Acta Obstet Gynecol Scand 2003; 82: 48–52.
7. Philips Z, Barraza-Llorens M, Posnett J. Evaluation of the relative cost-effectiveness of treatments for infertility in the UK. Hum Reprod 2000; 15: 95–106.
8. American Society for Reproductive Medicine (Practice Committee). Ovarian hyperstimulation syndrome. Fertil Steril 2003; 80: 1309–14.
9. Royal College of Obstetricians and Gynaecologists. Guideline on 'The Management of Infertility in Tertiary Care', London: RCOG, 2000. (downloadable at http://www.nelh.nhs.uk/guidelinesdb/html/downloads/infertility_tertiary_care.pdf).
10. Gerris J, Delvigne A, Olivennes F, Nygren K. Ovarian Hyperstimulation Syndrome Short Management Guidelines. Beigem, Belgium: ESHRE, in preparation. (downloadable at http://www.eshre.com/emc.asp?pageId=567).
11. Al-Inany H, Aboulghar M, Mansour R, Proctor M. Recombinant versus urinary human chorionic gonadotrophin for ovulation induction in assisted conception. Cochrane Database Syst Rev 2005; (2): CD003719.
12. Lainas T, Petsas G, Stavropoulou G, et al. Administration of methylprednisolone to prevent severe ovarian hyperstimulation syndrome in patients undergoing in vitro fertilization. Fertil Steril 2002; 78: 529–33.
13. Schwarzler P, Abendstein BJ, Klingler A, et al. Prevention of severe ovarian hyperstimulation

syndrome (OHSS) in IVF patients by steroidal ovarian suppression – a prospective randomized study. Hum Fertil (Camb) 2003; 6: 125–9.

14. Delvigne A, Rozenberg S. A qualitative systematic review of coasting, a procedure to avoid ovarian hyperstimulation syndrome in IVF patients. Hum Reprod Update 2002; 8: 291–6.

15. Schroder AK, Schopper B, Al-Hasani S, et al. Unilateral follicular aspiration and in-vitro maturation before contralateral oocyte retrieval: a method to prevent ovarian hyperstimulation syndrome. Eur J Obstet Gynecol Reprod Biol 2003; 110: 186–9.

16. Queenan JT. Embryo freezing to prevent ovarian hyperstimulation syndrome. Mol Cell Endocrinol 2000; 169: 79–83.

17. Germond M, Urner F, Chanson A, et al. What is the most relevant standard of success in assisted reproduction? The cumulated singleton/twin delivery rates per oocyte pick-up: the CUSIDERA and CUTWIDERA. Hum Reprod 2004; 19: 2442–4.

CHAPTER 25

Intravenous hydroxyethyl starch infusion and albumin administration: effective tools as adjuvants in the prevention of ovarian hyperstimulation syndrome

Oya Gökmen and A Zeki Isik

The induction of ovulation by gonadotropins can result in ovarian hyperstimulation syndrome (OHSS), which can be lethal in its severest form. Mild and moderate ovarian hyperstimulation are usually self-limited and require no further treatment other than observation. Severe OHSS, appearing in about 0.2–5% of cases undergoing induction of ovulation, is characterized by massive ovarian enlargement, ascites, pleural effusion, oliguria, hemoconcentration and thromboembolic phenomena[1–4]. Accumulation of extravascular protein-rich exudate in the peritoneum and in the pleura combined with intravascular volume depletion and hemoconcentration are essential characteristics of the syndrome and are related to an increased capillary permeability[5–7].

Primary and secondary preventive measures have been discussed in previous chapters. In this chapter, the value of the intravenous administration of albumin and hydroxyethyl starch (HES) is discussed in more specific detail.

INTRAVENOUS ALBUMIN ADMINISTRATION FOR THE PREVENTION OF OHSS

Two of its properties make albumin worthwhile both in the prevention and in the treatment of OHSS. First, albumin is the most abundant circulating protein, and responsible for 70–80% of plasma oncotic pressure. Second, it is the principal binding and carrier protein for a variety of substances including fatty acids, drugs, bilirubin and hormones[8]. Thus, albumin administration is able to prevent the fluid shift to the third space, and binds the above-mentioned factor or factors responsible for the major events in the development of OHSS. Human albumin also has an excellent record of both clinical and viral safety[9–11]. Therefore, albumin has been recognized as an effective volume expander in the treatment of severe OHSS[12,13].

The administration of intravenous (IV) albumin to prevent the development of severe OHSS was first suggested by Asch *et al.*[14]. Although no case of severe OHSS developed in this series, the study was not controlled, it had a small sample size ($n = 36$) and the embryo transfer rate was low, 15 transfers out of 36 cycles. Other prospective, randomized, controlled studies have given support to the effectiveness of IV albumin in the prevention of severe OHSS[15–18]. In the study of Shoham *et al.*, 31 cases with a mean serum estradiol level of 1906 pg/ml were randomized to receive, IV, either 50 g albumin or saline at the time of oocyte retrieval[15]. No case of severe OHSS was recorded in the albumin group, whereas four cases required hospitalization in the saline group. Shalev *et al.* also found a significantly higher number of severe OHSS cases ($n = 4$) in the control group than in the treatment group, who received a dose of IV albumin (20 g) after oocyte retrieval[16]. Isik *et al.* also reported a significant difference in favor of albumin treatment[17]. In another study, patients at risk of developing severe OHSS were randomized to receive IV albumin and transfer of fresh embryos or cryopreservation of all embryos[18]. Severe OHSS was not observed in any of the patients in either group. The results of these studies all confirmed that human albumin is an effective method in the prevention of OHSS.

Others have postulated that IV albumin given to high-risk patients is only beneficial in cases which do not conceive or carry singleton pregnancies[19].

In contrast, doubt was cast on the potential preventive effect IV administration of albumin on patients at risk of OHSS by Ng *et al.*[20]. In their cohort study, they stated that IV albumin does not prevent OHSS. The prospective, randomized, placebo-controlled, double-blind study of Ben-Chetrit *et al.* recorded four severe and five moderate OHSS cases in the IV albumin group ($n = 46$)[21]. In the control group, severe OHSS developed in one case and moderate OHSS in five patients. As no significant difference in the incidence of OHSS was found between the two groups, the authors suggested that albumin has no positive effect on OHSS rates.

Albumin as a potential preventive measure in OHSS was further investigated in a recent large randomized controlled trial[22]. Women undergoing *in vitro* fertilization (IVF) with > 20 retrieved oocytes ($n = 988$) were randomized to receive 40 g albumin IV or no treatment. No difference was found between the two groups in OHSS rates. Severe OHSS was observed in 5% of the albumin group and 4.7% in the control group. Although the study group consisted of patients considered at risk of developing moderate or severe OHSS, the standard protocol for controlled ovarian stimulation as starting dose was 225 IU/day of highly purified or recombinant follicle stimulating hormone (FSH) plus 75 IU/day of human menopausal gonadotropin (hMG), which was a fairly high dose for this group of patients. The high incidence of severe OHSS and the comment of the authors that albumin infusion on the day of oocyte retrieval was not useful for preventing the development of OHSS could be due to this high starting dose of gonadotropin administration, and to the absence of any other preventive measure against OHSS in this high-risk population. On the other hand, they stated that they did not see any side-effect in the albumin group, and albumin infusion did not seem to affect the IVF outcome.

A Cochrane review on the use of IV albumin to prevent severe OHSS enrolled 378 women (193 albumin-treated and 185 controls) from five randomized controlled trials[23]. The results of the meta-analysis pointed out a significant decrease in severe OHSS by albumin administration, with an absolute risk reduction of 5.5 (odds ratio = 0.28, 95% confidence interval 0.11–0.73). The details of the controlled studies using IV albumin versus placebo for the prevention of OHSS are listed in Table 1[24].

Isik *et al.* suggested a combined approach for the prevention of OHSS in high-risk patients by combining a late step-down administration of gonadotropins, a decreased dose of human chorionic gonadotropin (hCG) to trigger ovulation, IV albumin adminstration and progesterone use for luteal support[25]. The authors reported that this approach in their hands proved to be effective, and it has been supported by others[4,26]. The same group obtained extended experience using this combined approach in the prevention of severe to moderate OHSS[27]. The results for 87 high-risk patients managed by this approach were compared with those for 274 low-risk patients.

Table 1 Intravenous albumin for prevention of ovarian hyperstimulation syndrome (OHSS): controlled studies versus placebo

		No. of patients						
Study	*Type*	*Total*	*Albumin (IV)*	*Control*	*Albumin dose*	*E_2 level on day of hCG (pg/ml)*	*No. OHSS (albumin)*	*No. OHSS (control)*
Shoham *et al.*, 1994	Prospective randomized	31	16	15	50 g	1906	0	4
Shalev *et al.*, 1995	Prospective randomized	40	22	18	20 g	> 2500	0	4
Isik *et al.*, 1996	Prospective randomized	55	27	28	10 mg	≥ 3000	0	4
Ben Chetrit *et al.*, 2001	Prospective randomized	87	46	41	50 g	2724	4	1
Ng *et al.*, 1995	Cohort controlled	207	49	158	50 g	2724	2	10
Chen *et al.*, 1997	Prospective historical control	72	30	42	According to BMI	≥ 3600	4	14

In summary, the results of the studies can still be considered inconclusive, and the role of albumin in preventing severe OHSS in the eyes of these authors needs to be further clarified by multicenter, randomized, prospective studies. The routine use of albumin in high-risk patients must be judged by clinicians until large randomized trials give a definitive answer. When considering the data above, it seems that the use of albumin can be advocated, preferably in combination with other approaches rather than on its own.

PROPHYLACTIC INFUSION OF HYDROXYETHYL STARCH SOLUTION

Hydroxyethyl starch (HES) is a synthetic colloid, glycogen-like polysaccharide derived from amylopectin. It is an effective volume expander. It exists in different molecular weights: high-molecular-weight (MW) HES of 400 kDa; medium-MW HES of 200 kDa and low-MW HES of 50–100 kDa. These different HES molecules have different clinical properties. High-MW HES has a longer half-life, and it is associated more frequently with coagulation deficiencies (decrease in factor VIII, fibrinogen and von Willebrand factor). HES of MW 200, which was used in our practice, is associated less with such problems[36,37].

HES (MW 200) is used in several clinical conditions, such as hypovolemia associated with major surgery, circulatory shock or sepsis, and during and after cardiac operations[28]. HES provides volume expansion comparable to that of human albumin, and many papers have been published comparing albumin with HES in various clinical conditions. These studies were mainly anesthesiology- or critical-care medicine-related, and the authors in these series have concluded that HES and albumin have comparable efficacy[37]. Although it has been well known for a long time that HES is a cheaper alternative to human albumin, its use in the prevention and treatment of OHSS was not evaluated until recently.

Abramov *et al.* suggested that hydroxyethyl starch might be superior to albumin as a colloid solution for the treatment of severe OHSS. They have previously shown that severe OHSS is characterized by the leakage of albumin (with a molecular weight of 69 kDa) as well as immunoglobulins IgG and IgA (with molecular weights of 150 kDa and 180 kDa, respectively) to the abdominal cavity. No leakage of IgM, which has a molecular weight of 900 kDa, has been observed. IgA has been shown to leak more. It has been concluded that molecular weight is the most important factor determining protein extravasation. Therefore, low-molecular-weight human albumin solution for preservation of intravascular oncotic pressure in severe OHSS remains controversial[29,30].

The side-effects of HES treatment were anaphylactoid reactions causing pruritus and skin symptoms such as urticaria on the trunk, anus and legs[31]. Other reported complications related to high-molecular-weight HES included serum macroamylasemia, severe pruritus and, most important, bleeding complications and increases in prothrombin and bleeding time[31]. With the use of medium-molecular-weight HES, these complications are rare. The tendency toward bleeding in coagulation tests was found to be reassuring because of the state of hypercoagulation in controlled ovarian hyperstimulation. HES is removed from the circulation by two major mechanisms: renal excretion and redistribution. Renal excretion has two distinct phases. The first phase occurs upon administration, and a second phase of prolonged glomerular filtration ensues as HES molecules are metabolized. The duration of volume expansion with HES is approximately 24 h, with 29–38% of the colloid still available after this time.

The prospective study of Graf *et al.* compared high-risk patients (estradiol > 11 010 pmol/l and > 20 follicles) ($n = 100$), who received 1000 ml of 6% HES at the time of oocyte retrieval and

500 ml 48 h later, with control-group patients ($n = 82$) who were not treated with HES[32].

No reduction in severe OHSS was seen. In another prospective, randomized, placebo-controlled study by König *et al.*, 1000 ml of 6% HES was given after embryo transfer in a total number of 101 high-risk patients. It showed a significantly lower number of OHSS cases in the study group ($p = 0.031$)[33].

As HES is cheaper and carries no risk of viral or prion transmission of a blood product compared with albumin, it has been tested in the prevention of OHSS by different groups.

Gökmen *et al.* carried out a study in a large series to evaluate the efficacy of the prophylactic use of HES by comparing it with albumin, and a control group, in patients at risk of developing OHSS, in a prospective, randomized placebo-controlled trial[34]. In all 250 patients (cycles) considered at risk of developing OHSS in an IVF program were included in this trial. Criteria for inclusion were: serum estradiol value of > 3000 pg/ml or the presence of > 20 follicles of > 14 mm on the day of hCG administration. The characteristics of patients and treatment variables for the HES, albumin and control groups were similar with respect to patient age, serum estradiol level on the day of hCG, body mass index (BMI), the number of oocytes retrieved, the number of embryos transferred and pregnancies. The first group ($n = 85$) received 500 ml of 6% HES, the second group ($n = 85$) received 50 ml of 20% human albumin and the third group ($n = 83$) received a placebo. Table 2 presents the number and percentage of patients who developed moderate and severe OHSS in all patients receiving either HES ($n = 85$), albumin ($n = 85$) or placebo ($n = 83$). There were no severe OHSS cases in patients who received albumin and HES, whereas four patients who received a placebo developed severe OHSS. On the other hand, moderate OHSS was encountered in four patients in the albumin group, in five patients receiving HES and in 12 patients receiving placebo. The authors concluded that both HES and albumin significantly reduced the incidence of moderate and severe OHSS.

The same group further enlarged their study group and presented a randomized, prospective, placebo-controlled study of intravenous albumin versus hydroxyethyl starch for the prevention of ovarian hyperstimulation in an IVF program. This study was designed to assess the effectiveness of IV administration of 6% hydroxyethyl starch solution or intravenous 20% albumin versus a placebo group in the prevention of moderate and severe ovarian hyperstimulation (OHSS). Three hundred and twenty women who had a serum estradiol value of > 3000 pg/ml

Table 2 Comparison of incidence of ovarian hyperstimulation syndrome (OHSS) among groups of patients receiving hydroxyethyl starch (HES) or albumin for the prevention of OHSS

	HES group (n = 85)		*Albumin group (n = 85)*		*Control group (n = 83)*		
	n	*%*	*n*	*%*	*n*	*%*	*p Value*
Moderate	5	5.9	4	4.9	12	14.5	< 0.05
Severe	—	—	—	—	4	4.8	< 0.05
Overall	5	5.9	4	4.9	16	19.2	< 0.01

and/or > 20 follicles of ≥ 14 mm on the day of hCG administration were recruited and allotted to one of three groups: the HES group ($n = 112$) received 500 ml of 6% HES (Isohes; Eczacıbası/Baxter, Turkey); the albumin group ($n = 105$) received 50 ml (10 g) of 20% human albumin (Albumin Human; Octopharma/Berk, Turkey); and the placebo group ($n = 103$) received 500 ml of sodium chloride 0.9% solution, infused over a period of 30 min immediately after oocyte retrieval. The three groups were similar in age, serum estradiol level on the day of hCG, body mass index, number of oocytes retrieved, number of embryos transferred and duration of coasting (Table 3). Table 4 presents the number of patients who developed moderate, severe and overall (moderate + severe) OHSS in all groups. There was a statistically significant difference in the incidence of moderate, severe and overall OHSS among groups (p values < 0.05, < 0.05, < 0.01). Both HES and albumin significantly reduced the incidence of moderate and severe and the overall incidence of OHSS[35].

CONCLUSION

In conclusion, the combination of several effective measures of prevention of OHSS should be

Table 3 Baseline and cycle characteristics of the patients in a study of intravenous albumin versus hydroxyethyl starch (HES) for the prevention of OHSS[35]

	HES group (*n* = *112*)	*Albumin* (*n* = *105*)	*Control group* (*n* = *103*)	*p Value*
Age (years)	29.8 ± 4.3	30.0 ± 4.7	29.6 ± 2.8	n.s.
E_2 on hCG day	4975 ± 12.0	4556 ± 10.11	4940 ± 15.71	n.s.
BMI (kg/m^2)	22.1 ± 2.5	20.2 ± 2.1	2.3 ± 1.5	n.s.
No. of oocytes retrieved	15 ± 1.6	14 ± 4.7	13.2 ± 5.6	n.s.
No. of embryos transferred	3.4 ± 1.1	3.2 ± 1.1	3.0 ± 3	n.s.
No. of pregnancies	50.5% ($n = 136$)	44.1% ($n = 119$)	43.4% ($n = 117$)	n.s.

n.s., not significant

Table 4 Comparison of incidence of OHSS among the groups in the study[35]

	HES group (*n* = *112*)	*Albumin* (*n* = *105*)	*Control group* (*n* = *103*)	*p Value*
Moderate (n)	8	7	18	< 0.5
Severe (n)	—	—	6	< 0.05
Total (n)	8	7	24	< 0.05

assessed by more groups in order to reach a consensus on this issue, as no single measure can totally prevent OHSS.

In our experience, 500 ml of 6% HES of MW 200 kDa used during ovum pick-up is as effective as 50 ml of 20% human albumin to reduce the incidence of OHSS or blunt its clinical severity. Because its use carries no risk for infection with blood-borne agents and because it costs less than albumin, HES might be a more promising alternative to albumin for the treatment of OHSS.

REFERENCES

1. Navot D, Bergh PA, Laufer N. Ovarian hyperstimulation syndrome in novel reproductive technologies. Prevention and treatment. Fertil Steril 1992; 58: 249–61.
2. Al-Ramahi M. Severe OHSS – decreasing the risk of severe ovarian hyperstimulation syndrome. Hum Reprod 1999; 14: 2421–2.
3. Forman RG. Severe OHSS – an acceptable price? Hum Reprod 1999; 14; 2687–8.
4. Graf MA, Fischer R. Severe OHSS. An 'epidemic' of severe OHSS: a price we have to pay? Hum Reprod 1999; 14: 2930–1.
5. Chen CD, Chen HF, Lu HF, et al. Value of serum and follicular fluid cytokine profile in the prediction of moderate to severe ovarian hyperstimulation syndrome. Hum Reprod 2000; 15: 1037–42.
6. Albert C, Garrido N, Mercader A, et al. The role of endothelial cells in the pathogenesis of ovarian hyperstimulation syndrome. Mol Hum Reprod 2002; 8: 409–18.
7. Gomez R, Simon C, Remohi J, et al. Vascular endothelial growth factor receptor-2 activation induces vascular permeability in hyperstimulated rats and this effect is prevented by receptor blockage. Endocrinology 2002; 143: 4339–48.
8. Tullis J. Albumin 2. Guidelines for clinical use. JAMA 1977; 237: 460–3.
9. Horowitz B. Blood protein derivative viral safety: observations and analysis. Yale J Biol Med 1990; 63: 361–9.
10. Horowitz B. Specific inactivation of viruses which can potentially contaminate blood products. Dev Biol Standard 1991; 75: 43–52.
11. Grandgeorge M, Pelloquin F. Inactivation of the human immunodeficiency viruses (HIV-1 and HIV-2) during the manufacturing of placental albumin and gammaglobulin. Transfusion 1989; 29: 629–34.
12. Forman RG, Frydman R, Egan D, et al. Severe ovarian hyperstimulation syndrome using agonists of gonadotropin releasing hormone for in vitro fertilization: European series and a proposal for prevention. Fertil Steril 1990; 53: 502–9.
13. Meldrum DR, Wisot A, Hamilton F, et al. Routine pituitary suppression with leuprolide before ovarian stimulation for oocyte retrieval. Fertil Steril 1989; 51: 455–9.
14. Asch RP, Ivery G, Goldsman M, et al. The use of intravenous albumin in patients at risk for severe ovarian hyperstimulation. Hum Reprod 1993; 8: 1015–20.
15. Shoham Z, Weissman A, Barash A, et al. Intravenous albumin for the prevention of severe ovarian hyperstimulation syndrome in an in vitro fertilization programme: a prospective, randomized, placebo-controlled study. Fertil Steril 1994; 62: 137–42.
16. Shalev E, Giladi Y, Matiski M, et al. Decreased incidence of severe ovarian hyperstimulation syndrome in high risk in vitro fertilization patients receiving intravenous albumin. Hum Reprod 1995; 10: 807–10.
17. Isık A, Gokmen O, Zeyneloglu HB, et al. Intravenous albumin prevents moderate–severe hyperstimulation in in vitro fertilization patients: a prospective, randomized and controlled study. Eur J Obstet Gynecol Reprod Biol 1996; 70: 179–83.
18. Shaker AG, Zosmer A, Dean N, et al. Comparison between intravenous albumin and transfer of fresh embryos with cryopreservation of all embryos for subsequent transfer in prevention

of ovarian hyperstimulation syndrome. Fertil Steril 1996; 65: 992–6.

19. Chen CD, Wu MY, Yang JH, et al. Intravenous albumin does not prevent the development of severe ovarian hyperstimulation syndrome. Fertil Steril 1997; 68: 287–91.

20. Ng E, Leader A, Claman P, et al. Intravenous albumin does not prevent the development of severe ovarian hyperstimulation syndrome in an in vitro fertilization programme. Hum Reprod 1995; 10: 807–10.

21. Ben-Chetrit A, Eldar-Geva T, Gal M, et al. The questionable use of albumin for the prevention of ovarian hyperstimulation syndrome in an IVF programme: a randomized placebo-controlled trial. Hum Reprod 2001; 16: 1880–4.

22. Bellver J, Munoz EA, Ballesteros A, et al. Intravenous albumin does not prevent moderate–severe ovarian hyperstimulation syndrome in high risk IVF patients: a randomized controlled study. Hum Reprod 2003; 18: 2283–8.

23. Aboulghar M, Evers JH, Al-Inany H. Intravenous albumin for preventing severe ovarian hyperstimulation syndrome. Cochrane Database Syst Rev 2002; (2): CD001302.

24. Aboulghar M, Mansour RT. Ovarian hyperstimulation syndrome: classifications and critical analysis of preventive measures. Hum Reprod Update 2003; 9: 275–89.

25. Isık AZ, Kahraman S, Vicdan K, et al. Intravenous albumin combined with low dose human chrionic gonadotropin and late step down administration of menotropins are effective in prevention of severe ovarian hyperstimulation syndrome in high risk patients in an in vitro fertilization programme. J Middle East Fertil Soc 1997; 2: 238–42.

26. Hillensjö T, Wikland M, Wood M. Albumin in the prevention of severe OHSS [Letter]. Hum Reprod 1999; 14: 1664.

27. Isık AZ, Vicdan K. Combined approach as an effective method in the prevention of severe ovarian hyperstimulation syndrome. Eur J Obstet Gynecol 2001; 97: 208–12.

28. Shatney CH, Krishnapradad D, Militello PR. Efficacy of hetastarch in the resucitation of patients with multitrauma and shock. Arch Surg 1983; 68: 287–91.

29. Abramov Y, Naparstek Y, Elchalal U, et al. Plasma immunoglobulins in patients with severe ovarian hyperstimulation syndrome. Fertil Steril 1999; 71: 102–5.

30. Rabinerson D, Ben Rafael Z, Keslin J, et al. 10% HES for plasma expansion in the treatment of severe ovarian hyperstimulation syndrome. A case report. J Reprod Med 2001; 46: 68–70.

31. Warren B, Durieux ME. Hydroxyethyl starch: safe or not? Anesth Analg 1997;84: 206–12.

32. Graf MA, Fischer R, Naether OG, et al. Reduced incidence of ovarian hyperstimulation syndrome by prophylactic infusion of hydroxyethyl starch solution in an in vitro fertilization programme. Hum Reprod 1997; 12: 2599–602.

33. König E, Bussen S, Sutterlin M, et al. Prophylactic iv hydroxyethl starch solution prevents moderate–severe ovarian hyperstimulation in in vitro fertilization patients: a prospective, randomized, double-blind and placebo controlled study. Hum Reprod 1998; 13: 2421–4.

34. Gökmen O, Ugur M, Ekin M, et al. Intravenous albumin versus hydroxyethyl starch for the prevention of ovarian hyperstimulation in in vitro fertilization programme: a prospective randomized placebo controlled study. Eur J Obstet Gynecol Reprod Biol 2001; 96: 187–92.

35. Gökmen O, Akar M, Ozcan S. A randomized prospective placebo-controlled study of intravenous albumin versus hydroxyethyl starch for the prevention of ovarian hyperstimulation in IVF. Poster presentation at the Annual Meeting of the American Society for Reproductive Medicine, Montreal, October 2005.

CHAPTER 26

Ovarian hyperstimulation syndrome: summary and guidelines

Jan Gerris and Petra De Sutter

DESCRIPTION OF THE PROBLEM

Definition

The ovarian hyperstimulation syndrome (OHSS) is an iatrogenic complication of the luteal phase and/or early pregnancy after ovulation induction (provoking ovulation in anovulatory women) or after ovarian stimulation (in the context of intrauterine insemination or *in vitro* fertilization).

Essential characteristics

The essence of OHSS is cystic enlargement of the ovaries and a fluid shift from the intravascular to the third space due to increased capillary permeability and ovarian neoangiogenesis. Its occurrence is dependent on the administration of human chorionic gonadotropin (hCG). Without hCG, OHSS is extremely rare. Its impact on the general health of the patient may be very important. Fatal cases have occasionally been reported.

Early and late forms of OHSS

The early form of OHSS, although elicited by hCG, is related to an exaggerated ovarian response to gonadotropin stimulation, whereas the late form is mainly related to the secretion of placental hCG. The most recent definition[1] still relies on the underlying etiology, but makes a clear distinction between the early form (< 10 days after the ovulation-triggering injection of hCG) and the late form (≥ 10 days after hCG). Particularly those cases which are constituted by a combination of the early form followed by pregnancy are serious and long-lasting[2].

ANALYSIS OF AVAILABLE KNOWLEDGE

Incidence

Precise figures of incidence are unknown because of a lack of systematic registration. Mild ovarian hyperstimulation probably occurs in 8–23% of stimulated cycles, moderate forms in < 1–7% and severe forms in ~ 0.5% of stimulated cycles[3,4]. This causes severe OHSS to be viewed by individual gynecologists as a relatively rare complication. However, the total annual number of cases in the world is estimated to be in the thousands. The incidence has almost certainly increased over the years[5]. There are fatal cases, although these are never reported. Given the reason for treatment (infertility in young healthy women), each death is a disaster that should have been avoided.

Symptoms

Most frequent symptoms and signs

- Low-abdominal distension;
- Progressive increase in abdominal circumference measured at the level of the umbilicus;
- Ovaries enlarged up to > 12 cm;
- Nausea and vomiting preventing intake of food and fluids;
- Dyspnea and respiratory distress due to an elevated diaphragm and hydrothorax;
- Diarrhea;
- Quick weight gain.

More severe signs and symptoms

- Ascites;
- Hypotension;
- Pleural effusion (more and more frequently at the right side);
- Pericardial effusion;
- Adult form of respiratory distress syndrome;
- Oliguria and anuria;
- Multiple organ failure;
- Death (1/500 000 cycles)[6].

Biological findings

- Electrolyte disorders (hyponatremia < 136 mmol/l; hyperkalemia > 5.0 mmol/l);
- Hypovolemia;
- Hemoconcentration (hematocrit > 45%);
- Leukocytosis > 15 000/mm^3;
- Creatinine clearance < 50 ml/min; serum creatinine > 1.2 mg/dl;
- Elevated liver enzymes;
- Hypercoagulability;
- Hypoproteinemia and hypoalbuminemia (< 30 g/l).

Additional complications

Ovarian torsion This causes sudden, extreme abdominal pain and nausea. There is an incidence of 1/5000 stimulation cycles, but is more frequent if OHSS and pregnancy are present[7].

Ovarian bleeding This is caused by ovarian rupture or intraovarian bleeding as a result of pressure or bimanual examination. It leads to signs of acute hemorrhage (hypotension, nausea, sudden drop in hematocrit).

Thromboembolic symptoms Both venous (65.7%) and arterial localizations have been described; 83% of these occur in neck, arm or head veins (60%); thrombosis also occurs in arteries and veins of the lower body[8]; in 4–12% pulmonary embolism occurs[9]. Embolism has been described in the V. humeralis, subclavia, jugularis interna and cava, and arterial cases in the A. subclavia, ulnaris, carotis interna and cerebri media and in the coronary arteries.

Primary risk factors

- Polycystic ovarian syndrome (PCOS);
- Patients with some characteristics of PCOS:
  - High number of follicles in both ovaries at the quiescent state before stimulation (≥ 10 follicles of 4–10 mm in each ovary);
  - luteinizing hormone/follicle stimulating hormone (LH/FSH) ratio > 2;
  - Hyperandrogenism;

- History of OHSS;
- Young patients (less evidence);
- Lean women (less evidence);
- Allergic predisposition (less evidence).

Secondary risk factors

- Maximum serum estradiol > 3000–4000 pg/ml:
  - No clear cut-off value;
  - Relatively poor predictive power (max. 73%);
  - Estradiol itself is no mediator since OHSS is also possible with low serum estradiol values (stimulation with recombinant (rec)FSH);
  - The slope of the estradiol rise is the main risk factor and is of more importance than the maximum level (positive predictive value 77%);
- Number of follicles per ovary > 20–25;
  - No clear cut-off value (10–35);
  - Variation dependent upon operator and technique;
- Measurements of the absolute vascular endothelial growth factor (VEGF) serum concentration are not useful for individual prediction[10].

Pathophysiology

The pathophysiology of OHSS is increasingly better understood. The crux is an equilibrium between proangiogenic and antiangiogenic factors present in follicular fluid. The proangiogenic role of VEGF is beyond doubt the most important mediator of the syndrome[11,12]. High concentrations of VEGF have been demonstrated in follicular fluid, making the mediating role of ovarian VEGF in the development of OHSS very plausible. VEGF concentrations in ascitic fluid, serum and plasma of OHSS patients were shown to be increased[13–15]. The mRNA expression of VEGF in human luteinized granulosa cells is time- and dose-dependent on hCG, further underlining the role of VEGF in the development of OHSS[16,17]. Later, it was shown that two VEGF receptors exist (VEGFR-1 and VEGFR-2), both produced by endothelial cells, one of which exists in a soluble form, serum (s)VEGFR-1, acting as a *negative* modulator of the bioactivity of VEGF.

An excess of bioactive proangiogenic VEGF increases the risk for OHSS; an excess of antiangiogenic sVEGFR-1 (and other antiangiogenic factors) decreases the ovarian response and the risk for OHSS and is accompanied by a decreased pregnancy rate[11]. Absolute serum concentrations have no value in individual risk assessment because there are individual variations in the binding of VEGF to its receptors[10,12].

In rats, proof of concept was shown of a VEGFR-2 inhibitor (SU5416) to block hCG-dependent VEGF production (and ensuing neoangiogenesis)[18]. Also, in rats it was shown that ovulation triggering using LH instead of hCG results in lower VEGF production. This serves as the theoretical basis for ovulation triggering utilizing recLH in clinical situations[19].

The pathophysiological cascade of OHSS consists of: neoangiogenesis and increased capillary permeability of the enlarged ovarian and other endothelial surfaces, fluid shift from the intravascular space to the extravascular space (abdomen, pleura, pericardium), hemoconcentration, decreased renal clearance, oliguria/anuria, hyperviscosity of the blood, modification in coagulation factors and thromboembolic risks. Hemoconcentration leads to an increase of hematocrit, and of the concentration of platelets and leukocytes, creatinine, urea and liver enzymes in the plasma, as well as to hyperkalemia and acidosis. Serum albumin decreases as a result of extravasation of fluid and ascites formation[20]. The process is self-limiting as the hCG effect decreases, unless fetal hCG starts to be secreted.

Classification

The *quantitative* aspects of definition of the syndrome cannot exactly be measured: ovarian dimensions can be assessed to a certain extent using echography, but ascites volume is difficult to measure. Therefore, classification is not categorical and daily weighing and fluid balance assessment remain key elements of the clinical follow-up. The most frequently used classification system is the one proposed by Golan[3] (Table 1).

Subsequently, two further refinements were introduced: '*critical OHSS*'[4] and '*group C severe OHSS*'[21], which both describe the same life-threatening clinical entity: severe reduction in circulating volume, severe hemoconcentration, multiple organ failure (kidney, liver, heart) and/or thromboembolic symptoms. Both are considered as grade 6 in the modern classification of Golan.

It is essential to understand that these grades are not strictly separated entities and that a mild-grade OHSS can quickly evolve into severe OHSS. This should not be forgotten when deciding to follow-up a patient 'by telephone'. The foremost criterion of clinical seriousness implying immediate hospitalization is a *hematocrit > 45%*.

PREVENTION

Primary prevention

Patients who have a primary risk for OHSS should be exposed to gonadotropins as little as possible. This implies that all other more safe

Table 1 Classification of OHSS according to Golan *et al.*[3]

Grade	*Mild*	*Moderate*	*Severe*
1	Abdominal distension and discomfort		
2	Criteria of grade 1 + nausea, vomiting, and/or diarrhea. Ovaries enlarged 5–12 cm		
3		Criteria of mild OHSS + echographic signs of ascites	
4			Criteria of moderate OHSS + clinical signs of ascites and/or hydrothorax and respiratory distress
5			All of the above + changes in blood volume and viscosity, hemoconcentration, coagulation disorders and decreased renal output and function
6			Life-threatening form

treatments should have had fair trail: life-style changes (diet and exercise), oral ovulation induction, use of pulsed gonadotropin-releasing hormone (GnRH), laparoscopic ovarian drilling. This should especially be kept in mind when treating young women in their first assisted reproductive technologies (ART) treatment cycles, women with PCOS and women with a history of OHSS.

The identification of women with thrombophilia, those with a family history of thromboembolism and women with antiphospholipid antibodies should ideally be performed before starting gonadotropin treatment. When indicated, the lowest possible dose of gonadotropins should be used and treatment adequately monitored, which means frequent use of vaginal echography and serum estradiol measurements. All patients at risk should be informed verbally and in writing so that, at the occurrence of early symptoms, they should consult the gynecologist responsible and not an inexperienced physician.

In cases of high primary risk, prophylactic treatment with heparin has been proposed.

Secondary prevention

Cycle cancellation

In ovulation induction, withholding hCG prevents the early form of OHSS. Avoiding hCG and intercourse/insemination prevents both the early and the late forms. This decision is often psychologically difficult, especially in *in vitro* fertilization (IVF), because it may entail the loss of considerable financial expense in countries without reimbursement. In very severe cases with poor follow-up possibilities, however, it may be the only method to avoid disaster.

Coasting ('soft landing')

Principle When high-risk patients rapidly reach high (> 3000 pg/ml) serum estradiol levels with a large number (> 20 per ovary) of follicles during stimulation, gonadotropin administration can be decreased or stopped while maintaining GnRH agonist administration. This allows larger follicles to continue to grow, whereas intermediary and small follicles enter atresia. Based on the FSH-threshold theory, a number of follicles will no longer respond to the decreasing FSH levels, or become unresponsive to hCG[22]. Coasting causes down-regulation of VEGF gene expression and protein production as a result of increased apoptosis in the granulosa cells of all, but mainly immature, follicles without influence on oocyte quality and endometrial receptivity[23].

Although no randomized clinical trials have been conducted to assess its true efficiency, the method is very popular, and is followed by acceptable pregnancy rates[24]. It has the advantage that the cycle is brought to its expected end with the replacement of fresh embryos and that no additional technical procedures are needed.

Criteria for coasting Criteria for coasting are based on a relationship between the number of growing follicles and/or the serum estradiol level and the risk for OHSS. There are two criteria for decision: the serum estradiol level determines whether coasting is done or not; the echographic image determines when.

Serum estradiol levels Most authors use values between 2500 and 3000 pg/ml. *Continuing gonadotropins at a serum estradiol level of > 3000 pg/ml is considered not good clinical practice.* When using recFSH, estradiol values tend to be lower and the above criteria do not hold. It has therefore been suggested that the estradiol value should come into play only if at the same time there are > 20 follicles per ovary.

Number of growing follicles Coasting should not be started too early because follicle growth might come to a complete standstill. When < 30% of all follicles have reached a mean diameter of 15 mm, coasting will result in an abrupt stop in follicle development and rapid serum estradiol decrease. On the other hand, when the majority of follicles are > 15 mm at the start of coasting, a number of cystically enlarged follicles with decreased oocyte quality may ensue[25].

Hence, this leads to the *golden rule of the middle way*: coasting should start when ~50% of the follicles are ~15 mm in diameter and have become independent of further gonadotropin stimulation.

Duration of coasting It has been shown that a coasting period of ≥4 days (from the first day that the gonadotropin dose is interrupted or decreased) results in decreased pregnancy rates[26], but this remains controversial[25,27]. Further clinical research is desirable to assess the subtleties with respect to oocyte number and quality and endometrial receptivity.

Modification of the ovulation-triggering agent

Although good data are lacking, it is not impossible that lower doses of hCG than those usually utilized (5000 or 10 000 IU) may cause sufficient oocyte maturation while reducing the risk for OHSS.

The replacement of hCG by exogenous or endogenous LH as ovulation trigger could have a considerable impact on the incidence of (the early form of) OHSS. An endogenous LH surge can be provoked by the administration of a short-acting GnRH agonist[28]. This is only possible in cycles without pituitary desensitization by a GnRH agonist. The combination with an antagonist remains a possibility. The administration of exogenous LH (recLH) is another option, but for the time being there is no interest from the pharcameuticals industry to commercialize this (available) product for such an indication. Hence, it remains that the 50-year-old use of urinary hCG as ovulation trigger is much cheaper, but its impact on the incidence of OHSS is huge.

Administration of macromolecules

Albumin administration Prophylactic albumin administration is supposed to interrupt the development of OHSS by increasing the plasma oncotic pressure and binding mediators of ovarian origin. This effect could be counteracted by increased capillary permeability. Prospective randomized trials and one retrospective study with a control group show 39 cases of OHSS in 468 treated risk cycles (8.3%) versus 89 OHSS cases in 611 untreated risk cycles (14.6%)[24]. A Cochrane review also shows that intravenous (IV) albumin administration at the time of oocyte collection has a preventive effect in cycles with a severe risk for OHSS[29]. However, a recent prospective randomized trial of 488 cases in each arm of the study seems to prove the inefficiency of human albumin[30]. Two studies show a decreased pregnancy rate after the use of IV albumin[31,32]. Albumin administration also has side-effects: viral transmission, nausea, vomiting and febrile and allergic reactions, and it is expensive.

Hydroxyethyl starch solution (HES) Because of the risk of viral transmission with human albumin, some authors have tested the effect of a safer non-biological substitute with comparable physiological properties: HES. Three studies suggest a useful effect, but the cohorts are too small to draw definite conclusions[33–35]. Further clinical research seems warranted.

Cryopreservation of all embryos

Instead of canceling the cycle, it is also possible to administer hCG, to retrieve the oocytes and to freeze all embryos. This does not exclude the risk for the early form of OHSS, but it does exclude the late form (caused by pregnancy). The removal of a large number of granulosa cells from the follicles probably decreases the risk as well. A Cochrane review concludes that the present evidence is insufficient to consider this approach as the standard treatment[36]. It may be considered when coasting has not been applied when it should have, and when, at the time of oocyte retrieval, one finds oneself in a very high-risk situation for the early form of OHSS in a patient with a very good prognosis of becoming pregnant and, hence, who has a high risk for the late form of OHSS.

Summary

No method can prevent all cases of OHSS, apart from withholding hCG, still the ubiquitous ovulation-triggering agent, although other molecules exist (recLH) but are either not available or very expensive. In practice, in ART, coasting is still the most popular approach, which probably does have some preventive effect. The late form cannot be avoided altogether. Combinations of different preventive methods acting at different levels could give the opportunity to avoid OHSS completely[37]. Single embryo transfer after ART prevents multiple pregnancies but not OHSS[38].

CLINICAL MANAGEMENT

Criteria for hospitalization

- Hematocrit > 45%;
- Any sign of severe OHSS.

Elements of out-patient follow-up

- Daily fluid balance;
- Daily weighing;
- Increase in umbilical abdominal circumference;
- Instruction to contact the center at any sign of deterioration;
- Out-patient follow-up every 48–72 h with blood tests and ultrasound examination.

Elements of hospital follow-up

- Heart rate;
- Blood pressure;
- Daily fluid balance;
- Echographic assessment: ascites volume, ovarian dimensions;
- Radiography of thorax (if dyspneic) to diagnose pleural effusion;
- ECG (to exclude pericardiac effusion);
- Hematological examination: hematocrit, red blood cell count, white blood cell count, electrolytes, kidney function tests, liver enzymes, total serum protein and albumin, coagulation tests.

Treatment strategy

Maintain diuresis!

Fluid management

- Intravenous administration of Ringer's lactate solution;
- First 24 h: 1500–3000 ml; in order to avoid overadministration of fluid, some centers restrict total fluid intake (including oral) to 1500 ml;
- Subsequent days: fluid volume as function of fluid balance;
- Combination of Ringer's lactate + dextrose 5% solution or NaCl 0.9% + dextrose 5% (standard) solution.

Plasma expanders

- HES (hydroxyethyl starch) 6% solution in isotonic NaCl;
- Maximum daily dose: 33 ml/kg in 250–500 ml per day, drop-wise, utilizing slow administration to avoid lung congestion.

Albumin administration

- Is only started if hypoalbuminemia (< 28 mg/dl) is demonstrated because of the risk for hepatitis, overdosage with albumin, renal function disorders and high cost; should definitely be started when ascitic fluid is drained because this causes a huge loss of protein.

Anticoagulant drugs

Low-molecular-weight heparin preparations are preferably given primarily in all cases of severe OHSS with hospitalization, but certainly if:

- Clinical signs of thromboembolic complications;
- Documented thrombophilia;
- History of hypercoagulability or thromboembolism;
- Uncorrected hemoconcentration after 48 h of usual intravenous treatment.

As a prevention of thromboembolic complications, especially in patients who are immobilized due to obesity or other reasons, low-dose aspirin administration has been suggested. When ascites puncture is performed, this has to be weighed against the risk for bleeding. If available, thromboembolic disease (TED) stockings may be indicated.

Ascites drainage

This can be performed both abdominally and vaginally[39,40], but always under sonographic guidance. It is considered when there is severe abdominal discomfort and dyspnea, and results in rapid subjective relief for the patient. It also results in increased venous return and increased cardiac output, diuresis, creatinine clearance and lung ventilation. It should be performed gradually: a maximum of 4 l over 12 h. The removal of large quantities means losing huge amounts of protein, which must be substituted. One liter of ascitic fluid contains 3.0–3.5 g of albumin; daily administration of 30–50 g albumin is recommended.

Out-patient management of OHSS can only be performed following strict rules. When signs of deterioration occur, hospitalization should be considered, preferably in an expert center. Hospitalized patients must be visited frequently by the same physician, as the clinical picture may change quickly (over the period of a single day), and the clinician can and must recognize this. When critical OHSS exists, the patient must be admitted to an intensive-care ward. In very severe cases, the interruption of a beginning pregnancy should be considered.

Pregnancy after OHSS

The pregnancy rate in patients with OHSS is higher than average. This is because the patients are usually young women, in their first ART cycles, with many oocytes and good-quality embryos. Several authors have reported an increase in early pregnancy loss in OHSS patients[2,41].

CONCLUSIONS AND RECOMMENDATIONS

Although theoretically known, OHSS remains underestimated because the perceived incidence per gynecologist is low. The syndrome is very traumatizing for the patient and her partner. Subjective discomfort is very important, and objective changes may be dramatic. Although long-term sequelae are unusual, they are serious (thromboembolism). Although fatal cases are rare, they go unreported and thus may be underestimated, and they are never in proportion to the indication for treatment (infertility in young healthy women).

Essential recommendations, therefore, are:

(1) Gonadotropin treatment for ovulation induction should be considered only when all other options have failed after a sufficiently long trying time.

(2) If gonadotropin stimulation for ovulation induction is unavoidable, one should use 'friendly' stimulation regimens aiming at

'SOFT' (single ovarian follicle treatment): low-dose step-up regimen, step-down regimen, or antagonists, always utilizing blood and sonographic control of ovarian response.

(3) hCG as an ovulation trigger should be replaced by safer methods (recLH, endogenous GnRH surge by an agonist); recLH exists but is not commercially available.

(4) In IVF/intracytoplasmic sperm injection (ICSI) the principle of obtaining 'as many oocytes as possible' should be replaced by softer stimulation regimens aiming at fewer oocytes of good quality.

(5) In risk situations, the patient should be informed about possibilities such as canceling, coasting or freezing for subsequent replacement.

(6) When signs of OHSS occur, the patient must be completely informed and hospitalization should be proposed at the slightest deterioration.

(7) These patients belong in a hospital ward where the clinical picture is known and the personnel have expertise in its treatment and follow-up. Admission to an intensive-care unit is necessary when critical OHSS develops.

(8) Registration of all cases of severe OHSS and their outcome should become compulsory in all ART programs, as well as after ovulation induction.

REFERENCES

1. Mathur RS, Akande AV, Keay SD, et al. Distinction between early and late ovarian hyperstimulation syndrome. Fertil Steril 2000; 73: 901–7.
2. Papanikolaou E, Tournaye H, Verpoest W, et al. Early and late ovarian hyperstimulation syndrome: early pregnancy outcome and profile. Hum Reprod 2005; 20: 636–41.
3. Golan A, Ron-El R, Herman A, et al. Ovarian hyperstimulation syndrome: an update review. Obstet Gynecol Surv 1989; 44: 430-440.
4. Navot D, Bergh PA, Laufer N. Ovarian hyperstimulation syndrome in novel reproductive technologies: prevention and treatment. Fertil Steril 1992; 58: 249–61.
5. Abramov Y, Elchalal U, Schenker JG. Severe OHSS: an 'epidemic' of severe OHSS: a price we have to pay? Hum Reprod 1999; 14: 2181–3.
6. Brinsden PR, Wada I, Tan SL, et al. Diagnosis, prevention and management of ovarian hyperstimulation syndrome. Br J Obstet Gynaecol 1995; 102: 767–72.
7. Mashiach S, Bider D, Morano O, et al. Adnexal torsion of hyperstimulated ovaries in pregnancies after gonadotropin therapy. Fertil Steril 1990; 53: 76–80.
8. Delvigne A, Rozenberg S. Review of clinical course and treatment of ovarian hyperstimulation syndrome (OHSS). Hum Reprod Update 2003; 9: 77–96.
9. Stewart JA, Hamilton PJ, Murdoch AP. Thromboembolic disease associated with ovarian stimulation in assisted conception techniques. Hum Reprod 1997; 12: 2167–73.
10. Mathur R, Hayman G, Bansal A, Jenkins J. Serum vascular endothelial growth factor levels are poorly predictive of subsequent ovarian hyperstimulation syndrome in highly responsive women undergoing assisted conception. Fertil Steril 2002; 87: 1154–8.
11. Pellicer A, Albert C, Mercader A, et al. The pathogenesis of ovarian hyperstimulation syndrome: in vivo studies investigating the role of interleukin-1, interleukin-6, and vascular endothelial growth factor. Fertil Steril 1999; 71: 482–9.
12. Garcia-Velasco JA, Pellicer A. New concepts in the understanding of the ovarian hyperstimulation syndrome. Curr Opin Obstet Gynecol 2003; 15: 251–6.
13. McClure N, Healy DL, Rogers PAW, et al. Vascular endothelial growth factor as capillary per-

meability agent in ovarian hyperstimulation syndrome. Lancet 1994; 344: 235–6.

14. Abramov Y, Barak V, Nisman B, Schenker JG. Vascular endothelial growth factor plasma levels correlate to the clinical picture in severe hyperstimulation syndrome. Fertil Steril 1997; 67: 261–5.

15. Agrawal R, Tan SL, Wild S, et al. Serum vascular endothelial growth factor concentrations in in vitro fertilization cycles predict the risk of ovarian hyperstimulation syndrome. Fertil Steril 1999; 71: 287–93.

16. Neulen J, Yan Z, Raczek S, et al. Human chorionic gonadotropin dependent expression of vascular endothelial growth factor/vascular permeability factor in human granulosa cells: importance in ovarian hyperstimulation syndrome. J Clin Endocrinol Metab 1995; 80: 1967–71.

17. Neulen J, Raczek S, Pogorzelski M, et al. Secretion of vascular endothelial growth factor/vascular permeability factor from human luteinized granulosa cells is human chorionic gonadotrophin dependent. Mol Hum Reprod 1998; 4: 203–6.

18. Gomez R, Simon C, Remohi J, Pellicer A. Vascular endothelial growth factor receptor-2 activation induces vascular permeability in hyperstimulated rats, and this effect is prevented by receptor blockade. Endocrinology 2002; 143: 4339–48.

19. Gomez R, Lima I, Simon C, Pellicer A. Low dose LH administration induces ovulation and prevents vascular hyperpermeability and VEGF expression in superovulated rats. Reproduction 2004; 127: 483–9.

20. Delbeke L, De Neubourg D, De Loecker P. Het ovarieel hyperstimulatiesyndroom. Nieuwe inzichten en therapeutisch beleid. Tijdschr Geneeskd 1998; 54: 1463–73.

21. Rizk B, Aboulghar MA. Classification, pathophysiology and management of ovarian hyperstimulation syndrome. In Brinsden P, ed. In Vitro Fertilization and Assisted Reproduction, 2nd edn. Carnforth, UK: Parthenon Publishing, 1999: 131–51.

22. Fluker MR, Hooper WM, Yuzpe A. Withholding gonadotropins ('coasting') to minimize the risk of ovarian hyperstimulation during superovulation and in vitro fertilization–embryo transfer cycles. Fertil Steril 1999; 71: 294–301.

23. Garcia–Velasco JA, Zuniga A, Pacheco A, et al. Coasting acts through downregulation of VEGF gene expression and protein secretion. Hum Reprod 2004; 19: 1530–8.

24. Delvigne A, Rozenberg S. Preventive attitude of physicians to avoid OHSS in IVF patients. Hum Reprod 2001; 16: 2491–5.

25. Sher G, Zouves C, Feinman M, Maassarani G. 'Prolonged coasting': an effective method for preventing severe ovarian hyperstimulation syndrome in patients undergoing in-vitro fertilization. Hum Reprod 1995; 10: 3107–9.

26. Ulug U, Bahceci M, Erden HF, et al. The significance of coasting duration during ovarian stimulation for conception in assisted fertilization cycles. Hum Reprod 2002; 17: 310–13.

27. Delvigne A, Kostyla K, Murillo D, et al. Oocyte quality and IVF outcome after coasting to prevent ovarian hyperstimulation syndrome. Int J Fertil Womens Med 2003; 48: 25–31.

28. Emperaire JC, Edwards RG. Time to revolutionize the triggering of ovulation. Reprod Biomed Online 2004; 9: 480–3.

29. Aboulghar M, Evers JH, All-Inany H. Intravenous albumin for preventing severe ovarian hyperstimulation syndrome: a Cochrane review. Hum Reprod 2002; 17: 3027–32

30. Bellver J, Munoz EA, Ballesteros A, et al. Intravenous albumin does not prevent moderate-severe ovarian hyperstimulation syndrome in high-risk IVF patients: a randomized controlled study. Hum Reprod 2003; 18: 2283–8.

31. Shaker A, Zosmer A, Dean N. Comparison of intravenous albumin and transfer of fresh embryos with cryopreservation of all embryos for subsequent transfer in prevention of ovarian hyperstimulation syndrome. Fertil Steril 1996; 65: 992–6.

32. Costabile L, Unfer V, Manna C, et al. Use of intramuscular progesterone versus intravenous albumin for the prevention of ovarian hyper-

stimulation syndrome. Gynecol Obstet Invest 2000; 50: 182–5.

33. Graf MA, Fischer R, Naether OG, et al. Reduced incidence of ovarian hyperstimulation syndrome by prophylactic infusion of hydroxyaethyl starch solution in an in-vitro fertilization programme. Hum Reprod 1997; 12: 2599–602.

34. Knig E, Bussen S, Sutterlin M, Steck T. Prophylactic intravenous hydroxyethyl starch solution prevents moderate-severe ovarian hyperstimulation in in-vitro fertilization patients: a prospective, randomized, double-blind and placebo-controlled study. Hum Reprod 1998; 13: 2421–4.

35. Gökmen O, Ugur M, Ekin M, et al. Intravenous albumin versus hydroxyethyl starch for the prevention of ovarian hyperstimulation in an in-vitro fertilization programme: a prospective randomized placebo controlled study. Eur J Obstet Gynecol Reprod Biol 2001; 96: 187–92.

36. D'Angelo A, Amso NN. Embryo freezing for preventing ovarian hyperstimulation syndrome: a Cochrane review. Hum Reprod 2002; 17: 2787–94.

37. Isik AZ, Vicdan K. Combined approach as an effective method in the prevention of severe ovarian hyperstimulation syndrome. Eur J Obstet Gynecol Reprod Biol 2001; 97: 208–12.

38. De Neubourg D, Mangelschots K, Van Royen E, et al. Singleton pregnancies are equally affected by ovarian hyperstimulation syndrome as twin pregnancies. Fertil Steril 2004; 82: 1691–3.

39. Padilla SA, Zamaria S, Baramki TA, Garcia JE. Abdominal paracentesis for ovarian hyperstimulation syndrome with severe pulmonary compromise. Fertil Steril 1990; 53: 365–7.

40. Aboulghar MA, Mansour RT, Serour GI, Amin T. Ultrasonically guided vaginal aspiration of ascites in the treatment of ovarian hyperstimulation syndrome. Fertil Steril 1990; 53: 933–5.

41. Raziel A, Friedler S, Schachter M, et al. Increased early pregnancy loss in IVF patients with severe hyperstimulation syndrome. Hum Reprod 2002; 17: 107–10.

Index

Printed and bound by CPI Group (UK) Ltd, Croydon, CR0 4YY
23/10/2024
01777689-0003